LAST RIGHTS

Death Control and the Elderly in America

Barbara J. Logue

Lexington Books

An Imprint of Macmillan, Inc.
New York

Maxwell Macmillan Canada
Toronto

Maxwell Macmillan International
New York · Oxford · Singapore · Sydney

This book is published as part of the Lexington Books Series on Social Issues,
George Ritzer, general editor

Library of Congress Cataloging-in-Publication Data

Logue, Barbara J.
  Last Rights : death control and the elderly in America / Barbara J.
Logue.
    p. cm. — (Lexington Books series on social issues)
  Includes bibliographical references and index.
  ISBN 0-669-27370-8
  1. Life and death, Power over—Moral and ethical aspects.
  2. Frail elderly—United States—Death—Moral and ethical aspects.
  3. Frail elderly—Care—United States—Moral and ethical aspects.
  4. Right to die.   I. Title.   II. Series.
  R726.L6   1993   92-39452
  179′.7—dc20   CIP

Lexington Books
An Imprint of Macmillan, Inc.
866 Third Avenue, New York, N.Y. 10022

Maxwell Macmillan Canada, Inc.
1200 Eglinton Avenue East
Suite 200
Don Mills, Ontario M3C 3N1

Macmillan, Inc. is part of the Maxwell Communication Group of Companies.

Printed in the United States of America

printing number
1   2   3   4   5   6   7   8   9   10

Contents

Tables

Preface

A journalist calls a Texas hospital to question officials about the man who came in and killed his sick wife; the hospital spokesperson asks, "Which one?" Family members disconnect the machine keeping their father alive and physically prevent hospital staff from reconnecting it; no indictment follows. A husband of forty years smothers his critically ill wife with a pillow, cuts his wrists, and lies down beside her to die. Elsewhere, spectators in a Long Island courtroom weep and cheer as the jury acquits a young surgeon accused of murdering his patient. An advertisement in a major national newspaper urges "Protect yourself." The organization is not selling burglar alarms or advocating seat-belt use, but promoting "living wills," whereby citizens can "protect" themselves from doctors and hospitals, not thieves or drunk drivers. Meanwhile, despite condemnation of assisted suicide from many physicians, lawyers, and ethicists, "Dr. Death" and his "suicide machine" elicit widespread approval from the public at large, and a how-to suicide manual tops the *New York Times* best seller list.[1]

What is happening in America? Why do these people, and uncountable others, want to die or help others to die? Why do they seem to think that the medical establishment is "the enemy"? Is this new behavior? If so, what social forces underlie and explain it? Will the trend continue? Where will it all lead?

New realities—our aging population, the tremendous power and tremendous weakness of scientific medicine, the fragmentation, gaps, inefficiencies, and cruelties inherent in the American system of long-term care, and unprecedented burdens of morbidity for individuals and their families—underlie the attitudes and behaviors reflected in the examples just listed. As the long history of scientific endeavors in medicine and public health illustrates, human beings have always tried to minimize sickness and postpone death. But, more recently, growing recognition of limits to both curing and caring—the extent to which disease, disability, and suffering can be alleviated with the means now available—has fueled a growing demand that the individual's right to choose to die be respected. In other words, when a "good life" is no longer possible, many contend that the individual is entitled to a "good death." Citizens have the right (and, some add, the responsibility) to control the timing and circumstances of their death, and, if necessary, others may act on their behalf.

The dilemmas of long-term care provision are frequently raised in the popular media, and growing numbers of families are gaining personal experience of the issues by witnessing the extreme frailty and prolonged dying of friends and relatives. Clearly, choices about death affect everyone and have a public component that goes beyond individuals and their families. This book delineates the issues and explores possible solutions to some of the most perplexing questions of our time. Chapter 1 introduces the concept of "death control" and provides an overview of aging trends and their growing impact, explaining how death control options are especially salient for those who are both old and frail. Chapter 2 places issues of frailty and death in historical and cross-cultural perspective to show that current problems are not entirely new. Moving forward to the contemporary situation, in Chapter 3 I review the circumstances of the frail elderly in modern industrialized nations, using experiences in the United States for illustration. The argument is that in many ways modernization is irrelevant to the status of the frail elderly while in other ways it worsens their plight. In particular, changes in the medical sphere have exacerbated their plight as potential victims, either unduly hastening death (through abuse, neglect, or inequities in access to care, for example) or delaying it by medical means without due regard to the quality of life.

Three preconditions are necessary in any society for increased resort to death control to occur: *acceptability* of new ideas and behavior, *advantages* to them, and adequate *means* for achieving the new goals.[2] A variety of evidence, such as survey data since the 1930s, documents the growing acceptability of death control in the United States today. Groups having a stake in the legitimation process include patients and their families, medical professionals, the media, the courts, government agencies, ethicists, and religious leaders. The meaning of death and its proper timing and circumstances are rightful topics for societal debate; controversy is healthy and absolutely essential for bringing key issues into the open and directing social change in line with citizens' wishes. Hence I also describe the views of those who oppose death control. These are the topics covered in Chapter 4.

Chapter 5 continues the discussion of preconditions by analyzing the advantages of death control. The United States is characterized by low fertility, which means fewer siblings to share parent care, and increasing family disruptions due to migration, divorce and remarriage, and the development of alternative roles for women, particularly in the paid workforce. As a result, the supply of family caregivers is constrained even as the demand for elder care increases, and a need arises for community-based and government-sponsored services. But a slow economy, competing social obligations, and fears about runaways costs and a growing population of highly dependent old people constrain formal service provision too. Moreover, despite all the money, personnel, and effort poured into it, the health care system, in the eyes of many Americans, seems unable to improve the lives of the very frail, and in fact often victimizes them. Collectively, these forces lead individuals, families, and other social groups to consider the advantages of death control. In Chapter 6, I discuss modern means of communicating one's end-of-life preferences through the use of advance directives, reviewing their advantages and drawbacks. Then I contrast the means that *can* be used to terminate lives with those *actually* used in the United States and with those typically employed in premodern societies.

Chapters 7 and 8 focus on the feasibility of possible alternatives to death control, their risks and shortcomings, in the informal and formal care sectors, respectively. Can more money, more and better caregivers, better training and more supportive services, better nursing homes, more stringent rules and regulations eliminate a demand for death control? Is better pain management the answer? Is an improved caring environment enough? Are our current goals realistic or achievable? What factors hinder end-of-life care of such commendable quality that it can deter choices for deliberate death? The scarcity of reliable caregivers is particularly problematic, and the disproportionate burdens borne by women and minorities as a result of our current approach to long-term care are cause for grave social concern. Equally distressing is the apparent inability of systemic improvements to substantially alleviate the suffering of the most vulnerable or to do so without causing undue suffering to others.

Chapter 9 delves into a compelling topic only touched on in earlier chapters—differences in vulnerability *within* the frail elderly population. It explores the risks of premature death and delayed death as they may vary among class, sex, and ethnic groups—risks that we have barely begun to recognize. It is clear that death control itself, as an emergent solution to newly perceived problems, inevitably brings other problems in its wake.

Finally, Chapter 10 leaves readers with some inescapable questions that only they can answer—questions that call for weighing the risks and benefits, rights and responsibilites, advantages and shortcomings of death control versus the considerable drawbacks of the current system, the pros and cons of deciding for oneself versus leaving it to others. Clearly, critical thinking is called for. Since the problems facing frail elders today are everyone's problems, and will be our personal problems if we live long enough, we cannot decline to choose. That is the most dangerous choice of all.

Writing a book on old age, sickness, and death can be an immensely trying experience. I was fortunate that many people helped to make the task lighter. I am grateful to Judy Treas, who provided the initial opportunity from which this book has resulted. Phil Brown, Anthony Glascock, and Ann Dill offered advice and shared their expertise in the book's critical early stages. Series Editor George Ritzer and several anonymous reviewers made valuable suggestions for improvement during the later stages. Beth Anderson proved herself a skillful editor whose enthusiasm not only kept me going but added considerably to the book's readability by challenging me to clarify concepts and illustrate them with concrete examples. To Pat Savard, who listened and cared, my warmest thanks.

The professional staff at the Jackson State University/ Universities Center Library helped in tracking down hard-to-find materials. Dottie Canzoneri and Monica Edwards were extremely capable typists. Special thanks are due to Patsy Brown, who provided skillful research assistance and carefully supervised the mechanical aspects of putting the book together; more important, however, her generous sharing of her experience, insights, and sense of humor have enriched my work. My friends and colleagues at the Mississippi State Institutions of Higher Learning contributed lively commentary on an ongoing basis, as well as moral support. Finally, my husband, Larry, filled many roles: patient listener, gentle critic, and best friend, but, most of all, a constant reminder that life is good and full of possibilities.

Introduction

Death control is deliberate behavior that causes a quicker death for a person suffering from an incurable condition, or complex of conditions, including the degenerative symptoms of old age. It encompasses self-deliverance (suicide or autoeuthanasia), where the individual terminates her own life, and assisted suicide (euthanasia), in which a mentally competent person makes the decision to die but receives help in implementing his plan. For instance, a friend may purchase a gun for someone too sick to get it himself, or a physician may advise as to the appropriate lethal dose of various drugs. The assistants must always be motivated by compassion and the "best interests" of the person and act at his request. Thus euthanasia is always voluntary on the part of the recipient.

Death control, however, encompasses more than euthanasia, because it includes deliberate choices made by substitutes for persons unable to choose for themselves, especially those who failed to leave any reliable instructions while they were still competent. Although it is likely that if the patient had foreseen her present circumstances, she would have chosen euthanasia, neither the proxy nor anyone else can be absolutely sure of this if she left no instructions. Whether proxy choices are invariably motivated by compassion for the decedent is also unknown. Certainly we hope that they are. But whether or not it is accurate to call these decisions euthanasia, connoting both voluntariness on the patient's part and merciful motives for the assistants, clearly they are death control. Hence, deliberate choice and a wish for control over the timing and circumstances of death are paramount in death control, but the identity, and possibly the motives, of the controller vary.

Insofar as possible, I avoid the term "mercy killing" because "mercy" and "killing" are contradictory words to many and hence paradoxical in their simultaneous suggestion of victimization and altruism. I also prefer to avoid the confusing, inaccurate, and increasingly strained, but still commonly made, distinction between "active" and "passive" euthanasia, sometimes characterized as "acts" versus "omissions."[1] If behavior is deliberately intended to speed the arrival of death, and in the absence of the behavior life would continue, it is properly called death control, and perhaps euthanasia. There is nothing passive about it. Suicide and aid-in-dying provided by loved ones or medical personnel are forms of exerting control. Decisions to forgo treatments that merely prolong the dying process, or to withdraw them once initiated, knowing the likely result is death, are other forms of deliberate control, regardless of who makes them. In a few cases, of course, such as the administration of large doses of drugs with the intent *only* to ease pain, not to facilitate death, there is no death control, even if death occurs as a direct result of the drugs. But since some experts maintain a distinction between "active" and "passive," this book will use the terms in quotation marks to remind readers that there is no general agreement that any meaningful distinction exists.

Death control hastens death. With its emphasis on mercy and altruism, euthanasia is a special, benign form of death hastening. For instance, antibiotics may be withheld from a dying cancer victim when a severe infection occurs, on the rationale that the infection will kill her sooner and more gently than the cancer will. But death hastening also encompasses neglect, abuse, contempt, derision, discrimination, exclusion from socially valued roles, and criminal victimization, all obviously nonaltruistic. These forms of behavior may encourage decisions favoring deliberate death, by affecting the recipient's will to live, for example. Such a death might well be premature.

Since there are many parallels between death control and birth control, and since birth control is a concept most people are familiar with, I draw analogies between the two behaviors whenever possible. Birth control refers to deliberate attempts to influence the number, timing, and circumstances of births, not merely to prevent them. If the intent is something else, the term "birth control" is inaccurate. For instance, if a couple uses condoms during intercourse solely to prevent HIV infection, with no conscious intent to prevent pregnancy, condom use is not birth control, but merely has that unintended side effect. As with death control, the deliberate intent to influence an outcome in a particular direction is paramount in defining the behavior.

A common theme linking the two concepts is the desire to exercise personal control over fundamental life events. The decision to have a child, especially the first, transforms one's daily existence drastically and irrevocably. It is the single most important commitment many of us will ever make. It demands our attention, our energies, our financial and psychic resources. It links us to future generations and the human community. To elect to have no children has tremendous implications too; life may be just as happy or unhappy, but it will assuredly be different than if we had a child.

In today's crowded, polluted, and often dangerous world, each new life also has repercussions for everyone else—not just our immediate family, but our neighborhood, our town, our nation, and our world. When an act is this important, when it has such an enormous impact on our lives, we owe it to ourselves to think carefully and decide wisely. The fact that our private choices have serious repercussions for others' lives too reinforces the need to choose wisely. So who should tell us when, or whether, to take so momentous a step? Who should weigh the pros and cons and decide what to do? The history of birth control is quite clear on this point: most people, in most times and places, have wanted to decide for themselves. Unless they were ignorant of the fact that they *had* a choice, or their freedom to choose was restricted by powerful outside forces, they have tried, more or less successfully, to actively direct their fate.

Avoidance of preventable suffering is a powerful motivator underlying resort to both birth control and death control. Before anesthesia and antibiotics, for example, a complicated pregnancy could very well be a death sentence for a woman. She was also endangered by too many pregnancies, those that came too close together, or those that occurred when she was too young or too old to withstand the demands on her body. The family's existing children, and the parents themselves, would suffer if there were too many mouths and too little food. Too few children, on the other hand, could endanger the very survival of the group. So it is easy to see how a desire to ward off physical, psychological, and economic distress could lead people to try to control their reproductive capacity. Similar motivations—the urge to manipulate significant life events to suit oneself and to avoid unnecessary suffering—underlie the current move toward death control.

Both those who control births and those who would control deaths distinguish between two critical concepts: having a life (a *biographical* concept) and being alive (a purely *biological* notion).[2] If being alive took precedence, parents would not care how many children they had; they would not concern themselves about the child's characteristics or its welfare. But parents do not typically think so narrowly. They want their children to have a biographical life—to learn, love, and laugh, to work and play, to have hopes and dreams and see at least some of them fulfilled, to be aware of themselves as unique individuals, to interact with others, to contribute to their community. To have a life in the biographical sense obviously requires life in the biological sense, but the reverse is not equally true. This is the logic that guides the thinking of death control proponents. Being alive is not enough; one must have a life and, as long as one does, there is an absolute prohibition against ending it. The corollary is that if one's biographical life is over (if one is permanently unconscious, for example), there is no point in having a biological life.

Just as "there is no inherent contradiction between love of children and desire for reproductive control," however, there is no necessary inconsistency between love of life and a desire to end it.[3] In fact, love of children and concern for their well-being encourages most couples to keep their family small. Those who choose death typically fight long and hard to postpone it; they are not lacking in courage. It is only when they can fight no more, when all the things they value about life are gone, that they close the door, or a compassionate relative, friend, or physician does it for them. An earlier death is a choice no one truly wants to make. But since it must be made, they want to make it themselves.

Like reproductive decisions, the need for hard choices about when and how to die affects us all. For example, everyone's heart will stop beating at some point. So, since cardiopulmonary resuscitation (CPR) techniques were developed in 1960, there is a time when everyone could potentially be resuscitated.[4] CPR is aggressive, "heroic" medicine—a violent, messy, and invasive procedure that may prolong one's life, or prolong one's death, because its outcome is never certain. We will have to choose ahead of time whether to take the risk, or someone else, perhaps a stranger, will decide for us. Doing nothing is a choice too, and has important consequences in both arenas—an unwanted child or an "undignified" death, for example. For a sick person, there is no limbo, no neutral ground; he is treated or not, resuscitated or not, and each has consequences.

Although we may not realize it, outsiders typically play a large role in seemingly individual choices about birth control and death control. Physicians prescribe "the pill," insert and remove intrauterine devices, and perform vasectomies, for example, and courts and legislatures set limits on the availability of legal abortion; cultural influences about the "right" time to start a family and "appropriate" family size also come into play. So too do social and cultural influences affect the definition of a "good" death and the "right" time to die. Like choices about family size, decisions about death and dying typically extend beyond the individual to involve negotiations with relatives, the medical establishment, and the larger society. Only the individual dies, of course, but dying is inevitably a social act as well: every death affects others and is affected by them. Controlling the timing and circumstances of death, moreover, almost always requires the active cooperation of others. Their opinions and needs influence our choices, assuming we remain mentally competent to the end. For the incompetent, others must both make and carry out end-of-life decisions.

A patient's right to refuse life-sustaining treatments is equivalent to the right to choose death when continued life is possible. Every year, for example, about one in seven of the 80,000 patients on artificial kidney machines voluntarily quits dialysis, knowing death is imminent. Their right to do this is now beyond dispute in the United States. Lawyers, health care professionals, and policy makers agree that treatment refusals by dying patients should be honored even when death is certain. Moreover, courts have sanctioned the choices made by guardians for incompetent patients, as well as for competent patients who might have continued to live for some time if they agreed to accept treatment. Of the 6,000 or so deaths in the United States every day, the American Hospital Association estimates that seven in ten are negotiated, with medical technology withdrawn or not applied, following discussions among medical personnel, family members, the patient (if possible), and other interested parties. Suicide is no longer illegal in any state. Helping another to die, however, is illegal, although courts and juries have been very lenient to defendants in the few cases that have come to trial.[5]

Since death in advanced industrial societies is concentrated at the older ages, death control is most salient for the elderly; hence I chose to focus on them. This is not to deny that death control is a serious issue for younger people. Choices about death in the case of multiply handicapped newborns, AIDS victims, and young cancer patients, for example, pose similar dilemmas for individuals, families, doctors and nurses, and society. Decisions in these cases and decisions for the elderly influence and reinforce one another, helping to legitimate death control, but the elderly, especially the oldest and frailest among them, remain the single largest group affected by such choices.

The desire to end useless suffering is timeless and universal, and euthanasia has a long history. The increasing acceptability and resort to death control in the late twentieth century, however, stem from the great social, economic, and cultural changes that have occurred since the Industrial Revolution, especially the development of a modern biomedical industry. They are not attributable to a devaluation of human life or a diminished desire for longevity, but reflect conscious choices by individuals who see important advantages in choosing death and find no acceptable alternative to that choice. The means of ending life have always been easy to devise, but harder to implement in the absence of strong motivation. That new attitudes and forms of behavior have developed and that they persist in the face of disapproval by some key social institutions— such as the medical establishment, some religious groups, and the law—attests powerfully to the strength of individual motives. Striking parallels are found in the history of the birth control movement, wherein social institutions also followed the public in enlarging the scope for personal choice over fate and nature, rather than leading the way.[6]

Human aging, death, and dying are universal concerns, not limited to any particular place, time, or culture. In this book, I review the medical, social, ethical, and legal issues associated with death and dying and put current problems in historical and cross-cultural perspective. This provides the necessary background to enable us to interpret today's world more knowledgeably, recognizing that neither the problems nor the range of possible solutions are entirely new. For the current situation, I incorporate studies from a variety of disciplines, including gerontology, sociology, psychology, medicine, and bioethics, to explain why death control is necessary, why it may be advantageous, and why it may be hazardous.

This book is not a treatise on morality or a set of instructions about how Americans should die. (Many such books have already been written.) Nor do I intend to advocate death control, in any form, as a solution for any individual or social problem. To assert that powerful forces in our society are propelling us toward increasing resort to negotiated death is not to suggest blanket approval, since the forces exist independently of whether we condemn or condone them. Rather it is to describe our society as it is, and as it seems to be tending. Nonetheless, death control does have many benefits, albeit with significant risks. It is incumbent on all of us to learn about both, in order to make intelligent choices for ourselves and for one another. If this book encourages readers to think about the issues, to debate them with relatives, friends, and neighbors, to follow new developments as they occur, and to react intelligently to them, it will have accomplished its purpose.

The book's argument may be summarized as follows: Demographic, social, and economic conditions in the United States favor increasing resort to death control in its various guises, including "active" euthanasia. The potent forces already leading us in this direction—population aging, the increasing prevalence and burden of morbidity, changing requirements for long-term care, growing costs, and increasing constraints on care providers—are gaining strength, and they are increasing perceptions of advantages to death control and its acceptability. At the same time, the superficial appeal of possible alternatives (better "caring," for example) is likely to diminish as individuals gain more knowledge of and experience with their shortcomings. Furthermore, paralleling historical developments in the birth control arena, we may anticipate a shift to more effective, easier, and "pleasant" methods of inducing death. Lack of satisfactory alternatives to death control, combined with the coincidence of institutional goals of efficiency and cost containment in the health care sector with individual and family desires for a "good" death, will facilitate the diffusion of increasingly tolerant views. In short, for good or ill, tolerance for death control promises to grow and diffuse broadly throughout our society in coming years, as individuals and institutions become more aware of its advantages and as universal aversions to frailty and prolonged dependence at the older ages continue to influence values and behavior.

What are the preconditions that set the stage for greater acceptability of death control? Are some or all of them being met in the United States today (and in other advanced industrial nations as well)? What evidence do we have? What else do we need to know? Are there alternatives to deliberate death, and how viable are they? Are there serious risks or dangers? These are among the imperative questions that this volume addresses. We begin with an overview of the size, growth, condition, and increasing importance of the elderly population in the modern world.

Aging Trends

The world's population is aging, with the highly industrialized nations in the forefront. In 1900, one in every 25 Americans was 65 or older; by 1980, the proportion had risen to one in nine, and it is projected to exceed one in five by the year 2030 (Table 1-1). More important, the proportion of elders who are in the "oldest old" category (85 and over)—the frailest and most dependent group—has also increased substantially during the twentieth century. Currently about one elder in ten is extremely old, compared to only one in 25 as late as 1940; by 2010, the ratio will be about one in six. Then, as large cohorts of baby boomers swell the ranks of the younger old (ages 65 to 74), the proportion at the extreme ages will decline until, after 2030, the baby boomers themselves become the oldest old—over 15 million of these "senior boomers" are expected by the middle of the twenty-first century. All of these future oldest old persons have already been born, so the projected numbers are affected only by mortality trends, not by birth rates. Numbers at the older ages have been consistently underestimated in past projections, and death rates at the oldest ages continue to fall. Hence if actual mortality declines in coming decades exceed those anticipated, the number of people at the extreme ages will be even greater than Table 1-1 suggests.

Changes in health status with advancing age for American elders parallel those found in many studies in other developed nations. Population aging is more advanced and hence more compelling in highly industrialized nations, but it is of growing importance in even the least developed. By 2020, for example, China alone is projected to have in excess of 31 million octogenarians, an increasing proportion of the oldest old will live in Third World nations, and large cohorts will be approaching the extreme ages.[7] There is no reason to expect that these people will be less frail or needy than those now at the extreme ages, regardless of their nation's stage of economic development. As their populations age and modernize, developing nations will face constraints on care provision similar to those the industrialized countries are now grappling with, in addition to already critical resource shortages. In all countries, we can predict growing concern with cost containment as aging populations challenge the capacity of health care institutions to cope. Other nations will look to us for guidance with their own concerns, while trying to avoid the pitfalls we have inadvertently created.

The fact that most people now survive to old age, even advanced old age, is a tribute to centuries of economic and social progress, including the rise in standards of living and the achievements of scientific medicine. Most elders in the United States today are healthy, independent, and self-sufficient. But the elderly by no means constitute a homogeneous group, so generalizations must always be tempered with qualifications. For example, there are more women than men in the older population, and they have special characteristics and problems that bear on decisions about death and dying. The same may be said about elderly members of disadvantaged minority groups—a growing proportion of the total. Other compositional differences within the elderly population are important too. For example, the group aged 75 and over is now growing faster than the 65-to-74 group, a phenomenon re-

TABLE 1-1

Actual and Projected Growth of the Older Population:
United States, 1900–2050 (Numbers in thousands)

Year	Total population all ages	65 years and over Number	65 years and over Percent	65 to 74 years Number	65 to 74 years Percent	75 to 84 years Number	75 to 84 years Percent	85 years and over Number	85 years and over Percent	85+/65+ Percent
1900	76,303	3,084	4.0	2,189	2.9	772	1.0	123	0.2	4.0
1910	91,972	3,950	4.3	2,793	3.0	989	1.1	167	0.2	4.2
1920	105,711	4,933	4.7	3,464	3.3	1,259	1.2	210	0.2	4.3
1930	122,775	6,634	5.4	4,721	3.8	1,641	1.3	272	0.2	4.1
1940	131,669	9,019	6.8	6,375	4.8	2,278	1.7	365	0.3	4.0
1950	150,967	12,270	8.1	8,415	5.6	3,278	2.2	577	0.4	4.7
1960	179,323	16,560	9.2	10,997	6.1	4,633	2.6	929	0.5	5.6
1970	203,302	19,980	9.8	12,447	6.1	6,124	3.0	1,409	0.7	7.1

1980	226,505	25,544	11.3	15,578	6.9	7,727	3.4	2,240	1.0	8.8
1990	250,410	31,559	12.6	18,373	7.3	9,933	4.0	3,254	1.3	10.3
2000	268,266	34,882	13.0	18,243	6.8	12,017	4.5	4,622	1.7	13.3
2010	282,575	39,362	13.9	21,039	7.4	12,208	4.3	6,115	2.2	15.5
2020	294,364	52,067	17.7	30,973	10.5	14,443	4.9	6,651	2.3	12.8
2030	300,629	65,604	21.8	35,988	12.0	21,487	7.1	8,129	2.7	12.4
2040	301,807	68,109	22.6	30,808	10.2	25,050	8.3	12,251	4.1	18.0
2050	299,849	68,532	22.9	31,590	10.5	21,655	7.2	15,287	5.1	22.3

SOURCE: U. S. Bureau of the Census, Current Population Reports, Series P-25, No. 1018, *Projections of the Population of the United States, by Age, Sex, and Race: 1988-2080* (Series 14 - Middle Series) (Washington, D. C.: U. S. Government Printing Office, 1989), by Gregory Spencer. For historical figures (to 1980), see U. S. Senate Special Committee on Aging et al., *Aging America: Trends and Projections* (1987-88 edition) (Washington, DC:U. S. Government Printing Office).

ferred to as the "aging of the aged." By the turn of the century, those 75 and older will constitute 50 percent of the population of older Americans, up from 41 percent in 1986. The extreme aged segment, with its disproportionate needs, is growing especially rapidly: from 2.3 million in 1980, it is expected to increase almost fourfold, to 8.6 million, by 2030.[8]

The total number of frail elders is difficult to estimate because the distinction between "frail" and "independent" is based not on chronological age, but on health and ability to function, and definitions of disability vary from survey to survey. Demographic and health statistics are typically aggregated by chronological age rather than health status. But some of the extreme aged are in excellent health, whereas some chronologically younger elders suffer serious impairments.

If we define the frail as those who need help with the basic activities of daily life on a long-term basis, about 6.9 million older Americans fell into the category in 1988, or about one in five of those 65 and over; by 2000, their number is expected to increase to nearly nine million.[9] Many elders have conditions like arthritis or senile dementias, which can be extremely disabling but do not cause death directly. Some important questions bear on whether they are defined as "frail" in addition to elderly: Are they mentally alert enough to manage their affairs? Do physical disabilities or chronic illnesses preclude performance of the basic activities of daily life—dressing, toileting, and eating, for example? Do they need considerable help from family or professional caregivers? What is their quality of life? Their prognosis?

Our knowledge is limited because frail elders are typically very difficult to interview and their frailty is psychologically disturbing to many observers, and hence avoided. Such factors led one population specialist to describe the frail elderly as "statistical ghosts." They have also been called "the excluded twenty percent" because research efforts have concentrated on the rational, active, healthy aged, leaving the most vulnerable relatively invisible. In the United States, the existence of distinct subgroups within the older population was not recognized until recently. The difficulties of interviewing frail elders have not been overcome and are probably unsolvable, but at least now the problems are recognized and proxy interviews (with the patient's spouse or another relative, for example) provide some information, however limited. Another problem is the fact that well elders may enter the frail population at any time, sometimes literally overnight, while death may remove others just as quickly. Hence researchers must try to pin down a moving target. In one study, for example, 109 clients were interviewed at the outset. But only 43 could be interviewed at a follow-up twelve to fifteen months later. Some died, others' health had deteriorated so much that they could not be interviewed, and a third group was lost for other reasons.[10]

New Realities: The Growing Force of Frailty

For many years, we believed that falling death rates and gains in life expectancy meant that the population was becoming healthier. Now this confident assumption is being challenged by evidence that longer life is accompanied by *increases* in the prevalence of chronic illness and disability. Explaining this apparent paradox requires that we distinguish between *chronic* health conditions and *acute* conditions. The latter include the great epidemic diseases of the past—the Black Death and typhoid fever, for example—as well as the colds, flu, and appendicitis we are still familiar with today. Their onset is sudden and their duration short. Victims either recover quickly or they die; there are no gray areas of partial recovery or long lingering in some shadowy ground between life and death, in which one neither dies nor recovers completely to go on as before. Medicine has been quite successful in coping with acute conditions, and some, like smallpox, have been eradicated. But data from the National Health Interview Surveys show that population health is worsening because morbidity for many chronic diseases, such as heart disease and cancer, has been increasing. This is especially true for the older population. In other words, people seem to be living longer with, and in spite of, very disabling chronic conditions, which the health care system can "manage," but not cure.[11]

As we get older, the risk of becoming disabled and dependent rises dramatically, as Tables 1-2 and 1-3 show. Thus the "aging of the aged" is an important phenomenon because there will be proportionally more elders in the higher-risk ages. To illustrate, out of every 1,000 Americans aged 45 to 64, 254 have arthritis; the fig-

TABLE 1-2

Percentage of Community-Based Elderly with Difficulty in Selected Life Activities, by Age: United States, 1984

	65–74	75–84	85+
Difficulty in			
Walking	14.1	22.9	39.9
Getting outside	5.6	12.4	31.2
Getting in/out of bed or chair	6.0	9.2	19.2
Bathing/showering	6.3	12.3	27.9
Eating	1.2	2.4	4.4
Dressing	4.3	7.5	16.6
Using toilet	2.6	5.8	14.1
Controlling urination	6.0	10.3	17.6
Preparing Meals	4.0	8.8	26.1
Shopping	6.4	15.1	37.1
Managing money	2.2	6.3	24.0
Heavy housework	18.6	28.6	47.8
Light housework	4.4	8.9	23.6
Number (000s)	16,288	8,249	1,897

SOURCE: National Health Interview Survey, 1984 Supplement on Aging, calculated from data in Tables 38-44 in R. J. Havlik, B. M. Liu, M. G. Kovar, et al., "Health Statistics on Older Persons, United States, 1986," *Vital and Health Statistics*, Series 3, No. 25 (Washington, DC: U.S. Government Printing Office, 1987).

ure jumps to 437 per 1,000 for those 65 to 74 and to 555 per 1,000 for those over 75. The incidence of Alzheimer's disease, the chief cause of cognitive impairment at the older ages, also rises sharply with age, as do rates for other forms of senile dementia. Of people still living in their own homes, or in the home of a relative, nearly half those aged 85 and over are estimated to be afflicted with Alzheimer's, compared to only 3 percent of those 65 to 74 and 19 percent of those 75 to 84. Moreover, dementing illnesses

TABLE 1-3
Nursing Home Residents Aged 65 and over by Age and Functional Status: United States, 1985

Functional Status	65–74	75–84	85+
Needs help in dressing	70.2	75.9	81.9
Needs help in using bathroom	45.8	47.8	56.1
Difficulty controlling bladder	6.8	11.0	12.1
Difficulty controlling bowels and bladder	27.5	33.6	35.9
Can walk only with help	20.4	24.8	29.7
Chairfast	33.7	38.7	45.4
Bedfast	6.3	6.1	6.9
Needs help in eating	33.5	39.1	44.0
Vision partially impaired	10.0	14.2	19.2
Vision severely impaired or lost	5.6	6.1	11.7
Hearing partially impaired	7.4	14.8	25.3
Hearing severely impaired or lost	1.5	2.1	7.7
Number	212,100	509,000	594,700

SOURCE: 1985 National Nursing Home Survey, calculated from data in Tables 57 and 59 in R. J. Havlik, B. M. Liu, M. G. Kovar, et al., "Health Statistics on Older Persons, United States, 1986," *Vital and Health Statistics*, Series 3, No. 25 (Washington, DC: U.S. Government Printing Office, 1987).

are a major factor leading to institutionalization, so many nursing home residents are mentally impaired.[12] The elderly are disproportionate users of health and social services, and the oldest old are typically the frailest and most dependent of all, with many needing extensive help to manage their daily lives. They constitute the "truly old" population that many people stereotypically associate with old age.

Increasing age, of course, raises the likelihood that a heretofore healthy elder will become frail and dependent. As a person ages, existing health problems tend to worsen and new conditions often show up. A good example is Wallace Proctor's health history. In 1966, he was diagnosed with Parkinson's disease, a progressive, degenerative, incurable (but nonfatal) illness. He tried various drugs and increasing doses to manage it, but his health continued to deteriorate. Meanwhile, he experienced increasing pain from arthritis. Then, in 1977, he had a heart attack, which severely limited his independence and ability to do his favorite activities, like hiking and gardening. None of these health problems, though serious, killed Mr. Proctor. But nothing the doctors did cured him either. In his words, "each day seem[ed] to be a little less worth living," as it became more difficult for him to adjust to his limitations. Though he remained mentally alert and was not totally dependent, he saw helplessness looming and each day grew more fearful of becoming a burden on others.[13]

These are the kinds of elders this book is about: those with serious mental or physical health problems that the medical system cannot alleviate, those no longer able to do the things that make life worth living, those who cannot remember who they are or understand why they hurt, those tied into a bed or a chair "for their own good," and others like them. Not those who suffer a heart attack but can, with help, resume a reasonably normal life. Not those who have a stroke but can be rehabilitated to return to what is, for them, a tolerable existence. Not those who only need a cane or a wheelchair, a prescription, or a friend to have a decent life. None of these "helps" could help Wallace Proctor enough to keep him going. He killed himself. Likewise, a Florida man chose death when he asked that the respirator sustaining his life be disconnected, because "death can't be any worse than what I'm going through now." So did a couple in their late seventies, married over forty years, when they sipped their favorite sherry, took poison, and lay down to die, together still. So do countless others every day.[14]

Because chronic illnesses and disabling conditions, like those endured by Mr. Proctor, are unpredictable in duration, intensity, and degree of incapacity, they require large palliative efforts and restrict normal life activities in many ways. Although their biological

lives have been prolonged through advances in medicine and public health, elders' potential for a biographical life often becomes severely constrained. They may become dependent on medical
technology and on family and professional care providers. As
Tables 1-2 and 1-3 suggest, however, their greatest needs are often
not purely medical, but rather for help with the basic activities of
daily living, such as dressing and toileting. For example, about one
in seven noninstitutionalized Americans aged 65 to 74 has trouble
walking. Much smaller proportions have difficulty with other activities requiring mobility, such as shopping or getting to the bathroom, but may still be able to manage alone. Dramatic increases
occur with advancing age in the fraction reporting each type of
difficulty, however, and in the number reporting more than one
problem. Moreover, the *severity* of existing problems is likely to
worsen as the years pass. Impaired elders who remain in the community are able to do so because sufficient help is available, typically from family members; others must move to institutions and
rely on nonfamily care providers. Extreme frailty characterizes
many nursing home residents, as Table 1-3 indicates, and many
cannot manage without substantial assistance. About four in ten
suffer from some form of dementia and about 50 percent exhibit
serious behavioral disorders—agitation, confusion, screaming,
threatening others, and the like.[15]

Whether they continue to reside in the community or move to
institutional quarters, many frail elders require assistance for
years, not just weeks or months. Since the aged population is itself
aging, both more individual elders and greater proportions of the
aged as a group are expected to need help in decades to come.
Recent projections indicate a 31 percent increase by the year 2000
in the number of chronically disabled elders living in the community, compared to a less than 20 percent increase in the number of
nondisabled elders. In addition, the number of elderly nursing
home residents is projected to reach 5.2 million by 2040, up from
1.5 million in 1980, a growth rate faster than that of the older
population as a whole.[16]

Never before have so many old people been so sick for so long.
Never before have the elderly, their families, and society had to
bear the burdens of frailty for such extended periods. In earlier
eras, most sicknesses were brief, lasting eight weeks or less, and

were resolved quickly by either recovery or death. Medicine's ability to postpone death with the remedies available was sharply limited. Today, however, the costs (psychic and economic, public and private) of long-term care have altered substantially. Both the burdens of treatment (for the patient) and the burdens of care provision (for relatives, health care workers, and society) increase willingness to consider negotiated death as an alternative to continuous pain, suffering, or a life of unacceptable quality.[17]

Social institutions have been slow, even reluctant, to cope with changes in human longevity, especially the prolonged sickness, dependence, pain, and suffering that added years may entail. But, despite this lack of institutional preparedness, the population at risk is growing steadily. Even experts who are relatively optimistic about future morbidity patterns believe that "illness at the end of the life span will prove more refractory to treatment, more inevitable, less possible to cure, and increasingly less reasonable to treat."[18] Gloomier prognoses conclude that economic costs alone threaten to exceed even the highest estimates, whereas efforts to assess the subjective costs range from primitive to nonexistent. Thus the greater control over life and death that medical technology now allows has also raised critical questions about how to cope with new realities. The central problem is dealing with prolonged frailty of the elderly within a context of constraints. How will we relieve their suffering? Who will care for them? How will we pay for their care? In sharp contrast to past eras, frail elders are a significant group in today's world—their numbers are expanding and will continue to grow, their needs are costly and increasing, and they command far fewer personal resources than their healthier counterparts. For instance, they are more likely to be poor, having accumulated little or spent down their assets on daily needs, including health care, and are less likely to have surviving family members to look after their interests when they cannot. Their problems are often public problems too: since the vast majority lack long-term care insurance, taxpayers pick up much of the tab for their care.[19]

New Choices

New realities necessitate new choices. Perceived solutions to the predicaments of advanced age and extreme frailty, such as advocating a right to choose to die, legalizing physician aid-in-dying, rationing health care, or recruiting more and better caregivers also entail unforeseen difficulties of implementation and unintended consequences. The quality of life of frail elders "saved" by modern medicine is one such issue, because often they are neither fully alive (in the broader biographical sense of capacity for meaningful social relationships) nor quite dead, but somewhere in between. Defining, implementing, and paying for new choices are additional problems. The need for responsible choices in matters of long-term care, death, and dying is still unrecognized by many, and some people are unwilling to confront new realities because they are unpleasant or frightening. Many fail to appreciate that if they hesitate too long to make choices, others will inevitably do so for them, thus entailing the risk that their preferences will not be respected.

Frail Elderly in Nonindustrial Societies

Kin arrive and camp around the bed; relatives wash, massage, and comfort the patient, carefully attending to any special requests; shifts are rotated so that someone is always at the bedside; when death seems imminent, female kin weep and keen while clan elders sing traditional songs to guide the person's spirit back to its territory of conception.

This is how Janice Reid, in her study of the old in an Australian aboriginal society, describes a deathbed scene.[1] Her moving account is an excellent illustration of how, in simpler times and places, those who lived long were cherished for their contributions to society and respected for their exemplary lives and accumulated wisdom; when frail, ill, or dying, their needs were lovingly tended to by devoted members of the extended family, and their loss was genuinely mourned by the entire community. In many respects this better world has been irretrievably lost with the coming of the Industrial Revolution and its destruction of traditional mores. Yet even now in less complex societies, with their strong emphasis on filial piety, the aged are well treated. Close-knit families, grateful for their past contributions and continued presence, keep them safely enclosed in a warm, protective environment, even in the midst of poverty.

When was the generous "Golden Age"? Where are those compassionate societies where people are happy to share their resources, however meager, with frail, dependent relatives? Sadly, no one knows, for these are among the myths of aging—the romanticized nonsense and wishful thinking that many find so comforting in the face of rapid social change. Reid's account of death among the aborigines is true enough, but so are other facts she relates about the same society—stories of elder neglect and abuse, caregiver resentment, guilt, and feelings of burden. In her cautionary words, "the ideal is not always translated into reality." Nonetheless, relying on a false assumption that the past was somehow better than the present, the "primitive" superior to the "modern," many mourn the loss of what never really existed in the first place.[2]

The topic of old age itself became of interest to historians and anthropologists only recently. But even experts have often overlooked the fact that old people are not all alike. On the situation of the aged in preindustrial Europe and America, for example, historians have described a puzzling mixture of official respect and some real power, along with considerable degradation and derision. We read of elders who are kindly cared for by family or community, despite their infirmities; we learn of others, perhaps in the same society, who inspire prolonged disputes about who must accept responsibility for them, and still others who die of neglect or are literally auctioned off to the lowest bidder. There is benevolence and indifference, extraordinary solicitude and deliberate cruelty. "The old" seem to have been respected and loathed, loved and feared, supported and abandoned, in a confusing and apparently contradictory mix of attitudes and behavior, even within a single society.[3] Much of the confusion arises from the fact that, too often, writers neglect to clarify exactly which elderly are under discussion—the healthy and competent, the senile, those who are near death, or some other category. In other words, there has been a pronounced tendency to speak of "the old" as if they were essentially alike or as if differences among them scarcely mattered.

This tendency accounts for the apparently contradictory generalizations about their status that we have just noted. A major problem is the universal "invisibility" of some elders: those who are hard to interview, whose roles may seem so unimportant, uninteresting, or passive that observers see no point in documenting them, or whose condition is so distressing that they are avoided. Most ethnographers, in fact, do not distinguish frail from active elders in discussions about "the old." Some exclude the frail elderly from consideration because their sad lot is the same everywhere, or because a distinction is so seldom made by others. An exception is Charles Fuller's amply qualified description of roles for the aged among Southern African Bantu: "*Almost* every elder, in *most* Bantu tribes, *unless made incompetent through physical or mental disorder*, has a respected role as a wise counselor," and the eldest *responsible* male is consistently deferred to in traditional Bantu family decision making. The incompetent and irresponsible meet a different fate.[4]

Most nonsupportive treatment of the aged has gone unnoticed for several reasons. First, some researchers have confounded attitudes with behavior: by taking expressions of filial piety and respect for elders at face value, they erroneously concluded that people *actually* behaved the way they thought they *should* behave. In other situations, certain forms of behavior may be hidden from outside observers, so they see only a partial view of reality. Finally, many investigations are of relatively short duration (weeks or months, rather than years), so nonsupportive behavior may not have occurred while the researcher was observing the group or tribe. Hence, the fact that many investigators did not witness, or failed to record, particular behaviors, does not mean the behaviors did not exist.[5]

Since systematic quantitative data on the frail elderly—their numbers, condition, and treatment—are lacking for nonindustrial societies, past and present, the conclusions advanced here are necessarily tentative. However, as this chapter will show, we can be certain that individuals and social groups have invariably recognized that those who are "old" differ from those who are "decrepit." People everywhere seem to have no trouble separating the two categories, nor in directing different treatment at them. Behavior is very likely to change for the worse when the person who is merely "old" moves into the "decrepit" category. The latter are not just old, but too ill, too weak, or too senile to engage in normal social roles in their community. While they still live, such unfortunates are often singled out for special, negative treatments. Their death is anticlimactic, since they lived beyond their capacity for productive involvement in social affairs. Thus chronological age is not the primary factor that affects well-being in the later years of life. Rather, the extreme physical frailty, loss of mental acuity, and threat of prolonged dependence on others that may accompany advanced years determine one's status and how one is treated. In other words, even "primitive" societies distinguish between biological life and biographical life, between the physical body and the social persona. The body becomes insignificant once the personality and spirit have left it.[6]

Clarifying which aged are the reference group also confirms that, regardless of the impact of modernization on the competent old (especially those who remain both mentally alert and physically robust), attitudes toward the decrepit have been remarkably constant: though sometimes tolerated, they have never been valued and have often been mistreated. Continuity and change are considered in terms of four overlapping perspectives: the frail elderly as (1) asset or resource; (2) impediment, burden, or threat; (3) low priority; and (4) victim. Over the course of human history there has been more continuity than change for frail elders as resource, as burden, and as low priority. In the words of historian Lawrence Stone, "We are no more, and no less, anxious to have grandparents under foot than were our forefathers." Forms of victimization, however, have changed in important respects while remaining strikingly similar in other respects. Death hastening, which may be direct or indirect, and delayed death are the two major types of victimization discussed.[7]

Frail Elders as Resource

The claim that frail, dependent elders may be assets to family or community may seem incongruous to some. Factors that are universally important for the status and well-being of the elderly include the possession of important knowledge, control of family or community resources, the ability to continue useful and valued roles, and membership in an extended family. Of these, "material resources of economic value" are the most important predictors of deference to the aged in premodern societies. To guarantee their care, for example, old women in Rattan Garh, a traditional agricultural village in India, would keep their property locked up or bury jewelry and other valuables in secret places; in this way they let it be known that the relative most attentive to their needs would inherit these possessions. In seventeenth-century England, "parents had no illusions about how children might treat them if given the chance," so they took legal means to maintain sufficient control over their property to ensure good care in their waning years. Likewise in early America, legal documents, not mere verbal promises, specified in minute detail the obligations adult children had to fulfill if they expected to inherit parental property. Childless elders with property could exchange it for the care they needed; thus some turned land, livestock, and other possessions over to the community in return for board and lodging. The lot of those without property was grim—beggary, semistarvation, the humiliations and uncertainties of public and private charity. In the eighteenth century, for example, one aged couple became trapped between two Massachusetts towns: they were physically moved from one town to the other because neither town was willing to provide support.[8]

Elders must remain *actively* engaged in exchange networks in order to maintain their status and ensure their care. Many historians and anthropologists describe societies in which the aged serve as valued teachers, advisors, diplomats, religious leaders, and storytellers; they also perform essential domestic chores, such as child tending and food preparation. These lengthy lists of positive contributions clearly refer to the healthy and competent old, not those who are frail, dependent, or senile; in other words, they are people who help others, who contribute to community well-being, who provide something in return for services received. It is possible, nonetheless, that *frail* elders can be assets in some contexts. Although most of their resources may have been used up, relinquished, or appropriated, frail elders may remain sufficiently useful to kin or society to ensure continued good treatment. Their very neediness may command sympathy, and solicitous long-term care may reward providers with feelings of personal satisfaction as past debts are repaid and affection and love are demonstrated. Among the Semang people of Malaysia, for instance, an adult child will carry a fragile parent on his back when the group is moving camp. In Northern California, the Modoc Indians construct special housing for elders, with extra insulation for warmth, and keep the fire burning continually in the winter. Other caregivers may anticipate more tangible deathbed gifts in return for their services.[9]

Intellectual competence may be more important than manual abilities, since even physically frail elders may possess wisdom, humor, tact, and good judgment. Infirm aged whose only remaining resource is the control of expressive information (knowledge of family anecdotes or intricate kinship networks, for example) may continue to be supported for that reason alone. Frail elders may also be esteemed because they provide essential lessons to others by their piety, serenity, or the moral example of their lives. The dying may earn respect and admiration for their patient endurance of suffering and for helping others put life in perspective.[10]

Paradoxically, the "force of frailty" can be powerful. For example, reluctant offspring may be brought into line by the threat of embarrassment when parents complain publicly of neglect or mistreatment; the praise earned for good treatment may itself be sufficient incentive for good care. In some cultures, neglectful kin can be shamed by the threatened suicide of an aged relative and so provide care for fear of negative sanctions, even if the "neglect" is imaginary or highly exaggerated by the elder. Old Igbo men in Nigeria, for example, could demand care as their due; it was the person who failed to provide care, not the one who demanded it, who risked public scorn and ridicule. Cultural beliefs that elders have supernatural power to influence the health and prosperity of others, or to cause misfortune and natural disasters, may encourage younger kin to treat them well out of fear of retaliation from beyond the grave. Many societies share the belief that old people can more easily intercede with ancestors, since they will soon join them. Mental incapacity need not signal the end of valued roles either, because severe dementia may be confused with ritual power; symbolic value in religious rites is possible even for those too frail to be useful in more practical ways. Alternatively, the senile may be honored for past rather than current contributions.[11]

Thus derision, contempt, abuse, and neglect are not inevitable for the least powerful aged. Under some circumstances and in some cultures, the frailest continue to serve important social functions. But these are exceptions and do not invalidate the general conclusion that physically frail and mentally incompetent elders are seriously disadvantaged when it comes to resource control, and that only the rare family or community has relatively unlimited tolerance for decrepitude. The great majority of people who have

ever lived have been poor, the economically privileged a tiny minority in every society. It follows that most frail elders never had
much in the way of valued material resources in the first place or
consumed, sold, or lost them over a long lifetime. As for noneco-
nomic resources like wisdom, tact, and a good sense of humor,
these too tend to disappear with the onset of senility and the increasing severity of physical ailments.

The childless have typically been doubly disadvantaged because
they have to rely on more distant kin or on the charity of strangers.
The death of a highly dependent old woman in Kaliai (Papua New
Guinea) is an example. In attempting to kindle a fire, she fell into
the burning embers and lay there for some time before she was
found; days later she died of her injuries. The tragedy was due in
part to her lack of biological children to look after her: "The fact
that both of her stepchildren were responsible for large families
contributed to their resentment of the added burden of caring for
someone to whom they were but tenuously related." Among the
!Kung hunters and gatherers of Botswana, elders with no surviving
child are more likely to go hungry and be otherwise neglected than
their more fortunate counterparts; for aged Gusii women in Kenya,
to be sonless is to risk disaster. Childless elders in the Mexican village of Santo Tomás Mazaltepec continue to work even when they
are very feeble; when they cannot work at all, they must beg from
house to house. Childless or sonless old people among the Chagga
of Tanzania must also beg, often from people who resent giving because they have obligations to their own kin.[12]

Those whose children turn out to be vengeful, greedy, impatient,
or indifferent are often as disadvantaged as the childless. In the
same Mexican village, for instance, an old woman with three prosperous children rarely got enough to eat because "she spent for her
own diversions all the money which [her dead husband] had left
her, instead of saving it for her children. Now that she is ill and
penniless, they do not want to help her."[13] Other children may be
motivated more by community pressure or fear of neighbors' criticism than by love and affection, so they may meet the purely physical requirements of parents for food and shelter but overlook
important psychological needs. Alternatively, in any society, even
the best-intentioned child may be driven beyond endurance by the
demands of caregiving or competing obligations.

The weight of the ethnographic and historical evidence indicates limited tolerance for decrepitude and prolonged dependency in old age, as the next section shows. Frail elders are more likely to be perceived as burden than asset, their needs treated as low priority, and their status "gradually diminished, recast, and ultimately neutralized."[14] In many cases, if their dying promises to be too slow, kin and society will speed up the process, sometimes at the elder's own request.

The Frail Elderly as Burden, Impediment, or Threat

Every culture must deal with dependency: infants and children, the handicapped, the sick and injured are always with us. But the dependency of the frail elderly is a special case. Since the elderly have already lived long lives, since their condition will only worsen and their ability to make positive contributions will only decline, and since the burdens of providing care will only increase, elder dependency is less easily tolerated than that of other dependents. Among the !Kung people, for example, it seems that "if close family members have been seen to be caring for a decrepit elder for a very long period of time, a culturally acknowledged but unexpressed statute of limitations comes into play and abandonment is permitted."[15] They have done enough.

Certain characteristics of nonindustrial societies combined to make elder care less onerous than it is today in our complicated world. Many historians and ethnographers have discussed the significance of death and death rituals in premodern settings, but descriptions of long-term care and prolonged dying are exceedingly rare. The most obvious practical reason for this apparent neglect, of course, is that proportionately few people in nonindustrial societies lived to the ages when chronic diseases, such as cancer and heart disease, begin to take their slow toll. Death generally came quickly owing to the inability of medical knowledge to prevent it. At worst, then, frail elders were a short-term burden wherever death, and dependency, could not be prolonged by antibiotics, surgery, mechanical ventilators, feeding tubes, or other forms of human intervention.[16]

At the same time, the relatively high fertility of most nonindustrial societies resulted in more caregivers per elder; grandchildren in particular were often enlisted to do chores and provide companionship to the aged, as among the Chagga people of Tanzania. The traditional Navaho custom of giving grandchildren to grandparents is another good example; reports indicate, however, that these youngsters were ambivalent about their helping role and sometimes resented the restrictions on their freedom. In other societies, the burden of supporting the elderly was a community responsibility, thus easing the load on individual families. The forms of care that could be provided to frail elders were also much simpler—essentially the same as those directed to other dependents—food, water, comfort, and shelter. In the absence of modern medicine, little more could be done. Food and drink, for example, had to be taken by mouth or not at all, so no moral debates about artificial feeding were required. There was no expectation whatever "that medicine could significantly extend individual life or effectively combat the infirmities of old age." This attitude stands in sharp contrast to today's situation, when families do a great deal to extend elders' lives and combat their infirmities. For example, some relatives perform care routines so complex that even licensed vocational nurses are not permitted to do them in hospitals.[17]

Nor did geographic mobility and great physical distance hinder daily face-to-face caregiving in the past as they often do now, when families are split up as young adults migrate to cities for jobs, marrying and raising their children there while their aged parents remain behind. When most people, especially women, worked in or near the home, care provision was more easily handled than today, when work, for most, is at a distance from home. Compulsory schooling and many attractive leisure activities affect children's availability and willingness to aid frail, aged relatives. Without a wage system, the opportunity costs of providing care (to all dependent groups, not just the frail elderly) were less, though leisure time always has some value to individuals. Family financial sacrifices to pay for expensive medical or personal care needs were not required. For all these reasons, it would seem that simpler societies were better equipped to provide long-term elder care than our own. Yet we find evidence of considerable intolerance for prolonged dependency and even open resort to death hastening in traditional societies, suggesting that other values besides filial piety enter the picture.

History shows us, for example, that Western Europeans typically disvalued old age and were not tolerant of old people. Popular opinion in preindustrial France held that "old age was a horror and old people a great nuisance." In late-nineteenth-century Russia, as elsewhere, the ability or inability to work was what mattered, not age itself. The elderly were perceived as useful as long as they could work, even if the work was menial, but when they became too ill or infirm to work, they became burdens to poor peasant families or communes. Early Americans distinguished between a "green old age," with little or no restriction on activities, and decrepitude, which precluded work and independence; only those in the former category were respected, for their essential contributions. Similarly, respect and affection wear thin as elderly Eskimos, old Niueans in Western Polynesia, aging New Guinea tribesmen, and their counterparts around the globe are gradually transformed from active contributors to passive recipients of resources.[18]

Decrepit and competent elders are treated differently because of the value placed on *reciprocity*. A well-known anthropologist, Leo Simmons, wrote many years ago that "security and survival in senescence are not a boon of nature, nor a gift of the gods; they depend upon the contributions which old people can make or the rights which they can command." In other words, elders are valued in direct proportion to what they can do for others. One-way support for indefinite periods has not been tolerated in many nonindustrial societies because it creates strain for both parties and may threaten the welfare or even the survival of the group. Elders themselves may feel like parasites, unable to help their community or reciprocate for the services they receive. Time, energy, and other resources are finite everywhere, and even "primitive" societies may be quite pragmatic when it comes to resource distribution. A study of a Zapotec Indian village in Oaxaca, Mexico, in the late 1960s, for example, showed that villagers tended to accept death as inevitable when there was no money to spare for a doctor, implying that residents chose to spend what money they did have on other needs. Most important, the norm of reciprocity is universal, with certain exceptions such as early childhood, some phases of the childbearing cycle, senescence, and various crises. In all cases, the rule of reciprocity dictates that dependency is acceptable only for a limited time; once it runs beyond what the society expects, the individual becomes a burden—receiving support that cannot be reciprocated.[19]

There is considerable consensus that "excessive" longevity (survival beyond one's ability to make positive contributions to family or society) is universally disvalued. Attitudes and behavior change when it seems that illness will last a long time and the person will not recover. Continued support seems pointless or even counterproductive, if it hinders the person's transition to the next world. Relatives of a sick native woman in East Arnhem, Australia, for instance, became upset when a health worker offered her water, and her son threatened to knock the worker down. The woman died of thirst. Respect for an old person and a sense of responsibility for him may be seriously eroded as he becomes increasingly dysfunctional, eliciting a change in caregivers' attitudes from solicitude to indifference or resentment. The "living liability" of the decrepit old has often been confirmed. Among the Hopi Indians of the American Southwest, for instance, a son might remind his father, "you had your day, you are going to die pretty soon," and refuse to support the old man; as even the formerly powerful grow feebler, relatives might grab their possessions, scold them, or allow children to play jokes on them. And in an agricultural village in Japan, a man told an aged, dependent relative that "she might as well die" because she could no longer work and there was a serious food crisis. "The old woman brooded over the rebuke and not long after hanged herself," for which the man was severely censured by other villagers. This despite the fact that many may have secretly agreed with his assessment. The permanent disappearance of an ability to reciprocate services thus helps to legitimate poor treatment. But all societies seem to prefer passive to active forms of death hastening whenever possible, though outright abandonment and geronticide have been documented often enough.[20]

Fear of a personal transition from asset to burden keeps elders struggling against labels of "decrepit" or "useless," evidence that they too disvalue dependency. At the least, many try to accommodate to children's wishes in return for the necessities of life. Elders in primitive societies prefer any kind of social participation to complete idleness and the indifference of others. Among the Niue people of Polynesia, for example, those no longer capable of strenuous "bush work" may take over household chores or look for new roles such as "clown" or "storyteller," which are better suited to their declining abilities. A telling example of the struggle to remain useful is the case of an old woman in Mexico, observed by anthropologist Frances Adams: "Confined to her mat and lying on her side because of a painfully injured spine, [she] still shucks corn with her free hand." Similarly, to the Marquesans of French Polynesia, "the horror of senility or inactivity in dependent old age is obvious. One changes from being fully a person to being supported by others, being immobile, being evidently less than a fully competent person. [Thus] Marquesans expectably struggle against both being and appearing to be dependent." A continuing desire for self-respect and the respect of others, as well as fears of becoming a burden, underlie such efforts.[21]

The limited assets over which the frail elderly are sometimes able to retain control are easily outweighed by the perceived burden of their care and so influence how they are treated. Competing obligations and role conflicts are found in traditional as well as in modern societies and the childless (or sonless), as we saw earlier, have even less claim on the charity of others. In some primitive societies, frail elders may endanger group safety if food is scarce or rapid movement is required. Evidence of outright killing or abandonment of such elders was found in 20 of 95 premodern societies scattered throughout the world, ranging from the Kikuyu of East Africa to Fijians to the Shoshone Indians of North America. The decrepit aged may also have a negative impact on family and community morale, as vigorous youth and dying aged resent one another in a complex web of intergenerational tensions: the old resent the betrayal of their own bodies and the fact that the young flourish while they suffer, while the young resent the drain on their energy and limited resources, as well as the depressing image of the future the old present. The senility of frail elders may also be an embarrassment to kin or threaten their well-being by poor resource management, since mental acuity is important for the efficient use of land and other property; the unscrupulous in any society may take advantage of a parent's senility, endangering children's inheritance.[22]

Parents who seem to live too long may also frustrate children's efforts to control land, try innovative techniques (such as modern farming methods), or assume leadership roles. Among the Gisu people of Uganda, an ambitious son may kill his father and, in Ghana, the eldest son of a Tallensi man is often suspected of wanting to hasten the old man's death. In one case, in Papua New Guinea in 1982, mortuary rites were completed prior to a senile elder's physical death. "His family believed that his body was only a husk from which [his] vitality as a social person had gone," a fact that made him "physically irrelevant" although he had once been the village's most prestigious leader. The ceremony, in which the old man participated, defined him as socially dead, allowing his debts and obligations to be settled and his sons to become leaders in their own right. This case, while exceptional in some respects, is typical in its passivity, since the old man was not actually killed.[23]

The Frail Elderly as Low Priority

Every society, explicitly or implicitly, makes decisions about what constitutes "excessive" longevity, weighing the gains and losses of life extension and setting tolerable limits for resource provision. One way in which the "overaged" are tacitly helped to die is by making their needs low priority when life-sustaining resources are distributed. They may get insufficient food or food of low quality and little or no medical care. For example, the amount of money spent on a dying person in the Mexican village of Santo Tomás Mazaltepec varied with his or her usefulness to the family. The very old among the Gwembe Tonga of Zambia suffered first when times were hard. In preindustrial India, sick old men were left alone and without food all day when family members were busy in the fields. American colonial towns "warned out," or denied settlement to, people likely to become dependent, with older people, of course, more likely to be perceived as a threat; by 1750, as both population and needs grew, there was increased stringency in relief practices, and older people continued to be viewed as low-priority candidates because they had little to contribute. Everywhere, other social groups have been more worthy, other needs more compelling, scarce resources better spent than on the nonproductive old.[24]

In some instances where resources are plentiful, frail elders still do not get them because of the low valuation placed on their continued existence or because other values take precedence. A good illustration is the Polynesian island of Niue, where frail elders have been neglected despite the fact that their conditions were often treatable, physicians and nurses readily available, and all medical services free of charge. Elders likely to receive no care or only minimal attention included those who were disruptive, hostile, confused, or incontinent. One Niuean elder was seen lying semicomatose on the floor, "evoking rueful smiles from visitors and kin and comments about 'going out the hard way.'" Culturally regarded as obsolete and not-quite-human, such elders were not hindered in completing their transition to the next world.[25]

There is a long history of inadequate social institutions and grudging provision of funds to meet the long-term care needs of dependent elders, in terms of either quality or quantity. Historically, the chronic care facilities where many aged were consigned operated "on an inevitably lowest-cost-per-day basis," plagued by "constrained budgets, an almshouse heritage, and the dispiriting awareness that the brave new weapons of medical science were of little use in treating the victims of degenerative ills." This is not to suggest that the plight of the most vulnerable has been of no concern to philanthropists or policy makers, for concern has been expressed in a wide variety of historical and cross-cultural contexts. But the situation in late-nineteenth-century Russia seems broadly generalizable: despite expressions of sympathy, the assistance provided by charities and public relief programs did not begin to meet their most basic needs. Prescriptions for improvement have not been lacking either, but sufficient and effective *action* has been rare. Hence the conclusion that, explicitly or implicitly, the lives of the frailest are indeed low priority and that the community tacitly agrees that this choice is rational and necessary in the arena of competing needs.[26]

Victimization of the Frail Elderly

It is a small step from perceptions of burden and assignment to low priority to outright victimization of frail elders. They are the most functionally impaired group in a population and the least likely to have a protective family or social network. Many outlive children as well as spouse. They typically lack valued resources to exchange for the necessities and amenities of life. They may be too feeble to take effective action, or even complain, when they are mistreated, and few will speak for them. If frail elders are blamed for their own infirmities, or their afflictions interpreted as well-deserved punishments for wrong-doing earlier in life, as in the Polynesian society mentioned above, this too serves as sufficient rationale for abuse and neglect.[27]

Both cross-culturally and over time, behavior can be classified into two main categories, in both of which frail elders may be victimized: they may be helped or encouraged to die too soon (a premature death) or kept alive too long (a delayed death). Although admittedly these concepts are difficult to define, they are real and necessary.[28] The definitions preferred here, albeit somewhat subjective, are that a premature death is one that occurs while the individual still wants, and has a realistic potential for, social interaction (that is, a biographical life), whereas a delayed death is one that takes place after that point.

Dying well is a universal and timeless concern. For example, in Papua New Guinea

> A good death is usually the quiet death of an elderly person that takes place with his or her acquiescence. It is appropriate, it is under the dying person's control, and it permits time for the social connections that have bound the person to the community to be brought to satisfactory closure. . . . [It allows time to] settle debts and fulfill obligations, and bring both his social and economic affairs to a steady state before death.[29]

In contrast, sudden, unexpected deaths, as well as those that are lingering or "postmature," are deemed bad by most; rare exceptions include the rural Irish elders described by anthropologist Nancy Scheper-Hughes, who pray for "a slow, gradual, even painful death" but, significantly, one in which they remain alert and "in control until the bitter end." Deaths that occur on time—when one's affairs are in order and friends and relatives spoken to—are highly valued. Such "good" deaths allow individuals to die when they are ready and in their own unique style.[30]

Premature Death

Death hastening may be direct or indirect. Indirect forms include a variety of private and public behaviors that indicate limited tolerance for one-way support—contempt, derision, avoidance, exclusion from meaningful roles, "invisibility," negative stereotyping, residential or institutional segregation, and the like. Often, of course, these are applied to well elders too, but find their greatest expression in the case of the frail. Among the Yakut of Siberia, for example, children beat their decrepit parents, force them to leave their homes, and compel them to beg in order to survive.[31] Surely such treatment encourages a quicker death.

The power of the environment to influence how and when old people die has been shown repeatedly, and premature death is possible even in advanced old age if elders are influenced by what the community expects, or what they *think* the community expects. It follows that a definition of death hastening should include factors like ridicule or withdrawal that may encourage an old person to "let go" of life while he still has a desire and capacity for social interaction—for a *biographically* meaningful existence. The fact that death hastening is approved and openly practiced in many nonindustrial societies creates social expectations for individual compliance that would be difficult to resist had one so wished. Among Australian aborigines, for instance, the old and feeble may be deliberately isolated by their relatives, treated as if already dead. This breaking of lifelong social bonds strongly suggests the role that the frail person is expected, indeed compelled, to play. In consequence, he cooperates in hastening his own death by refusing medical aid, food, and water. In societies at every stage of development, derision, neglect, and all the concomitants of low-priority status, along with the suffering these entail, must also serve to encourage "letting go"—a socially induced "willingness" to depart from life graciously when the culture decrees that the time has come.[32]

In their scientifically rigorous study, anthropologists Anthony Glascock and Susan Feinman found some form of nonsupportive treatment, including direct death hastening, in 84 percent of a representative sample of small-scale nonindustrial societies with data on the treatment of the aged. Nonsupportive behavior included insults directed at old people, regarding them as witches, and confiscation of their property, as well as abandonment and geronticide. Moreover, when killing, forsaking, and abandoning were combined under the heading of direct death hastening, the elderly were "dispatched" in 50 percent of the societies reviewed.[33]

Suicide is an obvious form of premature death. Societies that encourage suicide for those who seem to have lived too long (sometimes complete with ceremonies in which the old person may be an active participant) circumvent the need for more open resort to geronticide. Live burial rituals, stress on the joys of an afterlife, belief in reincarnation, and the assignment of considerable prestige to an unflinching death are all functional for the timely removal of elders who are, or threaten to become, burdensome. Dying honorably and courageously provides a final opportunity to inspire the respect and admiration of others, so the individual's need for social approval encourages compliance with community expectations, minimizes resistance, and is convenient for everyone, including kin.[34]

In the preindustrial societies in which it has been documented, indirect death hastening and even outright geronticide seem to be accepted by everyone. Taking food and water away from the sick, for example, is openly discussed and commonly practiced by Australian aborigines and hastens death through dehydration; relatives may also insist that medical aid, such as antibiotics, be discontinued. In northeastern Siberia, frail old Chuchi are stabbed in the heart with a knife, usually by a son or daughter; in the Lau Islands off southern Fiji, the old one is abandoned in a lagoon, near a cave filled with the skeletal remains of those left there earlier. Another example is the "covering up" behavior engaged in by the Tiwi, a preliterate group in Australia. According to an anthropologist who witnessed one such incident, villagers dug a hole in a lonely place and put a frail elderly woman in it, with only her head showing above ground; in a day or two they returned to find her dead. It is important to note that these activities generally require the approval and active cooperation of relatives, and often the "victim" as well. Clearly, in all such instances, relatives' sense of burden or the futility of continuing care may coexist with their compassionate motives, and the frail may be *prematurely* deprived of their property, their power, and their lives. Since younger kin in all eras may be greedy, impatient, or torn by competing obligations, cultural prescriptions about the "proper" timing of death may disguise otherwise unseemly hurry. How truly voluntary such deaths were to the elders involved and what other options were available to them are not known, but the possibility of elder victimization through premature death must be admitted.[35]

On the other hand, some frail elders may have benefitted from death hastening if it allowed escape from intense suffering. In Samoa, for example, sickly elders have asked to be put to death, and welcomed the event as a relief from the problems of old age. Another way in which geronticide could serve beneficent as well as utilitarian purposes is live burial, which allowed elders to enjoy their own funeral celebration. For instance, a three-day feast preceded live burial for very frail elders among the Yakut people in Siberia. Cultural encouragement of geronticide or suicide may thus have allowed a dignified, timely end that is not easily attained when the dying are conveyed to institutions, surrounded by strangers and all the accouterments of modern medicine. But it is important to note that ceremonial means for "death with dignity" have been reserved for a few elite elders, especially men; for the many, over a wide range of cultures, death in old age has usually come "as a sad and trying experience."[36]

In all societies, then, those who appear to live too long may be victimized in a multitude of ways that contribute to their premature death: undertreatment for treatable problems, abuse, isolation, and the absence of a meaningful part in the life of the community deprive them of peace, security, dignity, and autonomy in their final years. Their continued existence, on the other hand, may exhaust and impoverish families or endanger the society if scarce resources are diverted to their needs, or it may deny them the very dignity they crave. In light of such considerations, deliberate choices for earlier death have been made in many instances where the option to await a more "natural" death was clearly available.

Delayed Death

Every society must deal with dependency in old age, and there seems to be remarkable consistency in how they do so: death hastening by direct means (geronticide, assisted suicide) is not preferred, but happens relatively often nonetheless, whereas more passive, indirect forms of death hastening are apparently timeless and universal. There is no ideal past or Golden Age to which we can return, nor are contemporary problems necessarily amenable to the solutions resorted to in simpler societies. If death is not premature for frail elders, ironically, it may be too long delayed—a form of victimization inadvertently made increasingly likely by modern medicine, but not unknown in premodern societies. For example, in Bariai, a small community in Papua New Guinea, euthanasia was requested by a woman who had suffered intense pain for a prolonged period; the community believed that if her son did not soon release her "spirit," contained in a bundle he held, "her ghost would retaliate against him for prolonging her suffering." In this case, the family delayed compliance not because they found euthanasia morally repugnant, but because a lengthy drought precluded their ability to provide a suitable burial feast; they were also reluctant to lose a loved one and hoped to find the sorcerer responsible for her illness and so prevent the death—reasons that families in many other cultures would readily identify with. We are not told what comfort all this afforded the dying woman, but local opinion held that the son waited too long.[37] Simple logic suggests that many elders throughout history must also have experienced a death too long delayed. Euthanasia requests that were ignored or denied surely occurred, but they are hard to document and writers seem to have been blind to them.

But prolonged dying on a large scale is a new phenomenon, produced whenever medical technology becomes highly sophisticated, the cause of death structure shifts from acute to chronic diseases, and key ethical questions remain unresolved. In nonindustrial societies, death occurred relatively quickly. No antibiotics staved off pneumonia or other infections, no respirators artificially maintained breathing, no "Code Blue" brought doctors and nurses running with special equipment when a heart stopped, no ethics committee met to debate the issues. Consider again the "ideal" death described at the beginning of this chapter, where kin gather, camp around the bed, and lovingly tend the patient night and day, elders sing the clan songs, and women weep. Could this happen *repeatedly* in this simple society? Would kin gather an indefinite number of times, elders sing again and again, women weep seemingly without restraint? Clearly the patience of participants in these "primitive" rituals has a limit.

Long-term care provision was simply not a compelling issue in the nonindustrial societies of the past and, when it threatened to become one, frail elders were often removed by one means or another—neglect, abandonment, killing. Yet in today's institutions of modern medicine, a patient can literally be brought back from the brink of death again and again. Relatives do gather repeatedly, do wait in dread for the phone call in the middle of the night, do prepare themselves repeatedly for a death that does not take place. The final crisis is averted. But the patient does not get well and return to a normal existence. Instead, she lives on to endure another crisis, another frantic rush to the emergency room, another summoning of relatives, and yet another postponement of the end. Recognition of a need to stop this cycle of potential victimization is slowly gaining ground, as the following chapters document.

Frail Elderly in
the Modern World

In the 1950s, in the remote Eastern Highlands of Papua New Guinea, a "wasting, shaking, demonic disease...was relentlessly picking off its victims." A degenerative disease of the central nervous system, described as "a galloping senescence of juveniles," kuru began innocently but made its victims helpless dependents after four months and killed them within a year. The disease was causing 50 percent of all deaths in the area and threatened to wipe out the Fore people entirely; panic and social disruption were considerable. The scientist investigating the kuru epidemic, D. Carleton Gajdusek, was impressed by the "hands-off" attitude of the people in regard to life-prolonging medical care. A preliterate group "living as in the Stone Age" in isolated mountain hamlets, the Fore conceded the good doctor's ability to cure pneumonia, for example, but they knew that kuru was beyond his magical powers; once fully incapacitated by the disease, they were inclined to reject further treatment and wished to die, at home, as quickly as possible.[1]

Most of kuru's victims were children or young adults, not frail elders. But the example is a nice illustration of two major themes of this chapter. First, decisions about when to "call it quits," avoid useless suffering, and let death occur are not restricted to advanced industrial societies; even "primitive" peoples can, and do, reject medical heroics. Second, the medical technology of the late twentieth century, with its ability to prolong existence but not necessarily enhance quality of life, has vastly complicated decision making, creating new uncertainties for patients, relatives, and doctors alike as they try one remedy after another, each more desperate than the last. In the case of kuru, for example, Dr. Gajdusek reported that, contrary to their own inclinations and in order to humor him and reward his strenuous efforts to help them, the Fore "haul litters over miles of cliff-faced and precipitous jungle slopes to bring the patients in for another shot at our therapeutic trials and experimental poking."[2]

For all its exoticism (it was once thought to be caused by cannibalism) and the fear and panic it incited among far-off mountain villagers, kuru is now safely extinct. But another mysterious disease, not unlike kuru in its effects on the human brain, is now at epidemic proportions in the United States and is predicted to grow much worse in coming years—nearly four million victims are expected by the turn of the century. With its irreversible and devastating effects on individuals and families, Alzheimer's disease "may well be the kuru of our society." In its later stages, the disorder is marked by disorientation, confusion, destruction of the personality, and utter helplessness, including urinary and fecal incontinence. The interval from first onset to death averages over eight years and, as for most dementias, the cause is unknown, there is no means of prevention, no cure, and no effective treatment. The worst aspect is that victims die *with* it, not *of* it: for years the sufferer may appear "wonderfully healthy" and "vibrantly alive," but "a short time in her company reveals a lost mind imprisoned in an active body." Due to its long duration and cruel symptoms, Alzheimer's disease has come to epitomize a "bad" death. Will patients and their relatives opt for more treatment? Will professionals cajole them on to further efforts? Or will they reject futile treatments and the kind of life that Alzheimer's offers, as Janet Adkins, a 54-year-old victim of the disorder, did when she killed herself with Dr. Jack Kevorkian's "suicide machine" in 1990?[3]

Chapter 2 explored attitudes toward and treatment of the frail elderly in nonindustrial societies from four overlapping perspectives: frail elders as resource, burden, low priority, and victim. The present chapter retains the same schema but changes the scene to the more technologically complex societies of the late twentieth century, especially the United States. A review of the evidence confirms that processes associated with modernization, especially in health care, have increased the risk of victimization for frail elders, by expanding their numbers, enhancing their vulnerability, increasing the duration of their dependence, and making care provision more onerous to both recipients and providers. Death hastening and delayed death are discussed in the modern context, and experiences in other nations are noted as appropriate. We will return to the kuru story periodically for illustration of important themes, focusing on continuities with technologically simpler societies and changes occurring with modernization.

Frail Elders as Resource

A similar lack of precision concerning "which aged" characterizes many discussions of the elderly today, as in the historical and ethnographic reports described earlier. Descriptions of "the aged as resource" seem especially prone to overlooking key distinctions among the old, along with changes in their characteristics with advancing age and ill health; they imply that old people are *always* resources, for example.[4] As with nonindustrial societies, it is more accurate to say that, depending on their functional condition, degree of dependency, and numerous other factors, elders may be both resource and burden to others, including their children, over their long lifetime.

Nonetheless, in modern industrialized nations, where dying is often prolonged due to advances in medical technology, frail, dependent, and dying persons may still be perceived as assets. For example, Tish Sommers, co-founder of the Older Women's League (OWL), used what she called her "deathbed power" to persuade donors to contribute to OWL projects that would continue after her death. And the essential lessons mentioned in Chapter 2 are still possible, of course. Lessons, like role models, may be positive or negative, and negative lessons may serve positive ends, as cautionary tales for participants and observers, for instance. How many children, having endured the prolonged dying of a parent, vow "I don't want to die like that"? In fact, many adult children who provided long-term parent care have informed their own children that they want other solutions for themselves. How many are moved to work for social change to ease the problems of care provision as a direct result of their personal experiences?[5]

Financial security is often highly significant in perceptions of frail elders as assets. A Hong Kong survey, for example, shows that children are more willing to live with aged parents who are economically independent and that parent-child relationships are more harmonious if elders can support themselves financially. And researchers in Quebec note that "there are many situations where an elderly relative is taken into a family because of the money he or she represents." Certainly these behaviors know no national boundaries.[6]

And elder care provides a wide variety of jobs, of course, ranging from nurses' aides to geriatrics specialists. In the United States, the health care industry employs millions, and expanding health-service industries have given a major boost to many local economies as other industries have declined; in Waterbury, Connecticut, for example, the proportion of workers in the health sector ballooned from 1.6 percent in 1970 to 12.6 percent in 1991, cushioning the impact of severe job losses in the brass industry. And in 1990 alone, more than 1,500 new firms began offering home care services, according to the National Association for Home Care. Many more potential workers are being trained in anticipation of a growing number of jobs in the field; stability or shrinkage in the industry would produce economy-wide impacts as established workers were laid off, competition for remaining jobs grew keener, or aspiring entrants found their options limited. Furthermore, drugs and medical equipment must be invented, manufactured, distributed, sold, maintained, and repaired—all contributing positively to employment rates and the gross national product. Sales of incontinence products, like disposable diapers for adults, are soaring as the American population ages, and this market is expected to double in the next five years. New medical technologies, in particular, have been accompanied by major expansions of training initiatives and career opportunities.[7]

Research on aging and disease processes may also benefit the young directly, or provide valuable clues that will enable future generations to enjoy better health when they become old. Hence the suffering of some can be rationalized on the grounds that others will eventually benefit. The frail and dying may still be altruistic, and the history of medicine is replete with tales of courage and unselfish motives for the betterment of other human lives. There would be a great loss to medical knowledge if every patient with a serious illness immediately committed suicide, as Janet Adkins did soon after being diagnosed with Alzheimer's disease. Researchers would never learn enough about the condition to prevent, postpone, or mitigate its effects, thus helping to extend lives of higher quality to future cohorts. Pushing at the frontiers of medical knowledge automatically entails risk and the use of unproven methods in hope of benefit, so without willing human subjects, many crucial areas of research may be forestalled. Of course, there is no social obligation compelling sick people to be altruistic for research purposes or the benefit of future generations, but some patients freely choose to prolong lives of poor quality for just such reasons. Many fellow citizens would praise their choice, while others would respect it, even though heavy costs are involved.[8]

Some care providers may feel fulfilled in that role, gaining satisfaction and happiness from helping others and welcoming the challenges of caregiving, even in the most difficult circumstances. Conforming to community norms and meeting the expectations of one's friends and neighbors provide gratification to caregiving relatives. Anticipated rewards in an afterlife motivate some, and others provide care because they expect to need help themselves someday. Medical professionals, of course, typically choose their careers precisely because they expect great personal satisfaction from their helping role. Opponents of death control believe that prolonged suffering ennobles the sufferer (and care providers as well) and helps preserve important family values. Others may perceive the same suffering as unnecessary and cruel and thus are inspired to work for social change as a result—witness the recent attention in many parts of the globe to quality-of-life issues, new definitions of death, and the right-to-die movement.[9]

The Frail Elderly as Burden, Impediment, or Threat

Citizens of modern nations typically make the same distinctions between frail and competent elders that more primitive peoples do, although they are less open about it. In 1975, gerontologist Robert Butler published a Pulitzer prize-winning book in which he described Americans' confusing mix of attitudes toward old people— images of "beloved and tranquil grandparents, wise elders, white-haired patriarchs and matriarchs" contrasted with opposite images which disparage the elderly, "seeing age as decay, decrepitude, a disgusting and undignified dependency."[10] The puzzle is resolved when one realizes that Americans, like other humans, respond selectively to old people in different categories, and their reaction to the same elder is subject to change over time as that person's condition changes.

Evidence of different treatments for different groups of elders is all around us. Even in otherwise optimistic accounts of the good treatment of old people in contemporary Japan, for example, "a theme of resentment and desire to abandon senile and incapacitated aged" is also evident. And cultural norms support, even encourage, suicide "to eliminate the self when it has become a drag upon others (family above all), when it no longer can contribute to their well-being." But it is unacceptable to speak openly about such matters, and those who do so risk censure, despite the fact that others may tacitly agree. Recent empirical work in the United States also suggests that an elder's condition is relevant for his/her relationships with kin: "vulnerable" aged in the community had *less* contact with children (though presumably they needed *more*) than the "nonvulnerable," and institutionalized elders had the least contact. Family visits taper off and relatives withdraw as a patient's condition deteriorates in a nursing home setting.[11]

Ironically, avoidance occurs even within the nursing home: the frailest elders may be shunned by their more intact neighbors. For example, one observer noted little interaction among residents: "Patients do not have anything to do with each other. To fraternize with other patients would mean to place oneself at their level, to admit that one indeed belongs" in the institution, an admission that is too threatening to be tolerated. The fact that, nationally, about 40 percent of nursing home residents suffer from dementia and about half display serious behavior problems certainly contributes to this aversion. Like the most primitive tribes, healthier residents make an intact/decrepit distinction and physically avoid the latter insofar as possible, in addition to distancing themselves psychologically. Intact clients know "who belongs where," and object strongly to any forced mixing with very decrepit, senile, or dying patients, although they may express sympathy with their plight. Such findings fit well with recent distinctions between "ageism" and "healthism" reported in a 1990 Canadian study—regardless of age, those in poor health were perceived negatively by respondents. Frail elders, of course, may suffer the "double negatives" of ageism *and* healthism.[12]

Societal ideals about how the old, the sick, and the otherwise vulnerable should be treated are still honored more in the breach than in everyday practice. Both individual and collective behavior indicate that frail elders are often seen as burdens, impediments, or threats to the welfare of others. In her discussion of medical decision making, ethicist Nancy Jecker notes that the old pose a threat to the "family commons" if their wishes "usurp all other considerations," including relatives' competing obligations. Many writers in the mass media and elsewhere have commented on what they perceive as the intolerable burdens that expensive overtreatment of intractably ill elders imposes on families. Daniel Callahan, a prominent medical ethicist, sees the elderly as a new social threat to other Americans; their expensive programs constitute "one of the great fiscal black holes, capable of consuming an ever-larger portion of tax revenues," and hence are unfair to other groups and ultimately dangerous to our society. Another prominent writer has described the graying of the American population as a serious obstacle to those working to lower the costs of medical care. Books such as Phillip Longman's *Born to Pay* popularize themes of intergenerational competition for scarce resources, maintaining that the well-being of younger generations is jeopardized by too-generous provision of resources to the old. All this despite the plight of millions of vulnerable elders who are underserved by public programs.[13]

Very dependent elders may not only be unable to make positive contributions to their society, but may slow or prevent the efforts of others by commanding their time, energy, and material resources for caregiving. The wife who leaves the workforce and exhausts her energy in providing care to her spouse, becoming poor and ill herself in the process, is transformed from productive worker to needy dependent. Or the daughter-in-law who, despite her credentials as a teacher, must stay home to tend her mother-in-law's needs may feel she is shortchanging her parents, her community, or the government that financed her education. Frail, needy aged may also have a negative impact on family and community morale. One 74-year-old nursing home resident, for example, wrote of the adult children, her own among them, who seldom visit their institutionalized parents because "today it's their parents, tomorrow it will be them. I see them peering into the rooms as they move along the corridors. I hear them exchange whispered words, 'Isn't it awful?'"[14]

In all advanced industrial societies, the phenomenon of population aging has been well publicized in recent years, primarily from a "burden" perspective. The emergence of the oldest old (aged 85 and over), in particular, has been viewed with dismay, as popular stereotypes cast them as overwhelmingly sick, depressed, alone, and extremely needy. Participants in a 1985 symposium discussed the importance of "positive" and "negative" migrant characteristics in defining the impact of elderly migration patterns on Sunbelt states. "Winning" states are "enriched" when elders who are healthy, active, and financially well-off move in; other states "lose in the exchange" if independent older people move out while those who are more dependent on health and social services—the oldest, the sickest, and the poorest—move back. In Japan, a nation whose population has been aging particularly rapidly, there are indications of widespread resentment against the caregiving burdens presented by highly incapacitated elders. Citizens, including old people themselves, lament the "ugly decline" during which elders are powerless, sick, and a burden to society. A survey of aged Japanese women found that "every informant stressed that she would do anything to avoid being a burden to the children"; the women prayed for a quick death, bypassing the bedridden phase. Hence cultural definitions of propriety in Japan, as elsewhere, assert that elders do not merit, or expect, unconditional support when providing it becomes socially destructive.[15]

In the United States and other modern societies, long-term parent care is becoming a more common stage of life for adult children, and more and more families are directly affected by the protracted illness of an aged relative. Other relevant developments include growing skepticism about medicine's ability to cure, increasing cost awareness, and a growing tendency to question the quality of life that additional health dollars are able to purchase, as well as constraints on the family's ability to provide long-term care.[16]

Today, as in the past, caretaking by relatives entails tensions and antagonisms as well as attachments and reciprocities. Recent research has challenged the assumption that adult children take care of their parents because of the emotional closeness between generations; instead, it is society's prescriptions of obligation and the penalties attached to noncompliance which foster the development of personal feelings of obligation. These feelings may be weakened by role conflict, geographic distance, gender, and parent type. When the young do meet their caretaking obligations, then, they may do so more from a sense of human decency, however grudging, than from love and affection. Elders' physical needs may be met while their equally important emotional and psychological needs are neglected, for example.[17]

As in premodern societies, the norm of reciprocity remains central, and one-way support for long periods is highly disvalued by all parties to the arrangement. In Anglo-American culture, past services do not obligate the recipient indefinitely, and old age is an acceptable excuse for dependency only if its duration is relatively short. One often-overlooked caveat is that if reciprocity is the basis for caregiving obligations, the bad must be considered along with the good: children who were ill treated by parents or the wife abused by her husband might owe nothing. In any case, if such obligations exist at all, there must be reasonable limits to them. But family members nursing frail relatives may be unable to withdraw from highly burdensome relationships for financial or emotional reasons, or lack of alternatives. Such situations not only compel involuntary caregiving but engender stress, tension, and perhaps ill health for providers while creating a potentially harmful environment for their vulnerable charges.[18]

Although few families today literally abandon or kill frail relatives, their sense of burden and limited tolerance for one-way support manifests itself in more subtle ways, such as psychological abuse, physical neglect, or open resentment of the elder's presence. For example, a recent survey in Shanghai showed that aged with little or no income received worse treatment from their children than those in better financial circumstances.[19] Neglect or abuse, such as the threat of abandonment or institutionalization, may affect the elder's will to live, hastening death indirectly.

Other key groups and institutions, including those specifically designated as "caring" personnel and "caring" institutions, openly disvalue the frailest. Health care practitioners often hold very negative attitudes about aging and the aged, in part because they deal with elders who are sick, not those who are well. In a novel based on his experiences as an intern, Samuel Shem refers frequently to the frustration, burden, and depression associated with caring for patients who cannot get well, referred to as "gomers" by staff. The term, an acronym for "Get Out of My Emergency Room," refers to "a human being who has lost—often through age—what goes into being a human being." The designation is typically accompanied by treatment that ranges from indifference to outright cruelty. For their part, nurses tend not to linger in the rooms of patients who are feeble, confused, or unaware of their surroundings, exiting as soon as their tasks allow; although time pressures are often blamed for impeding better care, nurses do not use their free time to intensify contact with such patients. While we may understand and even sympathize with such attitudes and behaviors by medical workers, clearly they are potentially harmful to vulnerable elders. Indeed, Shem's book has become a "must read" for medical students and the author is often invited to speak to medical audiences on how to achieve greater humanism in medicine.[20]

Institutions also use avoidance techniques. Nursing homes, for example, often choose to sidestep the burden that some frail elders present. Despite state and federal regulations prohibiting discrimination on the basis of health or financial status, preadmission screening often serves to exclude the sickest and the poorest, and those who use up their money may be discharged. In facilities run for profit (the majority), "proprietors have zigzagged through the maze of state and federal regulations, interpreting them the best they can to turn a profit. No sooner is a law passed than they jump to use every possible loophole." In the former U.S.S.R., medical institutions frequently refused admission to the terminally ill. For a variety of reasons, then, the medical establishment often retreats from (or mistreats) the most needy aged—those least likely to respond to their ministrations by getting better.[21]

Insurance companies too are anxious to keep clear of the expensive burden of aged who are or threaten to become frail on a long-term basis. Applications include questions on health and prior use of nursing homes, for example, and are usually sold face-to-face, so agents can screen out high-risk applicants; policies are seldom sold to those over 80. Few policies cover homemaker services, adult day care, or hospice care, and persons with long-standing but medically stable illnesses such as Alzheimer's disease often do not qualify for coverage. Partly due to reimbursement policies, even hospices selectively admit those who are expected to die soon (typically, cancer patients) in preference to those whose dying will be prolonged, such as dementia victims, who are often physically robust. Finally, governments everywhere typically seek to minimize their responsibility. Despite the millions of dollars spent annually on Social Security, Medicare, and Medicaid, American society traditionally has been reluctant to acknowledge a public role in service provision to citizens, leaving it to families, charitable institutions, and the private sector wherever possible; this is especially true of long-term care services. To the extent that societies must accept *some* responsibility for the most vulnerable, however, they do so by making their needs low priority.[22]

The Frail Elderly as Low Priority

Every society has limited resources and so must make hard choices about how to distribute them among many compelling needs. Rationing mechanisms may be difficult to perceive for what they are, but they are far more common in the United States than most people realize. Medicare rules requiring deductibles and copayments, for example, discourage poor people from using medical resources, and low physician reimbursement rates under Medicaid serve as rationing devices because many physicians limit the number of Medicaid patients they will see.[23] Some services that are very important to frail elders, such as home care, may not be covered at all, and services that are covered are often strictly limited. Sometimes health policy choices are unwise, misinformed, short-sighted, or callous, but they are made nonetheless and, once made, difficult to change. By common consent (or lack of public outcry), a variety of private and public behaviors indicate limited tolerance for one-way support of the most vulnerable elders. Contempt, derision, avoidance, "invisibility," ageist and healthist stereotyping, residential and institutional segregation are examples.

Occasionally, these behaviors are applied to well elders too, but find their greatest expression among the frailest.

Negative stereotypes of old age have persisted over time. Public attitudes toward death and dying in old age also suggest the stability of age-old views: that the older person is ready for death, or even longing for it, that death is natural in old age, that social loss is minimal when an elder dies, and that scarce resources are more appropriately directed to the young. In the British health care system, for example, it is axiomatic that care that saves or improves a child's life is more beneficial than those same resources targeted to an old person; prime-age adults with work and childrearing responsibilities also take precedence over the old. In other words, people generally think it is more sensible to extend the life of a young person than that of an old person, especially when health care is very costly. Similarly, mass media appeals for contributions to the care of senile or disabled elders, analogous to those we often see for a sick child, are all but inconceivable. The strong emotional appeal of cases where lives hinge on access to expensive health care clearly varies by age of the sufferer. Such prioritizing need not be based on current economic productivity or the potential for economic productivity in the future, but derives simply from weighing the gains against the costs when the patient is old. Seven in ten deaths in the United States occur to people 65 or older, and because life-prolonging terminal care ranks low on the scale of real human benefit, it is a likely candidate for cuts when rationing decisions are made. Indeed, in Britain, where health care budgets are far more strictly controlled than in the United States, physicians discontinue aggressive treatment for the incurably ill sooner than their American counterparts, and they assert that they would do so voluntarily even if resources were not constrained. Moreover, many Americans believe, with ethicist Paul Menzel, that "extending severely demented and senescent patients' lives should have lower priority even if their lives have no predictable limit."[24]

"Primitive" peoples prioritize in much the same fashion. Because the victims of kuru were primarily children or young women, many men were widowed or unable to marry (or remarry), and many children did not survive long enough to reproduce. Hence, the group's continuing existence was threatened and radical measures called for:

Desperately the Fore searched far and wide for cures. They placed guards on their boundaries to keep out people with malevolent intent. They called openly for confessions of sorcery and where the curse of kuru had been evoked to avenge an insult, propitiations were undertaken. Guilty clans were subject to savage acts of revenge; they were ambushed, stoned, or bitten, and...ritual murders were causing as many deaths as kuru.[25]

In sharp contrast, no case can be made that reproductive potential (in societies at any level of development) is threatened by the loss of frail elders. In fact, many now maintain the opposite—that their continued *existence* endangers group welfare. Reams of idealistic words have been written about care, love, duty, and the deservingness of the vulnerable old. Nonetheless, our collective *behavior* toward them meshes very poorly with those noble words, reflecting our real attitudes regarding their value. Thus a long history of inadequacies (of funds, of personnel, of time, of physical facilities) for meeting the long-term care needs of growing numbers of frail elders continues; both quality and quantity are lacking now as in the past.[26]

The nonacute care services required by many aged patients have been poorly supported by American society; such patients fit uneasily into a medical system attuned to very different expectations—that is, that the sick person will recover or at least improve. Because chronic conditions are irreversible, many physicians view chronic care as tedious, uninteresting, and an inefficient use of their time and talents. Nonmedical long-term care services (such as bathing, feeding, toileting) fare even worse. They do not convey the same sense of moral urgency that medical services do, so social obligations to provide them are not felt as keenly, and resource deployment may be minimal until a crisis intervenes; if disabilities are attributed to normal aging processes, less public effort may seem justified. Even physical pain, a major problem in long-term care, has been understudied for geriatric patients; leading textbooks of geriatric medicine devote scant attention to pain management, so many physicians and nurses lack sufficient knowledge for dealing with it. Hence it is not surprising that the care provided to frail clients in formal institutions emphasizes physical maintenance tasks that produce visible and measurable results (baths given, beds made, meals served) to the relative neglect of less tangible aspects of quality of life. Mental health needs, for instance, go largely unmet. In her study of long-term care for the elderly in several European countries, Betty Landsberger noted "universal dissatisfaction" with existing nursing homes, but most governments refrain from assuming responsibility for improvements.[27]

There is no denying that nursing homes—the institutions charged with taking up much of the slack in long-term care—face formidable obstacles in providing good care to profoundly needy patients. But few are as good as they could be. In the United States, care remains seriously deficient in many homes that receive federal funds; legislation passed in 1987, which set requirements for improving care and protecting patients' rights, has had limited impact and there is no consistent nationwide enforcement. While a plethora of regulations ensure that bedpans are counted and clocks are punched, no one seems to know how to measure quality of life, let alone produce it, for frail elders.[28]

Given much-publicized budget constraints and cost containment initiatives in recent years, chances for substantial improvements in nursing homes are slim. They are likely to remain low priority. Even increases in the supply of beds are unlikely, despite growing demand. Before facilities can be built or expanded, state permission—a "certificate of need"—is required if investors want the facility to be eligible for Medicaid reimbursement (something most investors want). But state governments are trying to restrict growth in the number of beds as one means of controlling total nursing home expenditures, which have been doubling every five years. Hence they frequently hold up or reject certificates of need to add more beds.[29]

Typically, it is the most vulnerable who are the first to suffer when cost considerations arise. The most explicit rationing efforts to date—those associated with Diagnosis Related Groups (DRGs)—are aimed at elderly Medicare patients. Enacted in 1983 under the Medicare program, the DRG prospective payment system was designed to contain costs by paying hospitals a fixed amount per patient, based on his diagnosis and other factors. If a hospital keeps a patient an unnecessarily long time or performs unnecessary tests, it loses money. Other incentives in the system encourage earlier discharge—"quicker and sicker"—and so entail a risk of inadequate care. Alternatively, since payment is the same for simple and complicated cases in the same diagnostic category, hospitals may cut corners or even refuse admission to sicker patients, whose costs of care threaten to exceed the payment rate. Most important, both Medicare and Medicaid are increasingly reluctant to finance long-term care, and nursing homes select against heavy care cases that are more costly in terms of staff time as well as monies. For example, when Frank Robinson tried to find a suitable nursing home for his ailing mother, the social worker told him, "Let's face it, nobody wants her. She's too heavy. They prefer the little skinny, eighty-pounders. And she can't go to the bathroom to relieve herself. She needs too much nursing." Hence the lives of the frailest continue to be low priority, and little community fuss is made about it.[30]

Within and outside our formal institutions, negative attitudes and stereotypes of elderly patients are common among health care professionals, and medical attitudes toward geriatric patients have been resistant to change. Articles on the health problems of older people, relatively scarce in general medical journals, fail to reflect the increasing use of services by this group. Physicians spend far less time with older than with younger patients and "continue to assume that extensive care for the old is economically unjustified and, ultimately, futile." Michael Wilkes and Miriam Shuchman, physicians themselves, claim that "chronologic age so colors the physician's view that the healthy as well as unhealthy older person is often denied medical options that are presented to others." For example, their cancers are routinely undertreated, and chemotherapy or radiation treatment may not be offered. Unnecessary suffering and an earlier death are likely results.[31]

The elderly are low priority in the national development plans of poor nations, and their social and health concerns tend to fall to the bottom of government aid lists. When the United Nations asked governments to identify major issues of concern for mortality and morbidity policy, none of 83 developing countries mentioned the aged. The focus everywhere was on the health problems of infants and children, women of childbearing age, and the working-age population. One observer's description of the Indian situation is typical: "There are so many persons in India who are not aged but are otherwise so gravely disadvantaged that one cannot envisage any welfare security plan for the aged without taking them into consideration first." For poor countries, such prioritizing is viewed as essential if they are to progress and compete in world markets. And, indeed, the need to prioritize is often mentioned in the growing literature on caregiver stress and burden in developing nations, echoing the concerns expressed in the vast body of literature on these topics in developed countries. Repeatedly, constraints on family ability to provide long-term care are noted; just as often, meager national resources, higher priorities, and government inability to provide services are lamented.[32]

But rich nations too continue to prioritize. Of 29 Economic Commission for Europe nations surveyed in recent years, for example, only Norway responded that the illnesses of the aged population were of special concern. The supply of medical personnel with expertise in geriatrics is seriously inadequate even in technologically advanced nations. In the United States, for example, the number of trained geriatricians is less than 3,000, and only 220 geriatric fellows are currently in subspecialty training. Barriers to recruitment include negative stereotypes of both the work and the workers and relatively low pay and prestige. Even comparatively generous provision of services, as in Sweden, a "model" welfare state, is insufficient to meet the growing needs of the very old.[33]

In rich countries as in poor ones, medical professionals distinguish between "treatable" patients—those capable of resuming social roles—and reject the rest, devoting minimal time and energy to their care. Health-care rationing decisions that use age, employment potential, family responsibilities, and other "social value" criteria exclude the oldest and frailest. When the probability of successful treatment outcomes and expected years of life to be gained are added to the equation, the frail elderly are indeed disadvantaged.[34]

Suicide among the elderly receives little attention. Although the seriously ill are highly vulnerable to suicide, suicidal elderly are poorly served by mental health facilities, suicide hot lines, and crisis intervention programs. Aggressive case finding and active outreach efforts are insufficient to locate and assist the suicide-prone. For their part, elders seldom seek out such services because most of those who attempt suicide "are deadly serious about killing themselves" and most succeed. Both the higher propensity of old people to kill themselves and the relative lack of social concern about it reflect longstanding attitudes that condone suicide as "more appropriate for the old, especially those who are physically ill or suffering intense pain, than for members of any other age group."[35]

None of this is to suggest a total lack of public empathy with the plight of the most vulnerable. Policy makers are seldom callous by choice, but they have other important things to worry about, such as the pressing needs of groups that are larger, more clamorous, and less negatively stereotyped than the frailest of elders. Those who do care—generally family members of patients—constitute a small, unmobilized, and relatively powerless group. Providers of home health care, adult day care, and respite services have not lobbied intensively for legislation favorable to the constituencies they serve. Lobbying efforts by advocates for the elderly and their caregivers for family leave legislation have been conspicuous by their absence.[36]

In the political arena, activists have been more concerned with promoting the welfare of the competent younger old than with the needs of the most vulnerable. Public policy measures employ standards of entitlement—age rather than need, for example—that enhance the lifestyles of relatively elite elders. Most programs under the Older Americans Act are not means-tested. Senior citizen centers, for example, which offer opportunities for social interaction, nutritious meals, and counseling services, are nominally open to all older people, but fail to reach the least advantaged. Those programs which *are* means-tested, such as energy assistance, are often susceptible to disproportionate budget cuts, so while better-off elders keep their benefits, the rest must struggle harder to make ends meet. Those 85 and older are poorer than other subgroups of the aged, ironically, while they are sicker on average; since illness necessitates additional spending on medical and personal care, they are doubly disadvantaged when budgets are cut.[37]

Common perceptions of fiscal crises related to elder care, an atmosphere fostered by the mass media, need not be accurate or real to be influential; so long as many policy makers *believe* that a crisis exists, they may enact cost-saving mechanisms that are not only harmful but unnecessary. But the problem is not just money. Even in prosperous times, families, governments, and dying individuals

may think it irrational to divert resources to those who can contribute little or nothing in return. For example, there are different
public perceptions of Medicare and Medicaid effectiveness in the
United States. The first program serves all those over 65, without
regard to need, whereas the second is aimed at poor people of all
ages, including the elderly. Both programs are costly, but Medicare
is seen as "medically successful," whereas Medicaid expenditures
on poor people have failed to produce health improvements of
similar magnitude. The latter program's negative public image is
due in part to the fact that "as the health insurance program of
last resort, [it] is forced to absorb the expensive problems that no
one else wants"—from crack-addicted babies to impoverished
nursing home residents. Beneficiaries may be perceived pejoratively
as weak, ineffective, and at least partly responsible for their own
problems—and hence undeserving. And despite a cost increase of
31 percent in just one year (1990 to 1991), the care provided
under Medicaid is often shoddy and inadequate. Hence economic
growth, full employment, and the reduction of inflationary pressures may well free up resources for elders in general with little or
no impact on the frail subgroup, owing to continuing negative
evaluations of their status and the assumed futility of
intervention.[38]

Public policy decisions in the United States will inevitably serve
as models (positive or negative) for developing nations. Their extreme poverty, for example, will compel most to avoid expensive
options like institutionalization. The complex ethical dilemmas of
modern medicine are the luxuries of the affluent, flourishing in the
United States only because we thought we could afford them. Such
dilemmas may never arise in poor countries, where it is well-recog-
nized that shortages of money, personnel, and equipment preclude
such niceties. Moreover, many would argue against the manifest
injustice of providing costly services to chronically ill and dying elders while children go hungry and workers cannot earn a living
wage. What lessons will developing nations draw from the "back-
tracking" now evident in American health policy for the aged—increased copayments and deductibles, for example, and the
incorporation of cost-effectiveness (historically not a consideration) in Medicare reimbursement decisions? What are the less privileged nations of the world to do when the richest say they really

cannot afford high-quality care for everyone after all? The lesson may be like that drawn by an Indian gerontologist: poor nations cannot afford to mimic the West, especially when the West itself finds its arrangements difficult to sustain. What course will they choose instead?[39]

Victimization of the Frail Elderly

Outright victimization of frail elders follows closely on their low priority status, and their victimization is strongly related to their frailty. For example, routine discrimination against *well* elders has diminished in recent years, owing to concerted efforts by the American Association of Retired Persons (AARP) and other advocates. Ironically, *frail* elders may be victimized by these well-meaning attempts to reduce negative stereotyping and ageism. One of the purposes of the AARP, with over 32 million members, for example, is to improve the image of aging. The organization's motto, "To serve, not to be served," coincides poorly with an explicit recognition of extreme frailty. The one demand, in fact, that AARP members "have most persistently presented to other Americans is for recognition of their consistent *lack* of demands"—they are responsible, independent people who find old age a positive and rewarding experience. The emphasis is on the aged as resource, and certainly not a burden. Hence organized efforts to "mainstream" the aged and to portray them as healthy, capable, and self-reliant are conducive to a greater propensity to deny the existence of the frailest and reluctance to admit their neediness. Indeed, remaining discriminatory tendencies are focused on elders with disabilities, with concern largely concentrated on long-term care costs.[40]

New popular stereotypes of the elderly as "greedy geezers" flourishing at the expense of younger generations or the "gray peril" whose political activism benefits only themselves and harms others can also work to the disadvantage of the neediest. Scholarly researchers have advanced the same themes: that the interests of the old are in conflict with, and deleterious to, those of the young, that elders are too expensive, and that children and younger adults suffer as a result. There seems to be an increase in societal propensity to scapegoat the aged, with an impressive list of social problems and economic woes linked to their assumed prosperity and selfishness. The rapid rise of health care costs is the major example, but expenditures on the aged have also been blamed for the nation's loss of global economic clout; even the poor school performance of American children has been attributed to the political power of older voters who are unwilling to finance education programs. Such thinking is often based on inaccurate or incomplete data and is dangerous because it diverts attention from elders who are poor, sick, or suffering from other forms of deprivation. Yet specific proposals to limit or deny health care to older persons are receiving serious attention in public forums.[41]

Owing to their high level of functional impairment, the frail elderly are relatively defenseless, unable to command sufficient resources or compel sufficient attention to their diverse needs. Many are poor; some never married, and more are widowed; some have outlived their children, as well as their spouse; their remaining relatives may be distant or indifferent. For those with relatives to assist them, it is unrealistic to assume that high-quality care is the norm. In fact, the quality of home care provided by family members is seldom investigated; it is more convenient, it seems, not to ask too many questions when the answers may be unpleasant or improvements costly. That studies are prone to uncovering disagreeable facts is clear from recent findings on elder neglect and abuse, much of which is perpetrated by relatives.[42]

The acute-care orientation of many national health programs and institutions also serves to victimize frail elders, whose chief needs are not medical, but social or personal (bathing, dressing, toileting, eating), producing a grave mismatch between the types of services needed and those available. The home health care industry does not lobby for more favorable legislation because it sees no substantial profits to be made in long-term care. Experts like Philip Brickner and his colleagues fully expect this bias against long-term care to continue. For example, they predict that most of the money allocated for home health services will continue to go to the acutely ill because it is cheaper to care for them at home than in the hospital; in contrast, those who are chronically ill will remain low priority until they become acutely ill. Then, when the acute episode is over, they will again be relegated to low priority status.[43]

Within the formal care system, elders are not always informed of treatment options normally offered to younger patients with the same chronic condition, or lifesaving treatments, such as kidney dialysis, are denied, as routinely happens in Great Britain. The frailest may also lack access to equipment that could reduce their functional disabilities because of the negative stereotyping and medical discrimination that classify such interventions as futile. Systems of health and social services that depend heavily on families to provide care, such as hospice, also severely disfavor the oldest, who are least likely to have kin available. Further, governments in countries at every level of development are reluctant to provide supports to family care providers, build more and better long-term care facilities, or finance community alternatives to institutional placement. In the United States, we have seen no major expansions of benefits to the aged since 1972 and there are no major new initiatives under way to help the most vulnerable.[44]

Legal guardianship is intended to protect persons at risk from exploitation, abuse, and neglect when they cannot adequately care for themselves or manage their property. Its use in surrogate decision making for the aged has been increasing in the United States, as population aging (and sometimes medical procedures) increase the number of incompetent elders. Thus guardianship is both essential and unavoidable. Elders' increased longevity may contribute to relatives' concerns, such as the need to pay their bills, to protect them from con artists, to shield other family members from financial liability for large medical and long-term care expenses, or to prevent the dissipation of an inheritance. But although four out of five guardians are relatives, we know little about the motives and behavior of family members in the guardian role. The fact that relatives seem more willing to serve as guardians in situations where a substantial inheritance is at stake, however, suggests a risk of financial abuse for some frail elders.[45]

Guardianship may also victimize elders if they are prematurely labeled incompetent and deprived of autonomy; they may become depressed, lose self-esteem, and lose their motivation to remain self-reliant. The great majority of guardianship cases involving older persons are full guardianships, wherein the ward essentially loses "all rights to convey property, enter into valid contracts, marry, manage financial affairs, select a domicile, or choose agents such as physicians or attorneys." Once lost, competency rights are rarely restored. It is unfortunate, then, that conclusive demonstration of the individual's incompetence is seldom documented in probate records; one recent study, in fact, showed that most wards were not overly incapacitated, either physically or mentally. Moreover, the same analysis showed that courts tended to rule in the interests of the petitioner rather than in accordance with the elder's wishes. And experts agree that appointment of a guardian is biased against elders who are simply eccentric or noncompliant rather than mentally incapacitated.[46]

Once granted, typically to an adult child, guardianship can be used for surrogate decision making on health and long-term care, including the use of life-sustaining treatments or changes in residence, such as from the community to a nursing home, which may accord poorly with the ward's preferences or best interests. The psychological impact on elders of unwarranted challenges to their competency and involuntary takeovers of their affairs is unknown, and perhaps impossible to measure. The potential for a variety of abuses is obvious. Financial reviews of guardianships are inadequate, for example, as shown in a recent Florida study where guardians who failed to file reports were not sanctioned (or even notified), and the court failed to audit the few reports that were submitted. Better judicial monitoring might prevent cases like the 92-year-old Miami woman found living in squalor, in a facility owned by her guardian, despite her $150,000 bank account.[47]

Frail elders may be afraid to complain about such mistreatment or unable to do so due to poor health; their complaints may be ignored, attributed to senility, or call down further mistreatment on the "troublemakers." Hence frail elders must often rely on outsiders to speak for them and look out for their interests—strangers who are paid to care. In their helplessness, the very frail risk both premature and delayed death.

Premature Death

Now as in the past, the social environment can strongly influence the timing and circumstances of death.[48] Vulnerable elders may still die prematurely—before their capacities for an acceptable biographical existence, on their own terms, are exhausted; this holds true even in extreme old age. Factors that encourage "letting go" seem to have changed little over time; modern industrial societies are more subtle in their death hastening, but contempt, labeling as burdensome, mistreatment, avoidance, and all the concomitants of low priority status, and the suffering these entail, certainly serve to encourage some elders to give up the fight.

How do advanced industrial nations hasten the death of frail elders and victimize them in the process? First, of course, the frailest are likely to bear the brunt of any negative stereotyping, discrimination, abuse, and neglect directed at elderly persons in general. Relegation to low priority and its potentially devastating physical, social, and emotional impact on the elder's quality of life and will to live are also relevant. Where retirement is compulsory, the oldest and frailest will have lived the longest in a devalued and dependent state and in so doing may be popularly thought to have used up any sympathy and gratitude they were entitled to on the basis of past contributions. Rationing of medical care is most disadvantageous to the oldest and sickest and carries the risk of premature death, as well as unnecessary suffering. When deaths of incompetent patients, especially those lacking close family members, are negotiated behind closed doors, employing uncertain criteria, as is currently the case in the United States, the possibilities for abuse are obvious.

Suicide, seriously undercounted for the elderly, is clearly a form of premature death. It is premature even for those who are terminally ill, because they must do it while they are still capable of acting; hence some "quality time" is inevitably lost because one is never sure of the moment when he or she may become incapable of self-deliverance. Elder suicide is sometimes difficult to recognize—drug overdoses, fatal mixtures of several drugs, or failure to take prescribed medications as instructed, for example, may all be deliberate actions, but difficult to document as suicides. Two major contributory factors to suicide among the elderly are hopelessness and helplessness, or the inability to control significant life events. Medical neglect and financial worries may contribute to such feelings, with tragic results. When a Colorado woman was released from the hospital in 1991, for instance, she received no pain medication (despite pain that was excruciating), no follow-up care, and no advice about how to finance her treatment. Fearing further bills, she refused the liver biopsy that would have disproved her preliminary diagnosis of liver cancer; then she killed herself.[49]

Little is known about suicide among elders living in institutions, but a fairly high incidence of both overt suicidal behavior and indirect life-threatening or self-destructive behavior has been documented.[50] It is difficult to believe that social attitudes and social priorities do not contribute to these suicidal feelings and efforts at self-destruction.

Home care comprises a variety of personal care services and domestic chores, such as helping an elder to bathe, dress, prepare meals, or clean house. Home health care, on the other hand, consists of purely medical services, such as changing a dressing or administering medication. Both are designed primarily as cost-saving alternatives to institutionalization, and both may inadvertently contribute to an elder's premature death. Agencies now offer increasingly sophisticated medical services and serve patients with more complex problems. But the work is often assigned to aides with limited training.[51] If a problem arises, expert help and equipment are not as readily available as in a hospital or skilled nursing facility. Thus delays or poor decisions by inadequately trained personnel in an emergency may contribute to premature death.

Institutionalization, of course, is no panacea. First, its many restrictions on most activities may be depressing and alienating. Residents typically cannot decide when to eat, sleep, or socialize, for example. Institutionalization may also be premature owing to children's refusal to provide care or to society's failure to devise community alternatives or reluctance to finance them. The continuing poor quality of long-term care institutions and the victimization of inmates are widely recognized in the United States. Inadequate care, malnutrition, "failure to thrive," and the overuse of drugs (for social control or to ease burdens on staff) are among the negative effects of institutionalization. Iatrogenic illnesses—those inadvertently caused or worsened by medical procedures—may also occur. An example is the patient who receives a tranquilizer because her agitated behavior makes caregiving difficult; the effects of the medication cause her to fall and break her leg.[52]

There are also many opportunities for crime in the nursing home industry, and employee theft, embezzlement of residents' assets, and other unscrupulous practices are widespread. According to one expert's detailed account, such crimes may account for the loss of hundreds of millions of dollars every year; the temptations are great and regulation is both difficult and costly. Given that staff members are often poor, and are poorly paid, the temptation to steal from weak, confused, or forgetful clients may be very difficult to resist, and relatives may be warned to remove a patient's valuables from the home. The psychic costs associated with residents' loss of enjoyment of what small comforts and luxuries remain to them, of course, cannot be measured. But such losses—the feelings of sadness, anger, and helplessness they inspire—can affect the will to live and so contribute to an earlier death.[53]

The oldest and most helpless patients, moreover, especially if mentally impaired, are those most likely to be victimized in institutions, as they are to be neglected and abused by their families. Since many aides are overworked, undersupervised, and minimally trained, it is unrealistic to expect that their reactions to debilitated or demented patients are either enlightened or humane in every case. Based on her work experiences inside nursing homes, for instance, anthropologist Maria Vesperi concluded that "staff members wish wholeheartedly for the death of incontinent or otherwise troublesome residents," suggesting that such patients receive less than optimal care. To busy aides a "feeder" is often an "object of scorn," and their heavy workload makes it "legitimate to stuff food down their throats." Mealtime becomes a nightmare as "food is served, forced into mouths, spat out, cleaned up, dropped on the floor, aides yell at patients, and patients scream in the hall, in their rooms, in their chairs, and then, silence again."[54] Should it surprise us that some elders prefer death to this kind of life?

More generally, another researcher noted, based on his personal observations, that abuse happened

> when a patient assaulted an aide or was perceived as deliberately making her job more difficult than it had to be. Kicking, biting, punching, or spitting at an aide were, in the aides' minds, inexcusable and punishable behavior. Likewise, a patient who defecated on the floor or in a wastebasket when, according to the aide, she was perfectly able to use the toilet, was liable to receive abusive treatment.[55]

Thus death may be hastened in myriad ways, directly or indirectly, within the walls of the "caring" institution. No prospective resident can know with certainty how she will fare within an institution's walls, but many assume the worst and some have committed suicide in their determination to avoid a nursing home existence.[56]

Few frail elders are acceptable candidates for hospice care. But even this highly touted care alternative, with its goals of preparing patients for death, controlling pain, and giving comfort to the dying, rather than effecting a cure, may hasten death unduly for some who subscribe to it. With its emphasis on palliative as opposed to curative therapy, hospice carries a risk of premature death for some patients, since prognosis is always uncertain and treatable (or even curable) disease may be overlooked; too-liberal use of drugs can also hasten death. In addition, "the termination of cure-oriented treatment, the encouragement of acceptance of death and the official pronouncement of time remaining may act to eliminate hope and undermine the will to live."[57]

Another factor that contributes to premature death is the fact that aid-in-dying is not freely available in the United States, and assisting a suicide is still illegal. Given the current confused social, legal and medical environment, death may occur too soon because elders diagnosed with a serious illness know that they must end their life while they are still capable of the necessary actions themselves, if they wish to avoid overtreatment (and *delayed* death) and protect survivors from prosecution for helping them. Others advanced in years may fear "demeaning deterioration and stultifying dependency," even if they are not yet terminally ill. Waiting too long, while one's health continues to decline, may make it impossible to implement a decision to die. It follows that if such persons were confident that aid-in-dying would be available when (and if) they needed it, their lives would be prolonged; quality of the remaining time might also improve as their greatest fears were removed.[58]

Victimization is not necessarily intentional. If patients are incapacitated, especially if they have not left specific instructions about their end-of-life treatment wishes, guardians or other surrogates must make decisions about the use of life-sustaining treatments, in many cases with little knowledge of the elder's preferences. Thus it is hardly surprising that proxies do not always decide as the patient would have. According to a recent study, for example, some proxies underestimated patients' preferences for treatment whereas others would have continued treatment when the patient would have stopped it; in cases where the proxy would ask for a do-not-resuscitate order, but the patient would not have made this request for himself, an earlier death is the likely outcome. Such discrepancies between proxy and patient preferences are sufficiently frequent to merit concern.[59]

An expanding population of frail elders provides no strength in numbers, for their poor functional condition deters collective action, and their relatives are disorganized and powerless. Growing numbers may in fact disadvantage the frailest by increasing societal perceptions of burden.[60] If cost-containment pressures in the health and social service sectors are heightened by increased emphasis on generational conflict and hence directed at the elderly, there is greater risk of death hastening, especially for the frail.

Recent popular and scholarly literature stresses the *obligations* of sick people to the rest of society. As citizens, they have responsibilities as well as rights, and their right to make health care choices is limited because society's resources are finite and other groups have rights too; the duties of citizenship extend also to those who make choices for others. As disproportionate users of health and long-term care services, frail elders are obvious targets when responsible decision making is at issue. Some, like former Colorado Governor Richard Lamm, suggest that elders have a duty to die. In other instances, older citizens are encouraged to arrange for self-disposition in case of terminal illness, in order to relieve others of the burden of care and the responsibility for making difficult choices. In this emotional climate, it is easy to envision a variety of circumstances in which suicide occurs too soon owing to a combination of social pressures, poor health, and weak resistance.[61]

In developing nations, poverty, negative stereotypes, and the low state of medical technology combine to victimize frail elders, resulting in unnecessary suffering and premature death. Health care financing is a serious concern, of course, and equipment and trained personnel are in short supply. Hospitals in most developing nations serve as little as 5 percent of the population, and there is a bias toward the urban elite; medical interventions and social welfare programs are typically prioritized in ways that benefit some groups—mothers and infants, workers, the more educated—and disfavor the old. There is a widespread assumption in poor nations that the traditional extended family cares for its aged members, and policy makers are quick to realize that this reliance on the family, however unrealistic, must continue indefinitely owing to the inability of governments to take over. Lives of continuous struggle make family care provision onerous, with the result that, in some cases, such reliance is likely to constitute "a gruesome and cruel experience of dependence, dearth, and degradation" for the aged.[62]

In all societies, then, those who appear to live too long may be directly or indirectly helped to die too soon. Others, wishing to avoid a delayed death, die too soon because we have not yet worked out acceptable policies regarding when and how life should end for the seriously ill. Presumably, many who die too soon weigh the relative risks and are willing to chance a death that is premature in order to avoid one that is delayed.

Delayed Death

"I am 82 years old, and I don't want this done," the still-competent patient told the medical team. Like her voice, Harriet Shulan's living will, filed in another state, was useless when she was hospitalized in Arizona. So "the life-sustaining tubes were inserted up her nose and down her throat and into her arms." While she was too weak to refuse consent, major surgery was performed; her condition worsened and she was placed on a respirator, while her continuing requests ("Please let me die") were disregarded because the hospital feared a lawsuit. When she tried to remove the tubes herself, her hands were strapped to the bed.[63]

In the past, the debilitated state of aged patients and small hope of success in restoring vitality discouraged experimental procedures by doctors, both for the patient's welfare and the physician's reputation. The average doctor did not wish to encourage public skepticism about his abilities or the efficacy of his remedies, and no one blamed him if a very old and very ill patient died without his intervention. Doubtless, ageism and practitioners' beliefs that interventions were pointless also played a role. Until recent decades in France, for example, the medical community virtually refused to consider therapeutic treatments for the elderly and focused instead on palliation.[64]

Thus a delayed death, like Harriet Shulan's, is a form of victimization inadvertently made possible, indeed increasingly likely, by the great advances of modern medicine. And, ironically, many people are now objecting to *over*treatment, suspicious of the physician's power to unduly delay their death. A good example is Frank Robinson's complaints about his mother's treatment: "I wanted her to go with God. God takes you in His way, but the doctors were fighting against nature, so how could she go?" Sadly, in many conditions "the preservation of life can only be bought by the prolongation of suffering," as the Robinsons learned. It is a price that growing numbers are unwilling to pay.[65]

Those who start on the road to technological dependence, whether deliberately or by being "saved" by paramedics in an emergency, are the worst off, since initiation of life-sustaining technologies often precipitates a continuous need for services. Further, it is precisely in such circumstances that patient self-determination becomes difficult or impossible. Thus developments in medical technology have created many of the current dilemmas of cost-effectiveness, quality of life, and patients' rights, which have helped bring right-to-die issues to the forefront of social consciousness. For most of human history and in poorer nations today, societies lacked the medical and human resources for extending life in old age. Nature controlled, for all of human ingenuity could not forestall death in most cases, and cultural norms functioned to remove other elders before they could be a burden (to themselves or others) for long. But continuing developments in scientific medicine gradually helped to create a conflict between the desire to prolong life with all available means and the growing costs (psychic, social, and monetary) and declining benefits associated with doing so. Technological changes have allowed many disabled persons to live on (to acquire yet more health problems that necessitate further care), when otherwise they would have died. To critic Ivan Illich, this "managed maintenance of life on high levels of sublethal illness" is the "ultimate evil" of medical progress. Modern medicine has undoubtedly postponed death and allowed individuals to avoid, postpone, mitigate, or cure a variety of diseases and disabling conditions. But by-products of the same processes have also made decrepitude more likely for more people for longer durations, at ever-increasing individual, family, and social cost. Eighty percent of all health care resources in the United States, for example, are now devoted to chronic disease. Increasing numbers of frail elders, especially dementia victims, are affecting more families and thus drawing more attention to the dilemmas of long-term care.[66]

Decisions to let die were simpler when fewer people (especially nonfamily members) and institutions had to be consulted and when little technological medicine or highly specialized skills were available to complicate decision making. In their evaluation of care to the terminally ill, for example, researchers found that as the number of professional caregivers increased, team communication decreased and adversely affected patient care.[67] With modern medicine and the numerous professionals who now attend to a single patient, once-private decisions have become more complicated and take longer to resolve.

The continuing emphasis on acute care in medical training, the "hospitalization of death," and the diverse values and beliefs of medical personnel have generally produced more conservative decisions (a bias to treat), tending to preserve life at all costs to avoid criticism, malpractice suits, and other legal battles. Other outsiders may also enter the fray; according to ethicist Daniel Callahan, for instance, if opponents succeed in restricting the right to cessation of treatment to only the most hopeless cases, many people who wish for a benign death will be kept alive, and in despair. This despite their avowed goal of protecting the elderly from *premature* death.[68]

Alternatively, a belief in progress and the well-publicized "miracles" of modern technology often leads to a desire by professionals and families alike to try out (or hope for the invention of) new therapies, hopes that are often unrealistic and make it more difficult to let the patient die. George Annas, an expert in the field of health law, suggests something worse: that dying patients are "fair game for use as teaching material" in medical training. As with premature death, victimization of frail elders by delaying their death may also be totally unintentional, caused by concerned people convinced that they are acting in the patient's best interests. How else can we explain a family's refusal to disconnect the respirator for an 87-year-old, in an irreversible coma for more than a year at a cost of nearly $1 million? And the fact that the doctors in this case sued for permission to disconnect, and lost? What would the patient have wanted? Who really knew her best interests? What other legitimate interests were at stake?[69]

When court orders, cumbersome legal proceedings, committee meetings, or complex consent forms are required to terminate treatment, or if there is disagreement among the parties involved, those who might rather die quickly must wait until a consensus is reached. For example, when a mentally competent 70-year-old suffering from five fatal diseases asked that his respirator be turned off, the hospital refused and the case went to court while the patient waited helplessly—on the respirator—for six months and, in fact, died before the court finally ruled in his favor. More generally, patients will be overtreated as interested parties debate whether there is "clear and convincing evidence" of their wishes. In other instances, relatives have insisted on futile or medically inappropriate treatments, contrary to the patient's expressed wishes or, as above, despite doctors' recommendations. Again, these are new forms of potential victimization of vulnerable elders, on a scale never dreamed of in simpler societies.[70]

Or, as in the kuru epidemic, a desire to please the doctor by trying his remedies may prolong dying; relatives may make such choices when the patient is beyond caring. Patients are first victimized by the disease and then by excessive medicine, some of which is authorized by loving relatives trying to act in their best interests. All this creates a situation where overtreatment (that which is unwanted or unbeneficial and simply prolongs suffering) is more frequent than undertreatment. In the case of kuru, Dr. Gajdusek

> tried every procedure he could think of, and every promising medication he could obtain. Kuru patients received aspirin, vitamins, antibiotics, drugs against roundworms, and others against parasites, detoxifiers in case of metallic poisoning, drugs then on trial for multiple sclerosis, drugs which would calm convulsions; . . . every one was useless.

The doctor admitted that some of his efforts were "based on the most remote chances of benefit" and caused pain, but he felt justified in trying them anyway. Despite the fact that the natives wished very strongly to die at home, their relatives were persuaded to cooperate with the doctor by bringing them to the clinic to "humor" and "repay" him for his efforts.[71]

Similarly, in today's medical contexts, the patient's *quality* of life and his personal perspective on his illness have been sadly neglected. "Successful" patients dominate in the media and treatment dilemmas are portrayed as simple mechanical problems, while ethical questions and the social components of illness, such as their devastating impact on families, are given short shrift or denied. A variety of legal and moral concerns inhibit assisted dying in most nations, with the Netherlands a prominent exception. But all the powers of medicine cannot restore frail elders to a reasonable quality of life either, so patients and families are left to cope as best they can within a system ill prepared to deal with the dilemmas it has fostered. Legal, moral, and medical systems have yet to determine what the most humane treatment is for growing numbers "who cannot express opinions, implement a plan for their own survival, or even recognize where or who they are." Thus scientific advances have unwittingly introduced new ways of victimizing the frail, by unduly delaying death and failing to resolve right-to-die issues.[72]

Implications

Modernization entails declines in fertility, fewer siblings to share parent care, the increasing geographic dispersion of family members in highly mobile societies, and the development of alternative roles for women, so that the supply of caregivers is constrained even as the demand for care grows apace. New opportunities and new goods, services, and leisure pursuits compete with family-oriented activities to fill the limited time available. Increasing longevity means that potential care providers as well as care recipients are old, retired, or suffer ill health. All these trends make direct care by kin more problematic and create a demand for government-sponsored services, including long-term care institutions.

The cost of living, especially in areas where un- and underemployment are endemic, combined with persistent ageism and fears about a growing aged dependency burden, may exacerbate concerns about the frail elderly as hindrances to family well-being, national productivity, or development efforts, and thus make their victimization more likely. Incidents of elder neglect and caregiver resentment have been reported among aborigines in Australia, some children in China are openly refusing to support their parents, elder abuse is becoming an important public issue in other Asian nations, and suicide and a right to die are debated in India. As their populations age and modernize, developing nations will face constraints on care provision in the last stage of life similar to those the industrialized countries are now grappling with. They are already learning that the Western model is a dangerous one, that they can ill afford care systems which even the wealthiest developed nations find unmanageable. In China, for example, experts are urging that the popular press be used to facilitate the acceptance and practice of euthanasia, in part because incurable disease "wastes limited resources of time and money—both private and public."[73]

Attitudes and behavior toward totally dependent elders have been remarkably consistent over time and place. Projections of the future size and composition of this population, its health care needs and related costs, continuing changes in the family that constrain its caregiving capacity, and severely limited public alternatives all suggest the likelihood of ever greater concern with health care rationing, quality of life, and the right to choose death in all nations, regardless of their level of socioeconomic development. The prevalence of dementias in particular will increase dramatically as populations age, and the victims will constitute the largest definable population of those who need long-term care, an average of 8.1 years from onset of symptoms to death.[74] Even with optimistic assumptions about the postponement or prevention of chronic illness in future generations of aged, most will experience a period of dependency prior to death. Those final years promise to be costly ones—in social, psychological, and economic terms—for all segments of society.

This chapter has argued that in many ways modernization is irrelevant to the situation of frail elders, while in other ways it complicates and worsens their plight. In every era, human beings must deal with dependency in old age. Questions of how much effort to expend on those who are aged, dependent, and infirm are not new, nor are related ethical and legal quandaries unique to Americans in the late twentieth century; what is vastly new and different, however, is medicine's ability to maintain life "beyond the point which many people think is reasonable."[75] Given the power of scientific medicine to sustain biological existence without regard to social capacity, an expanding population of frail elders highlights the need to confront difficult social questions. Already, there is widespread recognition that health care resources are ultimately limited, even in the most technologically advanced settings, that medicine is not all-powerful, and that life extension at any cost is not desirable. Meanwhile, the frail elderly retain their status as occasional assets, but they are more typically viewed as burdens or low priority, the quality of their lives diminished in many ways, and their death often quietly hastened. And some who would rather die linger on, or die with more suffering and less dignity than they would prefer, as families, legal systems, and strained economies struggle to come to terms with new realities.

4

The Acceptability of Death Control

A volume in my collection of works on population history carries the intriguing title *"A Dirty, Filthy Book."* Who could resist investigating its contents? A quick perusal reveals that the phrase is part of a larger statement, uttered in 1877 by Sir Hardinge Gifford, prosecutor in a notorious London obscenity trial. Sir Hardinge warned that "no human being would allow that book on his table, no decently educated English husband would allow even his wife to have it." What filth was this? What new dangers lurked between its pages? In fact, the infamous book was nothing more than a brief tract by an American physician, Charles Knowlton, described as "the first popularly written medical guide on how to prevent conception in the English language." When Charles Bradlaugh and Annie Besant tried to publish the little book in England, where the modern birth control movement began, their trial for "obscenity" was the immediate result. At almost the same time in the United States, an "absent-minded, puritanical Congress" passed the Comstock bill, which also defined information aimed at pregnancy prevention as obscene and banned the sending of any related material, advertisements, devices, or substances through the U.S. mail. Penalties for violations were severe—up to five years in prison and a fine of $5,000—an exorbitant sum at the time; thousands of "criminal offenders" were arrested and convicted under the law.[1]

In the nineteenth century, the idea of separating sexual intercourse from its consequences, pregnancy and childbirth, was offensive to many of those in positions of power. They saw birth control as a serious threat to family values and the very moral foundations of society and so roundly and repeatedly condemned it. Knowlton's writings are now considered absolutely innocuous, of course, since such information (and far more) is readily available in today's homes, schools, and public libraries. Indeed, even in the 1870s, the Bradlaugh-Besant trial ended with the exoneration of the two defendants, although in the jury's unanimous opinion the book in question did indeed threaten to deprave public morals.[2]

How quaint, we think. Birth control dirty and filthy? Couples forbidden to decide how many children to have, and when to have them? Doctors and publishers on trial for providing information to decent citizens trying to escape poverty and provide for their existing children? Letting nature, the church, or the government decide all-important questions of family size? The bitter fight for access to birth control is now over, and governments around the world are far more likely to promote contraception than to oppose it. Objections to birth control as "unnatural" or immoral and fears that its use would pave the way to worse abominations have also been laid to rest. So too the notion that the problems caused by unwanted births would, in time, take care of themselves, abrogating any need for deliberate human effort. We moderns are more likely to decry the blatant interference with private decisions that fueled the controversy than to condemn those who fought for personal freedom through social change. And nowadays it is the *failure* to learn about and use birth control responsibly that we label reprehensible.

The universal human desire to control fertility and a desire to control sickness and death are related. Population aging, in fact, is largely attributable to the substantial falls in fertility made possible by easy access to effective means of birth control. The agitation in some quarters over Knowlton's little book, and the unintended boost to the birth control movement occasioned by the resulting publicity, suggest that the ultimate outcome of similar current debates over death control will be greater acceptance of death by choice. For example, a number of "self-deliverance" guides, containing very explicit instructions on how to commit suicide, are now available in American bookstores. No real outrage, and certainly no trial, has yet resulted, though author Derek Humphry has described the "storm of controversy" in Britain and America over a similar publication in 1980, a storm whose chief outcome was large membership increases for euthanasia societies.[3]

In 1975, demographer Ansley Coale posited three preconditions necessary for a substantial resort to birth control in any society, all of which have important parallels in the present movement toward death control. First, couples must consider it *acceptable* to balance advantages and disadvantages before having a child—the concept of deliberate choice must not be viewed as immoral or unthinkable; second, controlled fertility must be perceived as socially and economically *advantageous*; and finally, effective *means* must be available, with sufficient knowledge, communication between spouses, and sustained will power to use them successfully. Clearly, most people weigh the advantages and disadvantages of having a child, communicate their feelings to significant others, and refrain from behavior they find morally repugnant. As the colorful history of birth control reveals, ordinary citizens are willing to challenge prevailing norms when they perceive advantages to doing so. Coale's framework is a useful paradigm for a discussion of death control in the United States today, helping us to understand the public's relatively tolerant attitudes toward death control when the positions of the various authorities—legal, medical, moral—are, at best, ambiguous. As this chapter will show, we have, for good or ill, come quite far along on the "acceptability continuum."[4]

For us, the importance of the Bradlaugh-Besant trial lies in the immense publicity it garnered, which, in turn, disseminated information on birth control to all segments of society and helped to popularize new attitudes and legitimize new forms of behavior by highlighting their advantages and providing role models. The significance of the mere *realization* by ordinary people that there was a solution to common problems—the hazards of childbirth, families too large to be fed, housed, clothed, and educated properly—cannot be overstated: although the specific mechanisms of the solution may remain obscure at first, the knowledge that there *is* a solution is the indispensable first step in social change. By the early twentieth century, even opponents of birth control in America accepted that "the practice was unstoppable. Public opinion spiraled: the more evidence of birth-control use became public, the more birth control became acceptable."[5]

This chapter explores the social context in which attitudes about death control have evolved in recent years in the direction of greater *acceptability* of death by choice, including suicide and assisted suicide. The following chapter focuses on perceptions of *advantages* to new behavior, from individual, family, medical, and societal perspectives. Since it would be unrealistic to ignore opposition to social change, the nature of the opposition and the grounds for their objections to death control are also explored. Finally, effective *means* of control, which encompass the forms of communication that relay the individual's wishes to other persons who must help in implementing her choices, as well as the implements themselves, are discussed in Chapter 6. The means for ending life quickly and painlessly in cases of extreme and incurable suffering are readily available today, awaiting only the will to use them.

As with birth control, economic and social changes are conducive to greater acceptability of deliberate human control over the timing and circumstances of death. These developments include growing skepticism about medicine's ability to cure, fear of the excesses of technological medicine, greater willingness to question the quality of life that additional health dollars (public or private) are able to purchase, and budgetary and other constraints on long-term care provision. New demographic realities combine with these other changes to focus more attention on life-and-death issues. Population aging, for example, means that a growing proportion of American families are directly affected by chronic illness and protracted dying, and that long-term elder care is becoming a common experience.[6] Hence, aided substantially by the mass media, the realization that problems exist, that current solutions are inadequate, and that innovations are necessary is diffusing throughout our society. As was the case with birth control, the spread of new attitudes and behavior seems to be class-related; innovation appears first among the higher socioeconomic groups and gradually diffuses to other segments of the population. Like birth control, death control in its various guises is now acceptable to many ordinary citizens, having been wrested from both nature and the doctors in the course of a revolution in public attitudes toward medicine and its appropriate goals.[7] The values and attitudes that underlie the growing acceptability of death by choice emerged in large part from growing recognition of new realities and the inadequacies of existing institutional mechanisms for coping with them. Many groups have a stake in the legitimation process and help to push it forward: patients and their families, the mass media, medical professionals, the judicial system, government agencies and policy makers, ethicists, and religious groups. Opponents, of course, also have a stake in hindering or halting change. These overlapping perspectives are discussed below.

The Public: Patients and Families

Popular interest in death and dying has grown immensely in recent years. The emergence of chronic diseases as the major causes of death, in a social climate where the frightening excesses of medical technology are well publicized, is largely responsible for new emphasis on the quality of life and patients' rights, especially the right to choose death. These concerns have been reinforced by growing public skepticism of the medical industry and the cost-effectiveness of dollars spent for medical care. Among the plethora of concerns, "dread of the power of medicine" stands out as the strongest incentive for death by choice. Public disillusionment began in the 1970s. Evidence was accumulating that the medical industry often caused harm and unnecessary suffering in the course of trying to cure, delaying death unduly with its heroic, yet futile, interventions. Many became uncomfortably aware of instances of excessive and unwanted medical treatment, sensitized by "horror stories" in the mass media and, increasingly, by the experiences of relatives and friends. As faith in medicine diminished, they came to see a need for patient empowerment to prevent abuses—painful and costly, yet pointless, overtreatment—by doctors and hospitals. To many, technological medicine now symbolized a modern form of torture, engendering fear and anxiety rather than faith and trust.[8] Clearly, it was time for change.

In 1975, 21-year-old Karen Ann Quinlan began to make legal and medical history. After apparently ingesting a mixture of drugs and alcohol, she suffered irreparable brain damage and lapsed into a permanent coma. When physicians refused to disconnect the respirator sustaining her breathing, her parents endured a long court battle to disconnect it, exercising Karen's right to discontinue futile treatment. They won their case in the New Jersey Supreme Court. But even without the respirator, Karen did not finish dying until 1985, ten years after her biographical life stopped. In the interim, she was unable to think or speak— "a comatose eighty-pound figure, curled in a fetal position and kept alive by intravenous feeding, . . . completely unaware of the outside world and completely dependent upon others."⁹

Nancy Cruzan enjoyed more years of biographical life than Karen Quinlan did. She was 25 when a car accident produced extensive brain damage in 1983. Unlike Karen, Nancy was never placed on a respirator. But each was sustained by a feeding tube surgically implanted in her stomach. In 1987, Nancy's parents petitioned a Missouri court to remove the feeding tube. The case went all the way to the U.S. Supreme Court, which ruled that while refusal of treatment is the individual's right, *states* should decide how that right may be exercised. So the decision to allow removal of Nancy's feeding tube eventually came from a Missouri probate court late in 1990. The young woman finally died after her remaining body functions gradually shut down, more than a week after the tube was removed.¹⁰

Although neither of these path-breaking cases dealt with elderly patients, both were highly influential in forcing Americans to confront the hard realities of modern medicine. In particular, they dramatized the central issues of death control debates: What is life, and when is it over? How far may one person go in helping another to die? What if the person whose respirator is disconnected or whose feeding tube is removed doesn't die? What if these actions cause additional suffering as the patient lingers on? How many weeks, months, or years should one wait for a "natural" death to occur? Who should decide? What constitutes sufficient proof of what the patient would have wanted?

Warned by the media drama surrounding the *Quinlan* case and, later, the prolonged dying of Nancy Cruzan, Americans now want to be protected against delayed death when circumstances seem hopeless. Opinion polls indicate that most people are aware of their rights in regard to medical care, including their right to refuse any and all life-sustaining treatments. In some instances, patients have threatened to refuse payment "for expensive treatments that promise no therapeutic benefits" and have gone to court over it. Everyone wants their preferences for future medical care to be respected; everyone wants assurance that if they become incompetent they will not be victimized by the whims, wishes, or self-interest of third parties, including relatives. Hence advance directives—living wills, Natural Death Act declarations, and durable power of attorney for health care—are increasingly sought and signed; many more people say they want such safeguards but have not yet enacted them. Americans today exhibit a growing awareness of the primacy of social components (the capacity to reason and to engage in social relationships, for example) for an adequate human existence. They are more willing to acknowledge their concerns about tradeoffs between the quantity of life and its quality, and to forgo the former for the sake of the latter. For example, "when people are asked to imagine themselves incompetent with a poor prognosis, they decide against life-sustaining treatments about 70 percent of the time." These wishes reflect the fact that those accustomed to exercising control over many other aspects of their lives want to maintain that autonomy to the end, keeping their destiny in their own hands.[11]

Such attitudes also help to reinforce popular notions that it is only fair, reasonable, and appropriate to aid the dying of the hopelessly ill, who have lived beyond their capacity to interact meaningfully with others. The knowledge that elders can now legally impose their treatment preferences on caregivers and thus, in theory, escape a delayed death, may be immensely reassuring. Like the "primitive" Fore of New Guinea, many today think that they can distinguish for themselves when medical efforts are justified and when they should be refused: while true medical miracles are appreciated, useless heroics are regarded skeptically and often rejected. The expansion of hospice programs in recent years attests to this growing tendency to reject aggressive end-of-life treatment in favor of palliative care. Since Medicare began to cover home hospice services in 1983, the number of hospice patients nationwide has more than doubled, to over 207,000.[12]

Increasingly, the average citizen supports the deliberate choice of death, a dramatic shift from earlier years. Table 4-1 indicates

TABLE 4-1

Public Responses to Survey Questions on Euthanasia and the Right to Die, 1937–1991*

Fortune Survey (Roper) (circumstances that justify euthanasia)
"Some people believe that doctors should be permitted to perform mercy killings upon...persons incurably and painfully ill. Under what circumstances would you approve this?"

1937	No circumstances	47.5%
	With patient's permission	11.6%
	With family's permission	4.2%
	With patient's and family's permission	10.9%
	With permission of medical board and family's and/or patient's	8.9%
	Don't know	15.2%

Gallup Polls (request by competent patient and family for aid-in-dying)
"When a person has a disease that cannot be cured, do you think doctors should be allowed by law to end the patient's life by some painless means if the patient and his family request it?"

Year	Yes (%)	No (%)
1947	37	54
1973	53	40
1978	58	38
1980	61	34
1985	64	33
1986	66	30

Harris Surveys (patient's right to instruct doctor)
"Do you think the patient who is terminally ill, with no cure in sight, ought to have the right to tell his doctor to put him out of his misery, or do you think this is wrong?"

Year	Put out of misery (%)	Wrong (%)
1973	37	53
1977	49	38
1981	56	41
1985	61	36

TABLE 4-1 (CONTINUED)

Roper Polls (physician aid-in-dying)

"When a person has a painful and distressing terminal disease, do you think that doctors should or should not be allowed by law to end the patient's life if there is no hope of recovery and the patient requests it?"

Year	Allow (%)	Do not allow (%)
1986	62	27
1991	68	23

General Social Surveys (NORC) (suicide/autoeuthanasia)

"Do you think that a person has the right to end his or her own life if this person has an incurable disease?"

Year	Yes (%)	No (%)
1977	38	59
1982	45	50
1983	48	48
1988	50	46

American Council of Life Insurance (the incompetent patient)

"A family ought to be able to tell doctors to remove all life support services and let the patient die if the patient is terminally ill, in a coma and not conscious, with no cure in sight."

Year	Yes (%)	No (%)
1983	70	17

Roper Poll (prescriptions for lethal drugs)

"As you know, lethal drugs are drugs, which can be taken either by mouth or by injection, that can end a person's life peacefully and quickly. Should doctors be allowed to prescribe lethal drugs to terminally ill patients who request them so that the patients can end their own lives, if and when they decide to?"

Year	Yes (%)	No (%)
1991	60	32

Roper Poll (lethal drugs for the incompetent patient)

"Some terminally ill patients lose their mental capacity. In these cases, if the patient had signed a Power of Attorney while still fully competent, giving a family member or friend the power to make the decision as to whether and when lethal drugs are to be given, do you think that should be allowed or not?"

Year	Yes (%)	No (%)
1991	68	26

TABLE 4-1 (CONTINUED)

Roper Poll (lethal injections)

"How about in cases where patients wish to die but are unable to take the lethal drugs themselves? Should doctors be allowed to give patients lethal injections in such cases or not?"

Year	Yes (%)	No (%)
1991	54	36

* Percentages may not add to 100 because responses like "don't know" are not shown.
SOURCES: Hadley Cantril, ed., *Public Opinion 1935–1946* (Princeton: Princeton University Press, 1951; Dennis A. Gilbert, *Compendium of American Public Opinion* (New York: Facts on File Publications, 1988), pp. 378–379; James Allen Davis and Tom W. Smith, *General Social Surveys, 1972–1988: Cumulative Codebook* (Chicago: National Opinion Research Center, 1988), pp. 246–247; Derek Humphry, ed., *Compassionate Crimes, Broken Taboos* (Los Angeles: The Hemlock Society, 1986), pp. 79–80; "1991 Roper Poll of the West Coast," *Hemlock Quarterly*, No. 44 (1991): 9–11.

changes in public opinion over time. Although questions were worded somewhat differently in the various surveys, it is clear that approval for the deliberate termination of life, one's own or an incompetent other's, has been rising steadily. Fifty percent in a 1988 poll approved of the individual's right to suicide in the case of incurable illness; in sharp contrast, only 12 percent in the same survey endorsed suicide for a person who was "tired of living and ready to die," and less than 6 percent approved for one who was bankrupt. Thus ordinary people see important distinctions among possible reasons for suicide. A 1991 Roper poll asked 1,500 respondents a series of questions about lethal drugs, finding that six in ten approved their use by terminally ill patients who requested them. Approval was higher (68 percent) for use of lethal drugs for incompetent patients, an indication of the lower valuation placed on continuing treatment for the mentally incapacitated. Approval exceeded 50 percent for lethal injections administered by doctors. These results should be interpreted with some caution, however, since respondents all resided on the West Coast, where attitudes on a wide array of social issues tend to be more tolerant. But, at the same time, West Coast residents are often trendsetters for the rest of the nation. Moreover, since poorly worded questions may precondition negative responses to death control queries, approval may be higher than polls indicate. Within the broad spectrum of support, indications are that persons of higher socioeconomic status and those with more liberal religious beliefs are more likely to favor death control, in all its forms.[13]

When it comes to themselves and their own relatives, however, people may respond differently than in the abstract case. They may believe that *their* relatives, *their* physicians, *their* hospital can be trusted even if those of others are suspect. Questions directed to samples of terminally ill patients, however, also show that a majority would forgo aggressive treatment when illness was incurable and pain intractable. In a California survey, hospital patients (mostly elderly) were asked "to suppose they had such severe memory loss that they could not identify people, were confused about where they were, and were unable to care for themselves, with no chance of recovery." Under these circumstances, over 70 percent said they would refuse intensive care, cardiopulmonary resuscitation, or a feeding tube to prolong their life. In a study of the medical care preferences of a sample of nursing home residents, participants were generally opposed to aggressive end-of-life treatments except those that would provide greater comfort or safety for the patient; treatment rejection reflected residents' personal experiences and was especially likely in scenarios involving serious mental impairment.[14]

A theme of what I call "responsible dying"—the notion that individuals owe it to themselves, their relatives, professional health care providers, and society generally to plan for their own disposition—has also emerged in recent years, in both the popular and scholarly literature. Patient passivity and the abdication of responsibility to others, including experts, are no longer acceptable. Individuals must plan for and document their treatment preferences before a crisis occurs, while they still have time to devote careful thought to the subject. An advice manual distributed by the American Association of Retired Persons (AARP) to its millions of members is replete with cautionary "shoulds" about the importance of advance planning; readers are asked to consider whether they "want to be kept alive by any means and whatever [their] condition," for instance. References to what "most people" want and reassurance that "patients removed from life support continue to be kept clean, comfortable, and free from pain" help diffuse ideas about what is acceptable behavior in the face of death. The AARP also offers free publications and provides the names and addresses of organizations that actively promote death control, such as the Society for the Right to Die, or that reject aggressive life prolongation, such as the National Hospice Organization. Similarly, a policy statement adopted by the Presbyterian Church USA in 1983 enjoins members to anticipate and plan conscientiously for the health care decisions they will face at the end of life.[15]

Significantly, the tone of such advice implies that people are seriously remiss if they postpone decision making until they are terminally ill. By then it is often too late because the illness, or the treatment, has impaired their decision-making capacity. Especially important for early decisions is the growing number of patients with Alzheimer's disease—victims are often physically robust for years, ensuring long survival, but in a mentally compromised state that requires constant and increasingly onerous forms of care. Because long-term care is financially costly too, patients need to identify treatments that are costworthy to them, weighing benefits to costs relative to other possible uses of their personal resources and considering the economic impact on their family. An individual who fails to make the necessary hard choices about forgoing or withdrawing treatment in timely fashion ultimately abrogates them to others, and this may constitute an unfair imposition on them. Hence preplanning is advocated not only for the individual's sake (to ensure that his preferences are respected), but for the sake of survivors: planning is an act of love, which can help families avoid disagreements about care arrangements, finances, and other difficult choices in a crisis. Finally, responsible dying is important in order to spare third parties, such as medical personnel, from the need to make hard choices on an individual's behalf.[16]

But many Americans, perhaps a majority, are understandably disinclined to make advance arrangements for their own demise, so experts are devising ways to circumvent their reluctance. A document called a "values history," for instance, is designed to encourage communication of personal values that will facilitate surrogate decision making when the need arises. Other experts have advised physicians to initiate discussions of end-of-life treatment options with their patients. Another suggestion is that at age fifty every citizen should be obliged to sign a legal directive as to his or her deathbed wishes, the penalty for failure to be exclusion from publicly financed health benefits. More controversial ideas include former Colorado governor Richard Lamm's contention that the terminally ill have a duty to die and ethicist Paul Menzel's argument that "allowing oneself to die to save resources can indeed be one's moral duty." Responsible dying is thus linked to dilemmas of cost-effectiveness, social justice, and perceptions of a societywide need to ration scarce resources. Whereas in the past, most Americans considered medical resources virtually unlimited, today that perception is vastly changed. In fact, health care costs are now generally perceived as having reached a critical level, and rationing "has become more palatable in the public policy debate surrounding health care."[17]

There are other indicators of social change. For instance, leaders have emerged, organizations have been formed, and legislation has been introduced in efforts to promote deliberate death as the answer to predicaments of death and dying previously thought intractable. The Euthanasia Educational Council was established in 1967 for the sole purpose of distributing information about death and dying. Membership rose to over 300,000 by 1975. The Hemlock Society was formed in 1980 because no other U.S. organization existed to support assisted suicide for the terminally ill, although such groups could be found in other countries; by 1991, there were 57,000 members and 70 chapters and, according to supporters, the movement was experiencing unprecedented growth.[18] The Hemlock Society actively uses the news media to advocate aid-in-dying and decriminalization of assisted suicide.

It is impossible to measure the collective impact of such concepts as responsible dying and a national crisis in health-care financing on individual decision making. But if patients do the rationing themselves, social institutions (the health care system, government agencies) will be spared a heavy burden. There is a danger, of course, that responsible dying will lead to deaths that are premature—contrary to the intent of death control proponents. Under the current state of affairs, when deaths are negotiated privately, with no uniform criteria to guide decision making, the possibilities for abuse are obvious. The public is not a homogeneous mass, as the section below on opposition to negotiated death will illustrate.

Different subgroups, such as women and minorities, also have a different stake, and face different risks, in the process of social change, a complex topic reserved for a later chapter.

The Mass Media

In the nineteenth century, the mass media, the courts, and concerned citizens interacted to diffuse both the idea of birth control and its practice throughout Western society. *Fruits of Philosophy,* the "dirty, filthy book" referred to in the introduction to this chapter, became enormously influential almost overnight, due in large part to the media publicity accorded the Bradlaugh-Besant trial. Earlier, in the author's home state of Massachusetts, the authorities had tried to limit distribution of the book—Knowlton was fined in 1832, prosecuted twice, and sentenced to three months of hard labor; from 1833 to 1877, only 40,000 copies were sold. Following the "obscenity" trial in 1877–1878, sales soared and Knowlton's tract became a best seller; more important, thanks to the publicity surrounding the trial, when the English press abandoned its previous reticence and covered the subject fully and impartially, attitudes toward birth control became more openly favorable. Contraception ceased to be a taboo subject and was well on its way to respectability. Citizens who had long seen and suffered the problems of too-large families would not be denied the necessary information for solving the problems; when a solution appeared, no court, church, doctor, or squeamish publisher could long conceal its existence or forbid its use. The trial also advertised the fact that many respectable people, unlike the authorities, did not think birth control an unfit topic for public discussion, nor did they consider its practice indecent or dangerous. Such perceptions went far to legitimate new attitudes and forms of behavior. More contraceptive manuals appeared in the wake of the trial; discussion of the trial and the issues underlying it was widespread outside England too and led to the establishment of the world's first birth control clinic, in Holland, in 1879. Later, in the United States, Margaret Sanger coined the term "birth control" and led the movement here; newspaper coverage of her speeches was copious and generally enthusiastic. The acceptability of deliberate family limitation as important, necessary, and praiseworthy behavior became firmly embedded in public consciousness.[19]

There are obvious parallels to the history of birth control in the late-twentieth-century shift to greater tolerance of death control. The mass media, with their great power to inform, persuade, and disseminate information to all segments of society, have played a large part in the evolution of public opinion. When dying individuals, or those who assist their deaths, become trapped in the legal system, for example, vital issues are publicized at a time when more and more families face similar hard choices for their own loved ones. Sensational "mercy killing" cases have been well publicized too and serve to raise consciousness about both the underlying problems and the motives for ending life. The fact that defendants are almost invariably treated leniently by sympathetic judges and juries, contrary to the letter of the law, cannot have escaped public notice either. In some instances, defendants have served as role models for others who copied their solutions for speeding the death of a relative after learning of them through the mass media.[20] Through their coverage of pivotal court cases like *Quinlan* and *Cruzan,* the mass media have provided valuable information and role models to the public, familiarizing us all with dilemmas surrounding the meaning of life and death, the horrors of uncontrolled medical technology, and the right to refuse treatment.

By the early 1970s, "Americans were embracing the subject of death and dying with a fervor that could not have been predicted ten or fifteen years earlier." Growing numbers of books, articles, television dramas, documentaries, and films depict death, dying, and the circumstances that lead some individuals to terminate their own life or assist another's dying. Popular treatments of euthanasia-related topics include such books as Andrew Malcolm's *This Far and No More,* describing a doctor-assisted suicide by a 40-year-old, Betty Rollin's *Last Wish,* an account of her mother's suicide in the face of terminal illness, and Philip Roth's *Patrimony,* which details his father's dying and his own helping role. A movie version of *Last Wish* aired in prime time on ABC in January 1992. Journalist Malcolm noted the immense response to his explorations of death-by-choice issues in the *New York Times*—a flood of mail indicative of "a desperate hunger for more information" from a public lacking direction from its major institutions; he has also written a very personal account of his decision to let his mother die. Television documentaries on such topics as Alzheimer's disease, organ transplants, and legal battles over aid-in-dying, such as a *Frontline* program on "The Death of Nancy Cruzan," are common. Analogous concerns about defective newborns and AIDS victims are also widely publicized.[21]

Expert advice to individuals on how to plan ahead to ensure that their last wishes are respected is also disseminated through the media. The advisability of advance directives, such as living wills and durable power of attorney for health care, is frequently discussed in newspaper and magazine articles. A *Newsweek* magazine cover in mid-1991 featured a "Do Not Resuscitate" bracelet—a way for individuals to convey their treatment wishes to emergency medical personnel. All serve to raise public consciousness in regard to critical life and death decisions and provide role models as well. Thanks to the mass media, most people now are aware of their rights as patients, including their right to refuse life-sustaining treatments. Nine in ten participants in a small study of elders' preferences regarding health care were aware of living wills, for example, and more than half of those said they learned of them through the newspaper, especially the "Dear Abby" column.[22]

This is not to suggest that people necessarily act on their knowledge—one may have full knowledge of the range of birth control methods, but choose not to use them, for example. Nor does it imply that all the complex issues surrounding death and dying have now been resolved. Many patients are incompetent in the last stage of life and some doctors still resent having their advice questioned, for example; other patients, or their surrogates, are afraid to ask questions, let alone challenge professional judgments.

By publicizing the views of leaders and the behavior of innovators, the mass media also help to crystallize coalitions and build constituencies for social change. The Hemlock Society's guidebook, written by its president, Derek Humphry, was the first U.S. manual on self-deliverance. Published in 1981 and available at first only to members, it is now openly advertised and available in many bookstores and libraries. A more detailed volume is *Final Exit,* by the same author, which incorporates advice from experts in the Netherlands, where physician aid-in-dying is widely accepted. Both books provide explicit instructions about lethal dosages of drugs for committing or aiding suicide. Like *Fruits of Philosophy* in the nineteenth century, and thanks to substantial publicity in the news media, *Final Exit* became a bestseller, and U.S. bookstores reportedly found it difficult to keep in stock owing to the high demand. Ironically, the opponents of death control helped publicize the book by calling for its banning; additional publicity accrued as the book became the subject of commentary by political cartoonists, editorial writers, satirists, and even comedians around the country.[23] It is safe to conclude that anyone wanting information on how to mercifully end a life can now get it quite easily.

The *Quinlan* case profoundly affected public opinion, rousing Americans to learn about and debate death control issues and work for legal changes. The case also greatly increased the demand for living wills—legal documents specifically designed to avoid dilemmas like Karen Quinlan's. The Euthanasia Educational Council handled well over a million requests in the eighteen months when the case was being resolved. More recently, the prolonged legal battle surrounding Nancy Cruzan's right to die further galvanized public opinion in the direction of a desire to be protected from excessive medical care. Concern for Dying, as the Euthanasia Educational Council was renamed, reported a large jump in requests for its version of the living will in the wake of *Cruzan*. The case also publicized the importance of a health care proxy for incompetent patients. A recent study in Boston found high levels of knowledge of famous court cases involving termination of treatment among both a sample of patients and the general public, knowledge that no doubt influences respondents' desire to have protective legal documents for themselves.[24]

Media influence is hard to measure and difficult to evaluate. All media efforts are clearly double-edged, however. Some of the blame for inflated public expectations in regard to "medical miracles," for example, can fairly be laid at the media's door. Admiring portrayals of heroic people who triumphed over adversity have often ignored or played down the negative side effects of treatment and the limitations of medicine, for example. So, to some extent, the current emphasis on medical excesses serves as a corrective mechanism as the pendulum swings back toward doubt and skepticism. "Scare stories" and "burden" tales about the elderly as, alternately, the greedy rich or the helpless poor, also form images in public consciousness that may be biased, ill informed, dangerous, and extremely hard to change once formed. Information is diffused, but so are attitudes and values, good and bad. Whether they intend to encourage preparedness, autonomy, and self-responsibility with cautionary tales, or simply sell a product, media reports inevitably have unintended or undesirable effects too—for example, encouraging premature death among overly sensitive elders.

Medical Professionals

The medical profession is not immune from a duty to adhere to the norms and values of the larger culture, or from a natural human desire to avoid negative sanctions for deviations from them. Hence the fact that most nineteenth-century physicians declined to provide contraceptive services to patients who requested them reflected their understanding of prevailing attitudes toward sex, women, and the family. But some doctors who publicly attacked birth control also helped individual patients in their private practice, knowing that such help was forbidden by law. Their actions reflected their realization that principles must be flexible, allowing for humanitarian motives in exceptionally difficult situations, as well as their trust in their own judgment. Physicians gradually modified their opposition and changed their behavior as they gained awareness of growing public support for family limitation, its practice by many couples, and more frequent requests from their patients for advice and assistance.[25]

Similarly, in the death control movement, one develops a strong sense that each group is waiting for someone else to take the lead, and the responsibility, for social change. Physicians await "permission" from the law or act in secret to protect themselves from liability; few openly challenge the system or campaign for social change. Those who make and enforce the law are guided by public opinion and the advice of medical experts. The media strive to give audiences what they want, often shaping opinions as they work to report them. Patients and their families—those who can least afford to wait—are tangled in the resulting webs of inaction, hesitation, fear, secrecy, and confusion.

Some concerns are timeless, of course: physicians in every era have come up against the limits of medical knowledge and, sooner or later, faced hard choices with their patients. Today the high price of longevity is increasingly discussed in medical circles, as topics previously shunned come out into the open. In the 1960s, for example, the majority of doctors were opposed to telling a patient that his illness was terminal, and few knew, or thought to ask, how dying patients felt or what they wanted from the health care system. Now, in contrast, some doctors are setting an example and urging their peers to initiate such discussions with their patients, instead of waiting for patients to take the lead. Sol Levine, a prominent medical sociologist, has commented on the recent redefinition of the doctor-patient relationship: from one in which "the doctor as scientific expert transmitted that knowledge to an ignorant but receptive patient who avidly and unquestioningly followed instructions" to a more realistic, dynamic view of active engagement by both parties. Evidence suggests that medical students tend to develop more egalitarian attitudes toward these "new consumerist patients" over the course of their training, in line with changing public attitudes about the doctor's role; in particular, many become "more skeptical of the value of physician authority and more accepting of patients' rights to have a voice in their own care." Levine has also discussed the recent emergence of "quality of life" criteria as basic to the evaluation of health interventions, defining "quality" broadly to incorporate "the more complete social and psychological being," encompassing the individual's social roles, mental alertness, sense of well-being, and relationships with others. Treatment decisions are not based solely on scientific or medical criteria. Although they may seem objective and rational on the surface, they are more appropriately viewed as "social decisions made by people playing social roles, guided by social values, and located in particular social settings." The medical community is compelled to acknowledge and respond to these social dimensions.[26]

The revolution in medical technology, along with increasing specialization and other changes in medical care delivery systems, have allowed doctors greater say in how and when death occurs. In the past, there was little the average practitioner could do to postpone death whereas today, ironically, she can often do too much. Patients today are often sicker, typically suffering from several chronic conditions, and are sicker longer, factors that may contribute to growing disillusionment of medical professionals with their traditional view of death as, invariably, "the enemy." Far better than most of us, physicians realize that cures for the ailments of the frail elderly are not within our reach, and will be slow in coming, if they come at all. In consequence, medical personnel have gradually shown a remarkably greater willingness to talk about what they do and the intricate problems of conscience they confront each day. Since 1968, when "the leaders of medicine fought doggedly to maintain their authority over all medical matters" and few wanted or sought public input into decision making, some physicians have come to realize that input from nonphysicians is essential if treatment is ever to be terminated in desperate cases. His interviews with physicians, for example, led journalist Andrew Malcolm to realize that many "sought some sign, even just a meaningful shrug" from family members indicating how aggressive or passive they wished treatment to be. Over time, too, medical workers are more attentive to the psychic toll on themselves as they share patients' helplessness and frustration and question their own continuing interference with the dying process.[27]

Organizations of medical professionals have taken firmer stands on death control over the years, in part because their leadership realizes that members cannot and should not bear the entire burden of end-of-life decision making. In 1973, the American Hospital Association approved the Patient Bill of Rights, a national policy statement that affirmed the individual's right to choose death by refusing treatment, even over the advice of physicians; in the same year, the American Medical Association (AMA) advised members to respect a dying person's wishes, but still officially condemned euthanasia. By 1984, a small group of prominent physicians was proposing a bill of rights for the dying, advocating that emergency resuscitation and intensive care should be provided sparingly, in line with the wishes of patient and family. Many doctors commended the proposals for their boldness in stating that aggressive measures should sometimes be withheld. Publication of the criteria in the *New England Journal of Medicine* allowed widespread dissemination of the new recommendations.[28]

Physicians, and medical personnel generally, thus share in the new skepticism about the benefits of medical heroics when additional efforts may not be in the patient's best interests, even if they will maintain her biological existence somewhat longer. In Minnesota in 1991, for example, a group of doctors sued for permission to disconnect the respirator of an 87-year-old woman in an irreversible coma, in opposition to the wishes of her family.[29]

Physicians are also more openly inclined toward deliberate death as public opinion tends in that direction. In 1975, "passive euthanasia [was] beginning to be cautiously considered as a viable social and medical practice under carefully controlled circumstances." Today, "No Code" or "Do Not Resuscitate" orders, formerly referred to only in furtive whispers, are topics of frank discussion among doctors, patients, and families. Veterans Administration guidelines introduced in 1983 allowed doctors in the nation's 172 veterans' hospitals to withhold life-prolonging medical therapy from critically ill patients whose heart and lungs failed; this was a reversal of 1979 guidelines prohibiting such practices; in 1986, the AMA affirmed that it was ethically permissible for physicians to withhold or discontinue all life-prolonging treatments for patients in irreversible coma, even if death was not imminent, as well as from dying patients. The term "imminent" was not precisely defined, thus leaving it to the physician's discretion. Nutrition and hydration were included among treatments that could be withheld or withdrawn. This is significant because the administration of food and water is an emotionally charged and hence highly controversial issue; nonetheless, 73 percent of physicians in a 1986 poll favored withdrawing them if the patient or family requested it; 12 percent were unsure, and only 15 percent were opposed. More generally, it is important to note that guidelines about treatment, like the AMA's policy statement, are *just* guidelines, not legally binding on either individual physicians or hospitals, though professional associations may discipline their members for violations. Nonetheless, such official "permission" is likely to influence attitudes and behavior in favor of earlier death.[30]

Doctors have been understandably hesitant about openly supporting physician-assisted suicide, given its questionable legal status. But recent opinion polls of physicians indicate that many would perform lethal injections if they were legal. When twelve physicians published a report on care provision to the terminally ill in 1989, ten of them agreed that it was not immoral for doctors to actively assist in the suicide of such patients. Other physicians have spoken frankly about their own practices, encouraging their peers to do so as well. In 1991, for example, Dr. Timothy Quill wrote in some detail in the *New England Journal of Medicine* about a suicide he aided, at his patient's request. In an editorial shortly thereafter, the *New York Times* called his action "courageous," praised his compassion and "exemplary procedural care," and concluded that physician-assisted suicide, if carried out with the same care shown by Dr. Quill, should be permitted in our society. Courage was certainly required, because assisting a suicide is still against the law in half the states. A similar situation obtained in the history of the birth control movement, when few medical men who privately favored its legitimation were willing to speak or act openly when state, church, and many of their peers objected to family limitation. A group of doctors, Physicians for Death with Dignity, has now organized to encourage others to talk about aid provided to the dying, representing yet another attempt to bring into the open practices that many are thought to engage in clandestinely.[31]

What further stake do doctors, especially those who work most closely with patients, have in deliberate death? First, of course, practioners want patients' trust and respect—something they must struggle to regain in the current climate of suspicion and fear. And they must walk a fine line in doing it. "Not even the most sympathetic [physician] wants a reputation as Dr. Death, the fellow who lets sick people go, perhaps too easily in the eyes of some." But neither does the doctor want to be known as one who tortures dying people needlessly by trying everything medicine has to offer, regardless of contraindications. Health workers want to be able to live with their conscience, knowing they did their best for the patient. They want some reassurance from patients, families, and the law that they acted properly, neither giving up too soon nor delaying death too long with excessive, futile treatment. Guidance from, and the approval of, their peers and professional organizations are also important. Finally, most would prefer to be able to act openly rather than furtively, with full confidence that they are protected from liability if they act in good faith.[32]

Medical practitioners have no desire to be society's rationing agents for scarce resources, yet they know that expensive overtreatment for some may preclude even minimal care for others—for example, the $93,000 spent on one 90-year-old patient in the intensive care unit of a New York hospital, whose prospects for survival were deemed poor at the outset, versus the needs of 37 million Americans with no health insurance. Physicians also worry about the possibility of malpractice suits, criminal prosecution, and damage to their careers if they appear to act inappropriately, and are concerned with the rapidly rising costs of malpractice insurance. In a litigious society, where patient silence and passivity can no longer be relied on, practitioners are coming to recognize that active involvement in decision making by patients and their representatives can protect professionals from legal repercussions. The great majority of states now have legislation that provides "immunity from civil and criminal liability to personnel and facilities which participate in good faith in withholding or withdrawing treatment...in compliance with a living will." Physicians are now legally and ethically bound by such patient directives. On the other hand, a physician who declines to comply with the instructions of a valid living will "may be held civilly liable for breach of contract, battery, and intentional infliction of emotional distress" to patient and family and can be sued for recovery of medical expenses resulting from unwanted treatments. Doctors who defy family wishes when the patient is incompetent are also at risk. For instance, when Edna Leach's family wanted to let her die and doctors insisted on treating her despite the fact that she was in a chronic vegetative state, her husband filed a $1.26 million lawsuit against both the hospital and the doctor.[33]

Hence doctors now have powers over life and death that many, for their own well-being, are understandably anxious to share. Practitioners can relax if major responsibility is turned over to patients and their relatives, especially if the law says that their wishes must be respected. Where there is doubt, or disagreement among family members or the medical team, such as for incapacitated patients, physicians will appreciate the opportunity to discuss treatment options with a surrogate, chosen by the patient, who has legal authority to give or withhold consent. The bottom line is that a potentially heavy burden for doctors is being transferred to patients and families. The primary physician, among all medical personnel, now has a strong stake in discontinuing or not initiating treatment, whereas for many years he was liable for failing to "do everything." Hence treatment cessation is a new form of defensive medicine. Like physicians, hospitals too now risk legal liability and loss of fees for aggressive treatments provided contrary to the wishes of patients or their representatives, so they too have a strong stake in determinations to stop treatment.[34]

But laws remain murky. Because many medical specialists are strangers to their patients, and so unfamiliar with their values and background, "it has generally seemed prudent to avoid legal problems by doing everything possible to keep a person alive."[35] Inadequate knowledge and fear of making the wrong decision, especially in an emergency, all too often produce a bias to treat. For patients who are both aged and very ill, this predisposition survives because of uncertain legal guidelines for termination of treatment (and the fear of prosecution this induces), as well as a natural human desire to put off difficult decisions. Automatic treatment in every case allows providers to sidestep the hard choices associated with that unique individual in those special circumstances. Thus, however commendable the guidelines currently endorsed by medical organizations, however clear the recommendations of hospital ethics committees, however many ethics courses are incorporated into the medical school curriculum, their collective impact is likely to remain relatively minor in the absence of definite direction from the law.

The stake of doctors, nurses, aides, and others who provide hands-on patient care is different from that of ancillary personnel with relatively little patient contact, such as radiation therapists and X-ray technicians, who do not work closely with the patient and never meet the family. Nurses are charged with carrying out the physician's orders, whether or not they agree with the course of treatment or have participated in decision making. Thus, of course, they are also vulnerable to criminal charges when things go wrong. As with guidelines provided to doctors by the AMA, those provided to nurses by the American Nurses' Association are also only recommendations, providing no real legal protection. Moreover, the recommendations are vaguely worded and may contain internal contradictions that inhibit interpretation of their intent. The Code for Nurses devised by the American Nurses' Association, for instance, states that "the nurse does not act deliberately to terminate the life of any person." But she is also enjoined to protect and support the patient's right to refuse or terminate treatment.[36] Obviously these instructions may conflict in any number of concrete situations.

At the same time, nurses are well acquainted with the day-to-day difficulties of suffering, pain management, and the undesirable side effects of treatment. As a thoughtful nurse described one such experience, "the doctors and technicians worked their miracles and walked away," leaving the nurses to deal with the resulting anguish of tubes and bedsores, pain and incontinence of a man who begged to die. Those closest to the patient "may be much more sensitive to the ravages that a drawn-out, terminal illness brings to the patient and to the family"; this emotional identification may make them more willing than physicians to terminate treatment. But, caught between the patient and family, on one hand, and physician orders, on the other, nurses may feel particularly helpless when a patient wishes to die and the doctor is unwilling to take the risk. Conflicting obligations are the order of the day for nurses working within a medical system that severely limits their contribution to decision making. Nurses (and other health care workers) are never entirely powerless, however. For example, they may have special knowledge about the patient or family and "enormous power to shape the communication that they transmit," deciding what information to relay and when to do so depending on their own assessment of the situation.[37]

Courts and Legislatures

Long before an organized social movement emerged to legitimate it, women and couples challenged the prohibitions on birth control. They sought information in defiance of the law, and passed on illegal information to others. Activists were arrested and jailed, but legal persecution always garnered publicity and inadvertently helped to spread the message. Eventually, like the medical establishment, the legal system came to modify its views because of the enormous changes in public opinion and public demand for birth control. The history of legislative change on Americans' right to choose death is also a story of growing tolerance and significant transformations over a relatively short time span. As with birth control, however, legislation has followed public opinion (and *de facto* medical practice) rather than leading the way; even judges have sought legislative guidance and urged that laws be passed to clarify the duties and responsibilities of physicians in terminating treatment.[38]

In a 1965 case, the U.S. Supreme Court first recognized the right to privacy as a fundamental constitutional guarantee; interestingly, *Griswold v. Connecticut* involved a dispute over access to contraception, and the expanded definition of privacy established in that case figured prominently in later right-to-die cases such as *Quinlan*. Almost a century earlier, the Bradlaugh-Besant trial attracted large crowds who gathered daily to follow the proceedings, making clear that their sympathies lay with the defendants. The judge was lenient, and the jury chose to exonerate the defendants from "corrupt motives" in publishing the birth control tract, but simultaneously regretted the book's assumed malign influence on public morals. The double-edged decision led codefendant Annie Besant to quip that the verdict amounted to saying, "Not guilty, but don't do it again," a summation that with equal accuracy could be applied to many "mercykilling" trials.[39]

Negotiated deaths are seriously underreported; the vast majority of cases remain undetected. Only 151 cases of "mercy killing" found their way into U.S. courts in the 65 years from 1920 to 1985, for example. Significantly, 70 percent of these occurred between 1980 and 1985, and most (64 percent) involved persons over 60. Only ten defendants were found guilty of criminal homicide and imprisoned; despite the legalities, even judges have been very understanding of defendants' humane motives. A case in point is that of 88-year-old Vahan Kacherian, accused of murder for plunging a knife into his wife's heart. When the court session was over, the defendant extended his hand to the judge and the prosecutor, who, in turn, wordlessly conveyed their sympathy to the fragile old man. All seemed to agree that his guilty plea was an admission that his act was illegal, but not immoral.[40]

What observers said of one court case could be said of many: that "the law connived with itself to give mercy" to the defendant.

Disregarding judges' instructions about the letter of the law, juries have reinterpreted laws and redefined "crimes" to fit the situation, tending to be extremely lenient with defendants. The public too has been overwhelmingly sympathetic to defendants in these cases, and the trials have served important educative functions. "Not guilty" verdicts in the United States have brought cheers from courtroom spectators, neighborhood celebrations, and help with trial expenses. A physician in the Netherlands enjoyed a 30 percent increase in his medical practice following his trial; when another Dutch doctor injected her ailing mother with a lethal dose of drugs, the people in her village formed the Society for Voluntary Euthanasia, now the largest euthanasia group in the world. Outside the tiny minority of sensational cases, negotiated deaths are carried out quietly, and no professional caregiver has ever been found liable for complying with a properly derived and adequately documented "Do Not Resuscitate" order.[41]

The history of efforts to legalize euthanasia in the United States makes it abundantly clear that courts, like other social institutions, have typically sought to avoid such issues, while doctors have cooperated in keeping cases (and themselves) out of the courts. The result was to leave vast gray areas where individuals, professionals and laypersons alike, have been forced to take matters into their own hands, helping dying patients clandestinely and risking prosecution for acts still defined as illegal. Others simply stifled their compassionate instincts and awaited a "natural" death for their patient or relative. The law has lagged well behind new realities and a need for new solutions; although legislation has been introduced repeatedly over the years, lawmakers have consistently preferred to sidestep the issues until forced to act. Nonetheless, a trend toward greater tolerance is apparent, as lawmakers feel their way along, taking due note of public sentiment along the way. Gradually, existing statutes are being expanded, as lawmakers learn from experience and realize that more permissive laws enhance freedom of choice without leading to any demonstrable abuse.[42]

The *Quinlan* case led to New Jersey's emergence to the forefront of the right-to-die movement. The case set a precedent in 1976 when the New Jersey Supreme Court allowed a respirator to be disconnected from the comatose young woman at her parents' request. The same court made three landmark decisions eleven years later, in 1987, expanding a patient's right to choose death; as with *Quinlan,* these rulings are likely to have continuing national impact as other courts look for guidance. Another precedent-setting case was a 1988 ruling by a Federal District Court in Rhode Island, which allowed a feeding tube to be removed from a comatose woman, causing her death a few days later. The president of the Rhode Island Medical Society praised the ruling for its support to doctors facing similar decisions in hopeless cases.[43]

A living will is a medical directive that instructs physicians in advance about the signer's wishes regarding life-prolonging procedures; the specific details about which treatments may be rejected and the circumstances under which this may be done vary from state to state. The concept was first advanced in the 1960s, and forms were distributed by churches and senior citizens groups, among others. But, although bills were introduced in fifteen states, they met with powerful opposition or insufficient backing, passing only in California. But by the mid-1970s, the Quinlan family's tragedy had given major impetus to right-to-die legislation in 38 states, in eight of which the bills were soon signed into law; more legislation followed, and living will statutes were enacted in 36 states by 1985. Now all but three states have laws covering living wills, durable powers of attorney, or both. Millions of living wills have been filed by ordinary citizens. While such wills are problematic, and physicians still justifiably hesitate to honor them, they are important indicators of growing acceptability of death control among Americans.[44]

A new federal law, the Patient Self-Determination Act, went into effect in December 1991; it requires all medical and health facilities serving Medicare or Medicaid patients to inform incoming patients of their right to make decisions about medical care and to execute a living will or durable power of attorney. The purpose of the new forms is to aid in implementing a patient's right to refuse any and all medical treatments, including those that might maintain his or her life indefinitely. Professional organizations, such as the AMA and the American Academy of Neurology, have endorsed such planning efforts.[45]

But the inconsistencies, idiosyncracies, and ambiguities of new case law have, as yet, failed to fully clarify the legal parameters of a citizen's right to choose death. The ruling in *Quinlan,* for example, led to a greater involvement of lawyers and judges in medical decision making, as cautious doctors and hospital directors thought it more prudent to go to court than to unilaterally terminate treatment. In 1986, Derek Humphry and Ann Wickett, cofounders of the Hemlock Society, wrote that "without the wisdom of the U.S. Supreme Court, which has so far refused to adjudicate in any such cases, there remains the absence of a binding standard and the absence of a constitutionally recognized right to die." By 1991, there was such a case, *Cruzan v. Missouri Department of Health,* but matters have hardly improved. The decision, fifteen years after *Quinlan,* still left murky the critical question of exactly what constitutes "clear and convincing evidence" of an incompetent patient's treatment preferences, leaving that to be determined by states. The burden is on the incapacitated patient and her family to "prove unequivocally that she would not want to be treated," while the state needs no proof to compel continued treatment. Public reaction indicated that most people believed that Nancy Cruzan should be allowed to die. Thus, to critics, the ruling "shows how far out of touch the Supreme Court has become with regard to how people think and behave."[46]

So although laws have been slowly changing toward greater tolerance of the right to choose death, ordinary citizens seem to be well ahead of both physicians and the courts in confronting difficult choices about when and how to implement that right; many cannot afford to wait until all legal niceties have been resolved. If it had passed in 1991, Washington's Initiative 119 would have been the first law in any state to decriminalize physician-assisted dying, the last bastion in the move to death control. National news media showed great interest in the measure, which derived from an earlier (failed) effort in California. Initiative 119 was significant because it explicitly acknowledged that the patient's right to choose death is often meaningless without physician cooperation, just as the individual's right to birth control is severely constrained if doctors are unwilling to prescribe the pill or perform surgical sterilizations. That efforts to pass legislation like Initiative 119 have only begun is indicated by the introduction of similar bills in four other states (New Hampshire, Iowa, Maine, and Michigan) in 1992.[47]

At the patient's request, "active" euthanasia is carried out quietly, without legislative sanction, in many nations, including England, Sweden, and Switzerland; in a number of Western European countries, there is a growing belief among physicians that they have a duty to perform euthanasia on a suffering patient who asks for help. The situation in the Netherlands, where death control is more openly practiced, is being imitated elsewhere; for instance, Dutch physicians receive calls from their peers in other countries requesting information on the best means of inducing death. Although Dutch laws have also lagged behind public opinion and medical practice, the courts have set standards for justifying aid-in-dying that serve as unofficial guidelines for physicians. Significantly, potential recipients need not be dying in order to request or obtain assistance, and both physical and nonphysical suffering (such as that associated with loss of personal dignity when one becomes highly dependent on others) are relevant.[48]

In contrast, the 1991 Michigan court case against Dr. Jack Kevorkian focused on the fact that he had assisted the death of a person not yet dying. Assisting a suicide was not then illegal in Michigan, as in many other states, so the case was dropped, but Kevorkian was instructed not to do it again. The presiding judge expressly noted that less culpability would attach to cases involving persons who are terminally ill, in irreversible coma, or suffering from incurable diseases accompanied by intractable pain or serious emotional distress. But judgments about the imminence of death and the severity of physical pain and emotional distress are notoriously difficult and inherently subjective. Where to draw the line that separates patients into two groups—those whose death may be aided and those whose may not be—is a question that no court case has yet satisfactorily answered. In 1992, Dr. Kevorkian was ordered to stand trial for murder because he aided in the deaths of two more women, further testing the law. Again murder charges were brought and later dismissed, but the prosecutor has vowed to appeal the decision. Charges were not filed in connection with a fourth assisted suicide, as authorities waited to learn the outcome of the earlier charges; as of this writing, four more women have been helped to die. The final outcome of charges against Kevorkian and the legislative changes now underway in Michigan may set a precedent for other states to follow. The doctor's precipitate actions with regard to persons not yet terminally

TABLE 4-2

Guidelines for Euthanasia in the Netherlands

1. There must be psychological or physical suffering that is said to be intolerable by the supplicant himself/herself.

2. The experience of suffering and the desire to die must be durable and persistent.

3. The decision to die must be established to be completely voluntary on the part of the patient/supplicant.

4. The supplicant must have a reasonable understanding of his or her situation and of the possible alternatives; he or she must be in such a state as to weigh the options and alternatives and must have completed this process upon requesting to die.

5. There is no other reasonable solution apparent to improve the situation for the supplicant.

6. There must be consultation with at least one other physician on the permissibility of a particular case of euthanasia.

7. Euthanasia must be administered by a physician, and the task may not be delegated to a nonphysician.

8. There must be no unnecessary suffering brought upon others involved.

9. With the decision to assist to die, as well as with the performance of the act itself, the greatest possible care must be involved.

10. Note of the fact that euthanasia occurred should be documented either in the death certificate or with the public prosecutor's office.

SOURCE: Carlos F. Gomez, *Regulating Death: Euthanasia and the Case of the Netherlands* (New York: Free Press, 1991), p. 62.

ill may also be a setback for the death control movement. The Hemlock Society and other organizations advocating law reform, for example, have criticized Kevorkian's behavior for "muddying the waters" and disavowed any association with him or approval of his behavior. There can be no doubt that if Kevorkian is eventually tried, the case will contribute enormously to the debate on death control and serve to further publicize the issues.[49]

The Netherlands appears to be well ahead of the rest of the world in both acceptance and practice of euthanasia, which it defines as "a physician's intentional killing of a patient at the patient's express request"; there is no artificial distinction between "active" and "passive" forms. The Dutch experience is worth commenting on in some detail because guidelines for euthanasia have become less restrictive over the years and because practices there may have a continuing influence on the American death control movement. The Dutch deny that they have legalized aid-in-dying, but physicians are not punished for assisting death; there is little public outcry against the practice, and recent polls suggest that a two-thirds majority of the population do not object to it. The Royal Dutch Medical Society, which in 1973 had a firm stand against any form of aid-in-dying, admitted in 1984 that euthanasia took place and that its legality should be quickly clarified. The guidelines, as set out by court opinions and the Royal Dutch Medical Society, are shown in Table 4-2. Although a government committee recommended legalization in 1985, such legislation has not yet been passed. The guidelines must be strictly adhered to, however—at least one Dutch physician has been sentenced to prison for carelessness and negligence in the performance of euthanasia, although he was credited with good intentions.[50]

Important goals of death-related legislation everywhere are to preserve individual rights; honor individual preferences insofar as possible; protect the vulnerable and the helpless from needless suffering and abuse (whether it be premature death or delayed death) and from their own hasty or ill-informed decisions, if necessary, with appropriate safeguards, such as a waiting period; protect those who help others to die solely out of compassionate motives; and punish transgressors. Legislation must recognize the need for uniform treatment of all citizens, not erratic or piecemeal case-by-case treatments, which have so far resulted in confusing and contradictory decisions. Legislation must also be practical, not so unwieldy, intricate, or vague that too much time is required for decision making.

The difficulties of implementing these goals are formidable. To illustrate, the Dutch guidelines shown in Table 4-2 are the best in the world. Yet consider how many vague and inherently subjective terms they contain. How many times, and in what ways, must one express a desire to die before it is deemed "durable and persistent"? How does one know when alternatives have been sufficiently weighed? When is there no other "reasonable" solution?

How do we ascertain that a decision is *completely* voluntary? What if physicians disagree?[51]

Different problems arise when patients are too incapacitated to decide for themselves. The Dutch guidelines, like the legislation that has been proposed in the United States, specify that only cognitively intact persons may opt for euthanasia. As one Dutch doctor put it, "If they cannot speak, they cannot die."[52] But what if the patient is too sick to ask for the release of a painless death and neglected to document his wishes ahead of time? The criterion of intact mental capacity obviously excludes many, if not most, frail elders. Only if doctors and families make good decisions will they be protected from both premature death and delayed death. And in order to decide wisely, we need solid data documenting what doctors do and what most people want when they cannot speak for themselves.

Consider next the obstacles to good record keeping, as illuminated by the situation in the Netherlands. Euthanasia is supposed to be noted on the death certificate or reported to the public prosecutor's office, but Dutch doctors rarely do either, despite the fact that the risk of actual prosecution seems negligible. Since no systematic records are kept, neither the number of requests for euthanasia nor the characteristics of recipients (such as their age, sex, or diagnosis) are known. Lacking such information, lawmakers cannot know what people want or what potential abuses to try to guard against through legislation. This is not to suggest wrongdoing in euthanasia cases, but merely to point out that we know too little to make any conclusive determination at all about the quality and circumstances of decision making. Nor do I mean to suggest that there are no good reasons for the secrecy surrounding euthanasia proceedings, either in the Netherlands or here in the United States. For example, discretion is important in order to maintain confidentiality between doctor and patient, to respect the patient's right to privacy, and to spare the feelings of the family during a time of much emotional trauma. In fact, the prime reason given by Dutch physicians for not contacting the prosecutor in euthanasia cases is consideration for the family's feelings, a desire not to intrude too far into their private affairs. Yet such intrusion is indispensable if vulnerable people are to be protected from *coercive*, involuntary death hastening. Clearly, adequate records *must* be kept and the particular circumstances of each case must be open to scrutiny. Recall that distrust of the powers of medicine—of life-and-death decisions made without sufficient input from patient or family—was instrumental in creating the movement for death control in the first place. If the timing and circumstances of death are to be determined by the individuals involved, the practice should be regulated. But how this can best be accomplished is no simple matter, and lack of guidance on the legal front is symptomatic of the enormous difficulties inherent in the undertaking.[53]

Most desirable is that death control decisions stay out of the courts entirely, remaining where they properly belong—with patients, families, and their doctors. But legal criteria to guide those decisions and legal sanctions to punish wrongdoing must be devised so that abuses may be prevented. In the case of life-termination decisions now, no party is sufficiently protected. Those most affected by the system's inadequacies are likely to be those least able to speak for themselves—the poor, the uneducated, the mentally incapacitated, whereas those who can manipulate the system will have the advantage. As with birth control, those with access to sympathetic doctors will get the death control they want. So too will those with loving relatives willing to challenge the law by following the aid-in-dying instructions in a "suicide manual." But others will be victimized by untimely delays, unwanted treatment, and unnecessary suffering, while still others will die prematurely because the secrecy surrounding negotiated deaths encourages fatal abuses.

Government Agencies

Government policies and regulatory efforts at all levels are, in theory, intended to promote the best interests of all the people, but particularly the weakest. In the health care arena, government agencies must be concerned with the quality and quantity of health care institutions, the people who work in them, and paying the bills when patients and families cannot. Ethical considerations, such as minimizing suffering and helping to assure an equitable distribution of health care resources among various segments of the population, also enter the picture. Since 1968 the federal government has assumed a key role in setting ethical standards through the appointment of a number of national commissions charged with investigating pressing issues in medical ethics; the most influential is the President's Commission for the Study of Ethical Problems in Medicine and Biomedical and Behavioral Research.[54]

Government regulations also set many of the constraints within which individuals and health care institutions must operate— through Medicare reimbursement mechanisms or rules for nursing homes that receive federal funds, for example. What forms of care are reimbursable and the level of reimbursement inevitably affect who gets what in the health care system. Since government finances a greater share of the health care needs of the old than of the young, government cost-control efforts are now being directed to later-life medical and long-term care expenditures. The budgetary pressures resulting from the aging of the American population will compound those generated by increased Social Security outlays, the reduced tax revenues collected from a relatively smaller working-age population, and widespread public resistance to higher taxes.[55] Lobbying efforts can influence decision making in all these areas but, as we have seen, lobbying by and for the frail elderly is extremely limited. Given the great scope of modern government and its power to influence all facets of life, it is surely a mistake to think that government prioritizing does not influence the thinking of ordinary citizens as to what is important.

The deliberations of ethicists, lawyers, and judges regarding medical matters and patient empowerment were not initially concerned with cost factors, let alone driven by them, and finances were rarely mentioned in earlier reports and debates. In 1966, when the Medicare and Medicaid programs were enacted, however, the federal government became the single largest purchaser of health services in the country and in so doing found an enormous stake in controlling the size of the health care budget. Now the extent of government obligations to the oldest and sickest is hotly debated, and the fact that individual treatment choices, especially for the aged, have a substantial impact on public costs is increasingly recognized as a valid consideration in treatment decisions.[56]

The present political climate, characterized by great and growing concern over health care costs, emphasizes a shift of major federal welfare responsibilities back to the states and the private sector, with a strong emphasis on the family. Current policies are thus oriented toward cost control, with considerations of need, access, and quality of care all of secondary concern. More worrisome to some is reaction to Daniel Callahan's 1987 book, *Setting Limits: Medical Goals in an Aging Society,* in which the well-known biomedical ethicist proposed age-based limits to government-funded health care. Once they have achieved a "natural life span" (say the late seventies or early eighties), elders should receive only palliative care—that is, help in alleviating their suffering and achieving a humane death; they are not entitled to endless, expensive, *curative* medical interventions, because this is both impossible to finance and unfair to other age groups. The book has received extraordinary attention in both the popular press and scholarly journals and, because some policy makers seem prepared to act on its recommendations, is helping to legitimize the concept of old-age-based health care rationing as a national policy. Callahan's proposal seems just the kind of thing that cost-conscious government policy makers can seize on to justify their prioritizing.[57]

The impact of health care costs on the growing federal deficit is also of grave concern. In 1970, spending on all health care activities in the United States totaled $204 billion (in 1989 dollars); in 1989, the figure was $604 billion. Despite efforts to control it, spending has been rising faster than the gross national product. In 1990, health spending accounted for 14 percent of the federal budget; by 1996 it is expected to comprise 19.5 percent. Regarding long-term care, a 1991 report from the Congressional Budget Office found "little basis for optimism" that these costs could be lowered significantly without restrictions on services.[58] Widespread perceptions of a fiscal crisis increase the willingness of governments to limit care to the aged in particular as they attempt to control costs, because old people are disproportionate users of health care resources. A logical extension is that greater tolerance will be accorded to deliberate decisions to terminate treatment by and for the elderly. Other government tactics may also promote greater tolerance for death control. Controlling bed supply in nursing homes, for example, is a common state strategy for holding down Medicaid spending that may affect propensity to elect death—however inadequate such institutions are, if waiting lists are long and there is nowhere else to go, some desperate people may see "death with dignity" as their best option.

Some hospices also seem to be selecting patients with an eye to Medicare criteria that determine what is reimbursed and set limits on reimbursement. Amendments to the Medicare bill in 1982 provide reimbursement incentives for palliation and management of symptoms in patients expected to die within six months; these incentives are substantially higher than reimbursement levels for treating their conditions. If some treatable conditions are in fact only "managed," there is a possibility of premature death. Hence the new reimbursement rules may exacerbate existing risks of premature death for some hospice patients. More generally, whether they are Medicare-certified or not, hospices must select "suitable" patients very carefully if they are to survive financially: those who live "too long" or cost "too much" threaten the viability of the hospice care alternative.[59]

The new Patient Self-Determination Act, effective in 1991, requires that all adult patients admitted to a hospital, for any reason whatsoever, be asked if they wish to plan for their death; for example, they may specify what treatments they would accept or reject and name someone to decide for them should they become unable to do so themselves. But the act is likely to diffuse more than just information about end-of-life treatment choices: it may also convey subtle messages that it is appropriate for frail elders to let go of their lives sooner rather than later. Reduced benefits or greater copayments under Medicare, changes in tax codes about definitions of dependents, and other government cost-containment efforts that make people more sensitive to the costs of long-term care, especially out-of-pocket costs, all will conceivably affect individual and family willingness to consider deliberate death as an alternative. Family responsibility laws, which exist in various forms in half the states, are attempts to control Medicaid expenditures by holding relatives financially liable for some or all Medicaid expenses incurred on behalf of a long-term care recipient. They are unpopular and difficult to enforce, and a return of major financial responsibilities directly to families through enactment or more rigorous enforcement of such laws is very unlikely.[60] But other efforts to shift care responsibilities to the family are more subtle. For example, if good-quality nursing homes are expensive, geographically distant, or have long waiting lists, relatives are forced to provide substitute care, even to the extent of giving up their jobs, so they are financially threatened indirectly by the absence, poor quality, or expense of alternatives. Hence government policies aimed at cost containment and family responsibility for elder care may support and facilitate death control. That is, maximizing individual rights by allowing refusal of or withdrawal from life-sustaining treatments will simultaneously help control costs because a quicker death is less costly than the alternatives.

Ethicists

The number of scholarly books and articles dealing with death, dying, and the complex ethical questions raised by right-to-die issues has increased dramatically over time. These topics were virtually ignored prior to the 1960s. But by the 1980s, one could find hundreds of citations to works in bioethics and several thousand to death and dying. Renée Fox, a well-known medical sociologist, has characterized the period from the mid-1960s to the mid-1970s as "the bioethics decade," which witnessed a huge outpouring of scholarly works, the appearance of new centers and programs, and the development of guidelines on a wide array of emerging bioethical concerns. Many of these new areas of inquiry focus on death and dying and the quality of life, and many receive wide media coverage. Bioethics now has a prominent place in the realm of medical decision making, a success largely attributable to its strong commitment to individual empowerment in confrontations with medical authority.[61]

The recent flurry of activity in bioethics does not imply that consensus is on the horizon; in fact, the efforts of ethicists may have clouded death control issues more than clarified them. Major ethical debates focus on whether a right to choose death in fact exists; how, when, why, by whom, and for whom it should be exercised; distinctions between "active" and "passive" euthanasia; possible abuses, especially if physician-assisted dying is legalized; and questions of distributive justice and generational equity. An early argument, articulated in 1951 by a leading Protestant ethicist, was that merciful motives distinguished euthanasia from murder, and that distinction makes all the difference in determining culpability or, more accurately, the lack of it. This line of thought has been much repeated in court cases since, and it is one that juries frequently fall back on despite judges' instructions to the contrary. But experts disagree sharply about "active" versus "passive" approaches to death, some maintaining that there is no distinction while others claim that there is a distinction between "killing" and "letting die" which is of supreme importance.[62]

Consider these hypothetical cases, all involving seriously ill elderly patients. In the first a nurse observes that Mrs. Smith's respirator is malfunctioning. Knowing that the patient has expressed a desire to die, she takes advantage of this fortuitous circumstance and waits quietly until the woman dies. In another room, Mr. Jones askes to exercise his right to discontinue unwanted treatment; his doctor disconnects the machine, and death soon claims him. Down the hall, Mr. Green's children request that resuscitation not be attempted if their father stops breathing; his breathing stops, nothing is done, and he is soon dead. Meanwhile, in the same hospital, Dr. White, a retired surgeon, knows that her death may be neither quick nor dignified if her respirator is turned off; to avoid this dilemma, she asks for a lethal injection and her doctor, an old friend and colleague, complies. In all these cases, the participants clearly intend to facilitate death. Whether their deliberate behavior is an "act" or an "omission," death is the predictable result. Is it really better in every case to wait "passively" for a machine to malfunction or a medical crisis to occur, as for Mrs. Smith and Mr. Green, than to "actively" disconnect the machine or administer the injection? In another situation, do decision makers really feel better about themselves if they "passively" allow an old woman to slowly starve herself to death than if they "actively" accede to her request to be killed quickly and painlessly with drugs? To date, ethicists have done a poor job of convincing the public that there is an "active"/"passive" distinction or, if there is one, that "passive" means are always more humane.[63]

There are some important contradictions in defining what is ethical that are particularly applicable to the frail elderly: in order to jusitify the receipt of *services* from others, the recipient must be truly in need of help, but a critical precondition for receiving *respect* from others is that one *not* be perceived as dependent or needy. This dilemma is only temporary for the acutely ill, but the seemingly endless needs of the chronically ill are much more problematic, raising questions of reciprocity, as discussed earlier. "In a society that treasures independence and autonomy, assuming the role of permanent patient is not likely to ensure the dignity and equality of those in constant need of medical treatment."[64] Yet a continuing bias to treat can maintain their disvalued lives almost indefinitely, while few ethicists openly espouse their right to suicide or "active" aid-in-dying either. "Permanent patients" are left in an awkward situation indeed.

Some ethicists stress the importance of individual responsibility for "disposition" instructions in the event of terminal illness— "responsible dying" to relieve others of burden. For instance, Paul Menzel suggests that "people have a personal moral duty to conserve resources in the courses of treatment they choose for their dying"—there is a duty to die cheaply, since the resources saved can be better used to help others; failure to do so may be a sign of moral weakness. In *Setting Limits*, Daniel Callahan argues that elders must understand and cooperate with government-imposed limits on their care, implying that failure to do so indicates a narrow-minded selfishness on their part. He also questions whether large expenditures on elder care are a wise use of resources even if funds are available. Callahan's ideas are significant because of his prominent position as Director of the Hastings Center—a New York-based organization that carries out research on ethical issues in medicine— and because his many books and articles have received widespread attention in both the scholarly and the mass media.[65]

Ethical concerns are now openly aired inside the medical establishment as well as outside it. In 1978, for example, virtually no U.S. hospitals had ethics committees (multidisciplinary groups including physicians, social workers, nurses, chaplains, and concerned citizens who work to resolve the complex problems inherent in modern medicine); now the figure is estimated at half to three-quarters of all hospitals and some nursing homes as well. The committees are not without their own problems, however. Important issues include the confidentiality of patient records, excessive bureaucracy, the legal liability of committee members and the institution, and diffusion of responsibility. It is unlikely that ethics committees can resolve death control issues satisfactorily; they may, in fact, add to the confusion, at least in the short run.[66]

In a democracy, the state may not regulate every aspect of the lives of its citizens, but only those that are hurtful to others. In other words, if no one is harmed when a sick person chooses a quicker death, the state has no grounds for restricting his right to do so. Hence one prominent ethicist, H. Tristram Engelhardt, Jr., has made a convincing argument to the effect that establishing any particular ethic regarding euthanasia is impossible in a society characterized by great diversity of beliefs: since there is no clear justification for states to prohibit euthanasia, it must be tolerated.[67] In our pluralistic society, it seems likely that this argument will have increasing weight over time. Some religious groups would disagree, however, as the following discussion suggests.

Religious Groups

There are no firm lines of demarcation between religious and ethical considerations. Since value judgments underlie death control choices, it is inevitable that conflicts will emerge, often reflecting religious convictions about the meaning and purpose of life. Religious beliefs undoubtedly influence individual receptivity to death by choice. For example, when elderly hospital patients were asked about their treatment preferences, those who wished to be treated under all circumstances were more religious than other respondents. But there is considerable diversity of opinion within as well as between denominations. As with birth control, religious affiliation alone is a poor predictor of negative attitudes toward death control. A good illustration is the suicides in 1975 of two well-known figures in American religion, both members of the Euthanasia Society, and one the former President of the Union Theological Seminary. According to one expert, the suicides reflected rational decisions to die rather than endure the pain and suffering of old age.[68]

Greater religiosity, rather than religious affiliation per se, seems to be positively associated with the belief that life, whatever its condition, must be preserved. In other words, the "sanctity" of life (its biological component) takes precedence over considerations of "quality" (its social components). In this view, only God can decide the proper time of death. On this point, however, adherents leave crucial questions unanswered, such as why medical intervention to *prolong* life is acceptable but intervention to limit suffering is not. When is *prolonging* life in opposition to God's will? How can one be sure, for example, that a patient's kidney failure is not God's message that his life is over? That resort to renal dialysis or a kidney transplant in such a case represents undue interference with God's prerogative?

Some groups consider catastrophic long-term illness a test of religious conviction: illness presents an opportunity to demonstrate their faith to others. For instance, the Archbishop of Seattle believes that older people need to be reminded of "the redemptive value of human suffering" and discouraged from seeking suicide to relieve their pain. And, according to a Roman Catholic priest who wrote a book on preparing for death, "Christians believe that pain is part of salvation and that it can be a healing thing and a force to bring people together." Bishop Joseph Sullivan, a well-known opponent of euthanasia, has expanded on this theme:

> If the suffering patient is of sound mind and capable of making an act of divine resignation, then his sufferings become a great means of merit whereby he can gain reward for himself and also win great favors for the souls in Purgatory .... Likewise the sufferer may give good example to his family and friends and teach them how to bear a heavy cross in a Christlike manner.

Those who live with an incurable sufferer have been given an important opportunity to practice Christian charity, according to the bishop.[69]

The strongest disapproval of euthanasia comes from more fundamentalist religious groups; within groups, opposition is more likely among those who attend services more frequently. For example, Catholics who attend services often are less approving than fundamentalist Protestants who attend once a year or less (48.7 percent versus 60.7 percent), whereas frequent attenders among liberal Protestants are less approving than low attenders among Catholics (48.7 percent versus 76.4 percent, respectively). Members of the Hemlock Society, whose avowed goal is legalization of aid-in-dying, are far more likely to identify themselves as agnostics or atheists than are Americans generally, although many were raised in one of the mainstream religions.[70]

The influence of organized religion on private attitudes, at least, seems to be on the decline, and the substantial hostility that some observers in the death control movement predicted has not surfaced. In the 1960s, a survey found that seven in ten Jews and Protestants, all of those who claimed no religious affiliation, but only 20 to 25 percent of Catholics, favored legalizing euthanasia for incurable adult sufferers who requested it; among Catholic physicians in another survey, disapproval of "active" euthanasia was virtually unanimous, but was approved by 10 to 15 percent of their Protestant and Jewish peers.[71]

Over time, however, there has been "a steadily increasing protest in all denominations against useless prolongation of life." The work of a leading Protestant ethicist, Joseph Fletcher, has been very influential. He maintained that there is no moral difference between "active" and "passive" euthanasia: "a decision *not* to keep a patient alive is as morally deliberate as a decision to *end* a life." Another Christian writer has argued that "it is a greater desecration to maintain a human being in a vegetable state or hopeless torment than to kill him." Although most Catholics in the 1960s opposed euthanasia as immoral and dangerous, some Catholic theologians began to distinguish between "ordinary" and "extraordinary" treatments for the incurably ill: religious doctrine did not necessarily enjoin the latter in every case and, in some cases, even "ordinary" measures could be discontinued on legitimate moral grounds. When Bishop Fulton J. Sheen was asked what he would do if he were kept barely alive by medical technology, he responded that "I would ask them to take them out. I find no moral difficulty in this."[72]

By 1985, a Gallup poll conducted in the wake of the *Conroy* decision by the New Jersey Supreme Court showed that almost the same percentage of Catholics as Protestants (77 percent versus 80 percent) approved the decision, which allowed artificial feeding to be discontinued for an 84-year-old incompetent woman. A 1986 poll querying public attitudes toward physician-assisted dying showed that 63 percent of Protestants, 59 percent of Catholics, and 71 percent of Jews agreed that the law should allow a physician to end the life of a terminally ill patient at her request—a convergence of attitudes that a reasonable person would have thought unthinkable just a few years earlier. Significantly, a similar convergence has occurred in the acceptability and use of "artificial" birth control, especially between Catholics and non-Catholics and in defiance of the strong and continuing disapproval of the Catholic Church.[73]

Jews and most Christian sects continue their official opposition to suicide and assisted suicide. But most religious groups have come a long way in their general acceptance of "passive" euthanasia (withholding antibiotics when the patient has pneumonia, for example) and some are sympathetic to "active" forms of aid-in-dying if the circumstances seem to justify it; still others prefer to leave the matter to individual conscience. The widespread condemnation of suicide in the religious world also seems to be weakening. In August 1991, for example, the General Assembly of the Church of Christ officially accepted suicide for the hopelessly ill, the first major religious denomination to take this step. Also illustrative of the vast changes in attitudes over a few decades is the fact that many ordained clergy from various denominations actively supported Washington State's Initiative 119; so did many Catholic laypersons, despite the opposition of their bishops. And, interestingly, most religious bodies now have a ready answer to questions of their position on euthanasia, something that could not have been said prior to 1976 and the stimulus given the issues by the *Quinlan* case.[74]

Widespread acceptance of self-deliverance and "active" euthanasia among religious groups is far from impossible. Biblical teachings do not explicitly condemn suicide. Hence thinkers like James Clemons at Wesley Theological Seminary believe that churches should review their opposition to it. Some ethicists maintain that "Thou shalt not kill" is a poor translation of the commandment's intended meaning. Better wording is "Thou shalt not commit murder"—that is, *wrongful* killing. In this interpretation, killing in a just war, in self-defense, and "active" euthanasia are not prohibited. A scriptural rationale for suicide and "active" euthanasia may be found as churches reexamine their attitudes. The fact that significant changes in other aspects of religious orthodoxy have occurred over time, such as growing acceptance of ordination for women and wide acceptance of contraception, suggests that further accommodations will be made in regard to death and dying. The need for flexibility has been well stated by the Reverend Alistair Bennett, a retired minister of the Church of Scotland:

> They [the writers of the Bible] could not foresee our situation and we can never go back to theirs. Like them we must have the courage

to form our own judgements . . . , responding to the situation in which we live. . . . We would be moral cowards and unworthy descendants if we tried to lean back and expect our ancestors to make our decisions.

In the interim, the willingness of individuals to differ with their church's official stance has already been amply demonstrated with regard to both birth control and death control.[75]

Opposition

As old as the idea of deliberate death itself is opposition to it. Opposition may or may not be grounded in religious beliefs but, although they may stem from different underlying moral perspectives, the arguments are similar. Despite the fact that survey results over the years indicate that a substantial minority of Americans disapprove of death control, open antagonism was rare before 1985, when several court decisions provided a rallying point for opponents. They fear a total breakdown of traditional family values, a devaluation of life, and a "slippery slope" toward involuntary killing of the helpless and needy. A recent collaborative statement signed by thirteen Jewish and Christian theologians, philosophers, and legal scholars, for example, asserts that "once we cross the boundary between killing and allowing to die, there will be no turning back" and "countless candidates for elimination" will be found.[76]

Additional fears are that a *right* to choose death may become an *obligation* to do so. In a political climate where cost containment is paramount, rejecting a quick and painless death may come to be seen as a selfish waste of resources; economic pressures to choose death may grow if deliberate death is more easily available. There is also concern that "suicide manuals," which are freely published in the United States under the protection of the First Amendment, will push those who are only "momentarily suicidal" into ending their lives prematurely.[77]

The most vocal protests against death control come from the Roman Catholic Church and antiabortion forces, many of whose members overlap. Leaders want to protect the elderly from the "slippery slope" they see represented by the prochoice movement on abortion and by decisions not to prolong dying for severely handicapped newborns. In their perspective, all available means must be used to extend and preserve biological life, and they are extremely suspicious of efforts to enhance individual freedom to terminate treatment.[78] Any built-in legislative safeguards for the vulnerable are viewed as dangerously inadequate.

Both secular and religious opponents of death by choice cite difficulties in truly ascertaining a patient's wishes, since ill health may make one unduly susceptible to suggestions from others or unreasonably pessimistic about one's chances. Otherwise competent patients who assess their quality of life as poor and hence choose to die are not to be trusted because their views are distorted by pain or anxiety.[79] Hence in this line of reasoning no one is *ever* competent enough to choose death.

In other situations, prior verbal assertions or even formal advance directives filed years earlier may not reflect the patient's wishes under the particular circumstances of the moment. In refusing to allow the withdrawal of a feeding tube for Nancy Cruzan, for example, the Missouri Supreme Court wrote that it is "definitionally impossible for a person to make an informed refusal of treatment" under hypothetical circumstances. Others, like former U.S. Surgeon General C. Everett Koop, emphasize the difficulties of accurately assessing another's quality of life, so that proxy decisions for incompetent patients are highly suspect. There is also concern that endorsing a unique need for euthanasia for the old would help legitimize the notion that "old age is a special time of lost hopes, empty futures, and personal pointlessness."[80]

Anti–death control attitudes are also found among the less educated, the politically conservative, and persons ideologically opposed to other forms of perceived "deviance," such as premarital sex, sex education, homosexuality, welfare, school busing, and permissive childrearing. Fears of genocide and concerns about unequal risk for members of certain ethnic or class groups, or other "undesirables," motivate some opponents. For example, Dr. C. Everett Koop worries that a "slippery slope" may lead to involuntary killing of the "sidewalk screamer," illegal aliens, "welfare queens," urban Indians, migrant workers, 12-year-old mothers, and 33-year-old grandmothers. And the National Legal Center for the Medically Dependent and Disabled—an organization with ties to the National Right-to-Life Committee but which, unlike organizations advocating death control, is financed by the Federal government—has submitted briefs in dozens of right-to-die cases, claiming discrimination against the disabled.[81]

Opposition to death control may come from those who profit from health-related and long-term care services. The pharmaceutical industry, insurance companies, manufacturers, suppliers, and distributors of medical equipment, and for-profit hospitals and nursing homes all have powerful legislative lobbies and strong incentives to increase profits. The recent boom in special wings in nursing homes for Alzheimer's patients, for example, seems to have derived primarily from perceptions of new income opportunities in the industry, since their effectiveness for residents has not been demonstrated. Unscrupulous physicians also stand to profit from suffering if they perform unnecessary tests, surgery, and other medical procedures that cannot benefit the patient. Presumably, easier access to deliberate death among potential customers would be viewed as a threat by those who think primarily in terms of profit and loss.[82]

Is the doctor's diagnosis of terminal illness a tragic mistake? Is a cure or significant mitigation of suffering just around the corner? Has the doctor seriously overestimated the speed of deterioration or underestimated the "quality time" remaining to the patient? Should a physician ever, under any circumstances, help someone to die? Many opponents of death by choice emphasize "the absolute importance of the medical profession's ethical commitment to the preservation of life," believing that suffering can usually be relieved. They worry that doctors might try to rid themselves of patients whose care is difficult, time-consuming, or otherwise unsatisfying. Doctors could also "bury their mistakes" more easily or work less aggressively to save lives, taking the "easy way out" with negotiated death. As one specialist on the intersection of law and medicine put it: "Deprived of an easy 'out', clinicians have had to pay attention to the symptoms, pain, and distress of these people to the end"; facilitating death would make everyone "less prone to linger in the room of the dying." Sadly, however, the claim that medical personnel now pay close attention to the dying is much exaggerated. We will return to these key issues in Chapter 8.[83]

On the patient's part, is a desire for an easier death merely an-other form of self–indulgence that society should discourage? According to Dr. Leon Kass, for example, assisted dying is a "con-venience," an "indulgence," or a form of "gratification" for the patient. As such, it is akin to cosmetic surgery undertaken for rea-sons of personal vanity or a vasectomy sought for nonmedical pur-poses, such as family limitation.[84] Are those who condone or assist another's suicide, including caregiving relatives and others with personal interests at stake, just selfishly trying to rid themselves of burden rather than acting in the sick person's best interests? Are relatives trying to assuage their own suffering in watching a loved one die? Will easier access to death control encourage suicide among the wrong people for the wrong reasons? Will patients shun a doctor who has helped others to die? Can modern methods of pain control and a supportive environment such as hospice sup-plant any need for deliberate death? These are other concerns that opponents have raised and that we will return to later.

Neither the right-to-die movement nor its opponents are mono-lithic; each has constituent subgroups embracing a variety of views, and internal conflicts sometimes occur. The Hemlock Society, for example, advocates "active" euthanasia, preferably with the aid of a physician, and has published advice books on self-deliverance. But Concern for Dying, which also espouses free-dom of choice in matters of death and dying, publicly condemned this sort of advice, fearing that it might be misused. Both the Euthanasia Educational Council and its politically active counter-part, the Society for the Right to Die, restricted themselves during the 1970s to endorsing "passive" euthanasia, although their founder's position embraced "active" forms as well.[85]

Different opposition groups also vary in the intensity of their concern. Some objected even to living will legislation, for example, and strongly opposed it during the 1970s. Interestingly, this attack became more muted in the 1980s, a fact that has been attributed to opponents' better understanding of the problems of modern medical technology. In other words, as they learn more about the great complexities surrounding end-of-life choices, some oppo-nents have voluntarily modified their position. Still, a few extrem-ists go to great lengths to register their objections. For example, a meeting of the Hemlock Society's Tucson, Arizona chapter was disrupted by a bomb threat, the first such experience for the Society. Overall, however, organized opposition is weak and divided against itself.[86]

As Table 4-1 shows, public attitudes have been shifting toward acceptance of more "active" termination choices over the years. The question asked in the Gallup Polls, for instance, incorporates a specific reference to legalization of physician-assisted dying, and shows approval doubling from one-third to two-thirds of respondents over the period 1947–1986. The Harris question also referred to physician aid-in-dying, but made no reference to the law; nonetheless, more than six in ten condoned such behavior in 1985. Approval is generally lower for suicide, but still grew from 38 percent to 50 percent in just eleven years. Public reaction to Dr. Jack Kevorkian's suicide assistance efforts—he has helped eight women to die—is telling. Instead of being horrified "by the rusty van in the parking lot" where the first woman died, for instance, a significant number of Americans had nothing but praise for the doctor, according to the head of the ethics committee of the Michigan State Medical Society.[87] Hence opponents face a formidable task if they hope to convince the public that deliberate death options are too dangerous and should always be rejected.

"Slippery slope" arguments have been made about social change in a wide variety of historical contexts. For example, birth control might encourage promiscuity, police protection might degenerate into brutality, torture, and oppression, and compulsory military service might heighten the risk of war and nuclear annihilation. There are some legitimate grounds for such fears, but societies have not generally allowed the risks to forestall a greater chance of benefit from social change. With strong arguments and justifiable concerns on both sides, consensus is not yet in sight. Support for "active" euthanasia and opposition to it may increase simultaneously, as those previously unaware of the issues, or undecided, learn more and take a stand. In the meantime, deliberate decisions to terminate lives deemed of low quality are indeed being made, with little public outcry, as values and behavior shift in response to new conditions. The long journey toward increasing acceptance of death control, including "active" forms, is now well along. Chapter 5 expands on the advantages that may be perceived by those who modify their behavior in response to changing circumstances.

The Advantages of
Death Control

"Sound of mind and body, I am killing myself before pitiless old age, which gradually deprives me of the pleasures and joys of existence and saps my physical and intellectual forces, will paralyze my energy, break my will power, and turn me into a burden to myself and others."

"I haven't the energy to go on. I'm getting so tired, I want out.... It's been a long fight."

An intelligent and dedicated school principal finds himself unable to complete the job application that would allow him to resume his teaching career. It is the beginning of a 15-year ordeal with Alzheimer's disease that encompasses several suicide attempts, more than five years of hospitalization, eight bouts of pneumonia, tube feeding, and the other concomitants of total care. Finally the man's family, nearly destroyed by his illness, decides that nothing more should be done to prolong his life. When pneumonia presents for the ninth time, they decline treatment on his behalf.

The son visits his 90-year old mother every few days, knowing full well there is nothing he can do for her: she lies in a fetal position and blinks uncomprehendingly as he talks to her. Her only sound is a shriek of pain when attendants turn her body from side to side in an effort to heal her horrible bedsores. She is incontinent and must be hand-fed. He asks, "Can't we put my mother to sleep?"

These statements, all from real people, are dramatic illustrations of the kinds of advajntages that individuals and families perceive in putting a deliberate end to life, their own or someone else's.[1]

In Chapter 4, I applied the first of three elements in the para-

digm for increasing resort to birth control in a society—acceptability—to the subject of death control. Here we move to the second
element: *advantages* accruing to innovative behavior. Although
people may accept the idea of judging whether or not a particular
life is worth living, and believe that taking deliberate steps to terminate it is legitimate behavior, they may not act on those beliefs
unless the anticipated benefits provide sufficient motivation.

This is not the place for an extensive discussion of people's motives for wishing to control the number and spacing of their children. Suffice it to say that motivation among individual couples
both preceded and encouraged legitimation of deliberate control
by larger social institutions—state, church, and the medical establishment. Couples perceived highly desirable rewards to successfully limiting family size: an improved standard of living, more
leisure time, the enjoyment of more goods and services, and hence
a more secure, pleasurable, and satisfying life. Motivation was also
negative: escape from poverty, drudgery, and crowding, for example. For women, there was avoidance of the anxiety, physical pain,
and risk of permanent illness or injury, or even death, associated
with repeated pregnancies, especially if they were unwanted or too
close together. As one prominent historian put it, "nine months of
gestation could mean nine months to prepare for death"; and
"women knew that if procreation did not kill them, it could maim
them for life," taking a toll on "their time, their energy, their
dreams," as well as their bodies.[2]

All these motives continue to operate today, of course. Both parents and the fewer children born when deliberate control is exercised enjoy the advantages and escape the penalties associated with
failure to control. Once restricted to the elite, the advantages of
family limitation gradually became apparent to other classes, and
by the early twentieth century the democratization of birth control
was well underway; innovators served as role models and the mass
media helped diffuse the knowledge that "bad" births (ill timed,
unaffordable, abnormal, or hazardous to the mother's health, for
example) could be prevented and "good" births facilitated by timing them to suit the parents' ability to raise a child. And, always,
those who believed that the advantages of a large family outweighed its drawbacks remained free to forgo the new forms of
control that were welcomed by the many.

Human beings also seek to facilitate "good" deaths and avoid "bad" ones. Like the struggle to legitimate birth control, the death control movement also has its innovators and role models, whose ideas and actions are widely disseminated through modern communication networks. Like its predecessor, the death control movement also represents the responses of individuals to perceived advantages accruing to behavior modification and, simultaneously, disadvantages attached to the maintenance of older norms. These cost factors, psychic as well as monetary, figure prominently in decisions to choose death. They can be viewed from four overlapping perspectives: the ill or dying patient; the family, especially those who are primary caregivers; professional care providers; and the larger society.

The illness trajectory encompasses more than just the patient's physical course of illness. It includes all the work that others must do to deal with the illness, as well as the consequences of the illness, such as its effects on social relationships, the quality of life, and family economic well-being. Over the many years of a chronic illness, for example, patients will typically cycle through hospitals, doctors' offices, home or nursing home, not once but many times.[3] Social roles and relationships undergo enormous strains during these processes. For those without families or whose families cannot or will not accept their culturally assigned roles as care providers, society is expected to take over. The illness trajectory of a single patient thus intersects at many points with the lives and well-being of numerous others—family members, medical workers, the community, the nation, and even future generations. Perceptions of advantages to death control are discussed first from the perspective of the individual.

Perceptions of Advantage: Individuals

Don and Betty Morris knew about nursing homes, including the fact that some provide excellent care. But both had had successful medical careers and had seen too many friends unhappily placed in an institution. Unable to bear the thought of finishing out their lives in such a place, they drank poison and lay down to die in each other's arms. Like the Morrises, many people know that in a good nursing home the surroundings are cheerful, staff are well trained, and a variety of pleasant social activities are provided for those able to participate in them. "Screamers" are quickly quieted, especially at night, the toileting accidents of the incontinent are promptly cleaned up, and dementia victims with a tendency to wander are protected by locked doors and an ever-watchful staff. The severely demented, intubated, or dying are inconspicuously transferred to a separate wing, which, as both residents and visitors know, is the final stop on the route to death.[4]

But for many, it is not enough to know all this about the good homes: they are as good as they can be, but not good enough. Many clients in even the good homes wonder why they have come to this, why their lives should end in such a place, why all their hard work failed to bring its just reward, why they should be "stuck" among the demented and the dying.[5] The Morrises' story helps to illuminate why some people, even those not yet terminally ill, may still choose death over the prospect of an institutional existence.

What can dying patients gain from hastening their own death? The first and most obvious benefit is avoidance of pain and suffering. Many people are terrified of dying slowly, as helpless victims attached to tubes and machines, with no one listening or really caring about their suffering, or equally helpless to prevent it. Experts speculate that fears of dementing illnesses and institutionalization, as well as physical ailments, may motivate suicide in older adults. The possibility of such suffering is sufficient to induce some to take their lives prematurely, fearing that when they are bedridden and helpless self-determination will not be physically possible. It is extremely difficult to commit suicide or help someone to end her life in a hospital or other institutional setting, where just the presence of alert staff can forestall an attempt and medical workers with their sophisticated equipment can prevent a death if it is attempted, as well as prosecute any assistants to the act. Studies of suicide attempts among the aged have also found that dementias "impaired the fatal completion of suicide by interfering with [the patient's] coordination, planning, determination, and awareness of reality."[6]

Although modern techniques of pain management can substantially alleviate physical pain for many, not all forms of pain and distress can be controlled; sedation to the point of unconsciousness *will* block pain, of course, but only by creating a deathlike state in which the person has no conscious experience, no significant communication with others, no joy, no movement toward personal goals—in short, no life. More crucial to death control decisions is the fact that pain relief is not equivalent to the relief of *suffering*. The latter encompasses psychological phenomena such as the frustration of not being able to do the things one enjoys, hopelessness about the possibility of returning to an acceptable quality of life, and the sense of being a burden to others. Pain medication cannot eradicate these nonphysical forms of suffering. Assuming the person remains mentally competent, no amount of psychological counseling or other caring activities may suffice to alleviate his suffering either. But such problems, as well as fears of loneliness, isolation, and abandonment by significant others if dying takes too long or too much of a toll on caregivers, are forms of suffering that a more timely death can forestall. Patients whose prognoses are similar may evaluate relevant facts quite differently, and they do not invariably see decisions to shorten life as difficult ones, especially if they have arranged their affairs and taken leave of loved ones.[7]

Most individuals wish to avoid a dying trajectory that is undignified, "degrading," or "disgusting" and to spare friends and relatives from watching it. These apprehensions too encompass much more than physical pain. Alzheimer's disease is a case in point, one that will gain rapidly in importance as the American population ages. Janet Adkins, who achieved posthumous fame as the first person to die in Dr. Jack Kevorkian's "suicide machine," was diagnosed as in the early stages of Alzheimer's. She had already lost her ability to read and play the piano. Looking to the future, she may well have seen herself, in columnist Anna Quindlen's poignant words, "incontinent, incompetent, incapable of knowing the difference between 'Tom and Jerry' and 'War and Peace.'" She chose to kill herself before that happened. Clearly others will also willingly forgo that kind of existence if an acceptable alternative is available.[8]

Elders have strong antipathies toward the prospect of moving in with their children. Preferences for self-reliance and independent living are characteristic of Americans, and dependence on others violates strongly held beliefs. Elders are seldom willing to interfere with their children's lives to the extent of coresiding with them. There is also a possibility of significant adverse consequences, such as decreased morale and life satisfaction, for elders who become dependent on their children or other family members. Many do not want assistance from kin, but see no alternative when their health is poor. Those who seem to "choose" family care may do so because formal agencies are not available or are an even less desirable alternative. If one wants love and affection and a sense of belonging from relatives but is instead merely tolerated by them, will a more timely death seem preferable? What of those who are abused or neglected? What of resentful or greedy caregivers? What happens when another option—physician-assisted dying at a time and place of one's own choosing, for example—is added to the current list? Will this new choice be welcomed or rejected?[9]

Institutionalization allows elders to avoid moving in with an adult child. But, as the ultimate form of dependence, it has long been, and continues to be, very negatively perceived. As one caregiving daughter noted, "My mother wanted to die rather than go into a nursing home. A nursing home is like the last stop." Hence it is not surprising that most elders strive to maintain their independence as long as possible. The mass media inundate us daily with the horrors of institutional life. A good example is Autumn Hills, the first nursing home corporation indicted for murder when two women patients died, apparently due to gross neglect. It matters little that such portrayals are not entirely accurate, that many homes provide decent care, since people often believe the worst and act accordingly: few voluntarily enter a nursing home. Most people believe that nursing homes are awful places, that even when they are clean, adequately staffed, serve decent meals, and provide interesting social activities, they remain too confining and prisonlike.[10]

Frail elders may reject the lack of privacy and personal autonomy that institutionalization entails, along with its "unyielding iron hand of regulations." They may also wish to avoid the indignities of "infantilization" and "toddlerization" that seem inescapably associated with long-term care, whether at home, in adult day care centers, or total institutions. Like children, nursing home residents may be talked about as if they were not present, addressed as "honey" or "sweetie," or have their legitimate requests ignored, trivialized, or misinterpreted. Aides frequently use baby talk with patients or dress them and arrange their hair in childlike fashion—practices that are frowned on by the general public. One nurse, well acquainted with elder care, exclaimed: "When I'm 80 years old I don't want a 20-year-old putting pink bows in my hair and calling me cute!"[11]

Institutional programs and activities are often aimed at the most cognitively impaired, whose bizarre behavior may be highly disturbing to nondemented clients. The literature on both adult day care centers and nursing homes is quite frank about how clients are "managed," their "acting up" tendencies kept under control with activities designed to keep them "pleasantly senile" rather than hostile or depressed. For example, lest an elder be upset by the departure of the family caregiver for the day, aides extend a hearty greeting as a distraction while she drives away. As with recalcitrant children, a "firm and positive attitude" and "calm, reassuring stance" are recommended to staff members as helpful management techniques for older adults.[12]

Planned activities encompass everything from discussions of current events to sing-alongs to birdwatching and include some, aimed at highly impaired residents, that readers may find disturbing. For example, one such list (addressed to the social director or her equivalent) recommends towel folding as beneficial for an elder's motor coordination as well as her "feelings of accomplishment and worth from focusing on a familiar household task." The writer adds that when this worthwhile task has been completed, the towels should be *unfolded* and stored for re-use.[13]

A closer look at the same expert's advice on baking cookies as a pleasant activity for dementia victims is also instructive. More cognitively intact patients may still be able to read the recipe or follow simplified verbal instructions. But as their condition deteriorates, it may be necessary for someone to steady the bowl or guide the patient's hand in stirring the ingredients. Later still, when she is confined to bed, she can still be "involved" in the activity if someone comes to her room, describes the baking project, and encourages her to smell the spices, whose scent may "trigger happy memories of previous baking experiences."[14] Now certainly if the only choices to be made are folding towels versus not folding towels or smelling spices versus not smelling them, most of us would probably fold and smell. But *are* these the only choices? How many people really want this kind of life? Why hasn't anyone thought to ask?

All of us, if we live long enough, are threatened with sufficient loss of health, functional abilities, or mental acuity to necessitate some form of institutional care. At current usage rates, about 43 percent of those living past 65 will spend some time in a nursing home before they die. No one knows how long this will be or how happy or helpless they will feel in those circumstances, but many imagine the worst. Can we assume that elders anticipate a long period of extreme frailty or senility with equanimity or a fatalistic attitude? What do they learn from observing the experiences of friends and relatives in the long-term care system? Should we take for granted that most will do nothing to avoid such miseries for themselves? As they grow frailer, elders see their options shrinking and the possibility of institutionalized dependency becoming more threatening. Some prefer the active choice of self-deliverance to such an alternative. This was precisely the choice Wallace Proctor faced in 1977. In a final letter to his family, he wrote of his repugnance at the thought of institutionalization and being a burden to others; then he killed himself.[15]

Uncertainty plays a large role in premature death. No one can "count on being lucky enough to have adequate warning of deterioration and enough time in which to deliberate while still free of impairment." No one can count on help being available if he postpones acting. As Percy Bridgman, a Nobel Prize winner in physics, wrote in his suicide note at age 80, following his doctor's refusal to help him die: "Probably this is the last day I will be able to do it myself." Similarly, those who find the prospect of institutional living abhorrent may resort to self-deliverance simply because they feel threatened, regardless of how realistic their fears are or the immediacy of the threat.[16]

Quality-of-life considerations may also induce suicide prior to a diagnosis of terminal illness. Persons of all ages and states of health, but the elderly in particular, fear both physical debilitation and the loss of self that accompanies dementia, as well as the surrender of independence and control they imply. For example, many moderately demented patients find that continued life in such a state is, on balance, no longer desirable in comparison with an earlier death; suicide rates for such patients have increased in recent years.[17]

The chronically ill for whom death is *not* imminent may simply not wish to settle for the particular level of functioning that is available to them, and fear further, less tolerable, declines to come; hence choices to "opt out of this life" can be eminently rational. Although statistics on opting out are rare, a study of patients' withdrawal from kidney dialysis is suggestive: of 1,766 patients who started on dialysis in the period 1966-1983, 155 (9 percent) discontinued treatment and died, when dialysis could have been continued. Older patients and nursing home residents were disproportionately represented among those who died. Half the decedents were clearly competent and made the decision to stop dialysis, knowing they would die within two weeks; the rest were incompetent and physicians and families made the decision for them.[18]

Suicide among the elderly has been increasing. Compared to community residents, institutionalized elders are at greater risk of suicide because they are older, sicker, and less likely to have concerned family members available. Research has uncovered instances of deliberate self-starvation by nursing home residents determined to die. Other forms of self-harm, such as refusal of medications, have also been reported. These are indirect forms of self-destructive behavior, as opposed to overt forms like slashing one's wrists, jumping out a window, or hanging. Indirect suicidal behavior may occur because people fear the stigma and guilt often attached to overt suicide, but there has been little research on the subject. It can also result from any of the myriad losses associated with old age and ill health—loss of a spouse, a familiar environment, independence, mobility, and so on. Institutionalized against her will, for example, one woman "confined herself to bed, spat out food and medicine, and refused to open her mouth." When respiratory complications occurred as a result, she was allowed to die. What we should now ask ourselves is whether these suicidal behaviors will change as suicide for the very ill becomes more acceptable. How many now refrain from suicide or postpone it (even past the point of their competence to carry out their intent) because they fear social disapproval? How many, like Percy Bridgman's doctor, are afraid to help someone die because they too fear social disapproval?[19]

Many old people trust their spouse or adult children to make decisions for them if they become incompetent, and see no need for formal advance directives, such as a living will, for documenting their end-of-life treatment wishes; even if they foresee disagreement among family members, some elders reason that relatives will work it out for the best. But not all relatives are trustworthy and not all old people have families. Generally speaking, very old patients are those most likely to lack a trusted other to make proxy decisions for them—no spouse, or even child, still living, or children who are aged and ill themselves, for example. People without families are more likely to execute advance directives than are those with close family members available.[20]

Many forms of advance planning have been recommended to elders to protect their survivors as well as themselves, as the discussion of "responsible dying" in Chapter 4 pointed out. Failure to do these things, the advice literature implies, is thoughtless at best, cruel and unfair at worst; doing them, presumably, creates feelings of gratification for elders who are able to tie up loose ends and do well by survivors. After assisting her mother's death, for instance, one daughter asked the dead woman, who had often expressed a wish to die but failed to act on it, some rhetorical questions: "Why did you put us both through this, why didn't you have the courage [to kill yourself]? Once again you have been totally dependent, once again you have left all the responsibility to others." Contrast this with the relief and gratitude of a husband whose wife had discussed her preferences with him and her doctor, with the result that "when she was so bad and had a heart attack, we let her go." Will even more personal gratification be thought to accrue from a quicker as opposed to a more lingering death? Cases like these suggest that it will.[21]

Insured or not, most patients are concerned about the financial aspects of their care. A growing number of reports cite the immense costs of life-prolonging treatments provided to some people in the last stage of life and the plight of families forced into financial straits as a result. It is questionable whether many patients would have wanted so much treatment if they had been forewarned about the expense or the small probability of benefit. Patients may decide that certain treatments are not sufficiently beneficial to warrant their high cost and may reject even those that promise substantial medical benefits, accepting an earlier death instead.[22]

Competent elders realize that neither long-term care services in the community nor their institutionalization necessarily reduce burdens on kin, financial or otherwise. They might wish to avoid impoverishing the family or dissipating their estate to pay for care, especially since costs are high and rising rapidly while the benefits are regarded with increasing skepticism. A husband may worry, for example, that his wife will not have enough money to live on following his death if their joint assets are largely expended on his long-term care needs. An aged father may see a choice between his own care and a grandchild's college education or a daughter's career plans. The monetary costs of alternative outcomes are surely weighed by individuals considering their end-of-life care options.

Bequest motives also enter into decision making. Understandably, those who struggled hard all their lives to have something to leave to their children may hesitate to spend it on long-term care, especially if the benefits do not seem proportional to the costs. Or, as one hospice patient reasoned, "Why should all my money go to health care if I'm not going to get better anyway? I'd rather give it to my sisters." Private funds, painstakingly accumulated, are not lightly spent. Changes in public policy that affect private costs may have untoward effects. For example, Stephen Moses has done extensive research on asset transfers by elderly Medicaid recipients. His research led him to recommend better enforcement of existing legislation allowing public long-term care costs to be recovered from a decedent's estate as one means of controlling the spiralling costs of long-term care. But such actions may threaten bequest motives and conceivably push some elders toward an earlier death to avoid diminishing their children's inheritance. The fact that elders do often transfer assets in order to qualify for Medicaid is evidence of their concern for survivors.[23]

Throughout their lives, people typically seek praise and avoid criticism. We all want others to think well of us. After death, we want to be remembered positively, and actions to ensure this are common. Praise for a good death, a timely death, one that takes account of the welfare of others can be a powerful motivator. Sociologist Michael Kearl reports that how one dies "shapes the quality of grief of significant others"—since the death trajectory makes great demands on them, "the utility of their sacrifices" is at issue. Equally powerful stimuli are desires to avoid negative labels like "selfish," "cowardly," "pitiful," or "undignified" in one's dying. Lingering deaths are generally viewed as highly undesirable, whereas dying "on time" is highly valued.[24]

Altruistic motives might encompass a desire to free public funds for more productive uses. Because many new life-sustaining technologies are both expensive and scarce, and because even the simplest long-term care needs are cumulatively very costly, they have consequences for the larger society and raise issues of distributive justice. Evidence of poverty, neglect, and preventable suffering is all around us—from drug-infested inner-city streets to unemployment to deteriorating housing stock, schools, and transportation systems. Some individuals will recognize and respond to these larger concerns, perceiving in a more timely death a final way to be useful. As ethicist Paul Menzel put it in his recent book, *Strong Medicine*, the knowledge that one is "parting with a small share of life for the benefit of others" helps make the last stage of life more meaningful; contrarily, clinging "to every last bit of one's life at great expense" may be "a selfish violation of the duty of mutual aid, the duty not to use up more than one's share of the pool of common resources."[25]

The advice literature implies that suicide (a voluntary and active choice) is preferable to death hastening which requires the direct action of others because it is more considerate of survivors, reducing their self-doubts and lessening their responsibility for hard choices. Also, although many elders apparently trust their relatives to make decisions for them should they become incapacitated, it is doubtful that relatives want that kind of responsibility. In his poignant account of his mother's dying, for example, Andrew Malcolm details his anxieties about allowing her to die and regrets that his efforts to ascertain her wishes while she was still competent were unsuccessful; her statements were vague and ambivalent, and he was "left to figure out," and agonize over, what she really wanted. The implication is that considerate elders will not want to burden loved ones in this way.[26]

Personal experiences with long-term care or the dying of others can predispose individuals to certain preferences regarding their own death. For example, a woman who cared for her invalid mother for fifteen years became so concerned about prolonged dying that she not only joined the Hemlock Society but "decided to take up every dangerous physical activity" she could think of, in hopes of avoiding a fate like her mother's. In the Netherlands, an 86-year-old man repeatedly instructed his doctor to administer euthanasia if he became demented; he had seen too many of his friends lose their minds, he said. Another man told his doctor that he preferred euthanasia to the prolonged dying he saw his friends endure. Both men got the help they wanted. In the United States, Edward Winter was less successful. The slow, painful dying of his wife led him to resolve "that nothing like that would happen to him," so he informed both his children and his doctor of his wish to be allowed to die; ironically, his preferences were not respected, leading him to file suit against an Ohio hospital in what is apparently the first "wrongful life" case filed by a patient. His case will doubtless serve as a cautionary tale to others—both patients and hospitals—as it is disseminated through the mass media.[27]

A frequent claim in the gerontological literature is that family caregivers provide care in part because they anticipate needing care themselves someday. But frail elders who earlier performed long-term care duties for others—a parent, for example—may *not* want their own spouse or children to do the same for them. Recollections of their feelings of burden, resentment, ambivalence, or role conflict can induce a wish to avoid becoming a similar burden to loved ones. In her exhaustive study of family caregivers, for example, Suzanne Steinmetz found that "many adult children, after the experience of providing care, have made it clear to their own children that they want alternative solutions" for themselves. They are emphatic in denying that they are accumulating credit for their own old age. As one caregiving daughter put it, "I worry. Is this the way I'm going to be? I don't want my children to have this." And the young son of an Alzheimer's victim, after witnessing firsthand the devastation caused by the disease, has vowed to commit suicide if ever diagnosed with it himself. If elders were neglectful or abusive as caregivers, they may fear mistreatment in turn. Even if their caregiving experience was gratifying, some elders will nonetheless prefer to avoid burdening others. We must also consider what elders expect of potential caregiving relatives who are themselves elderly, poor, sick, or overburdened with other responsibilities.[28]

We should expect that as knowledge of new problems and new alternatives increases, more elders will choose an earlier death. For example, many respondents in a 1985 survey (seven in ten of those over 65 and almost eight in ten of the general population) believed that Medicare would pay for an extended nursing home stay. As more people come to realize that this is not the case, patterns of decision making should alter. Similarly, public awareness of the immense caregiving costs (psychic and financial) associated with dementias is quite recent, but will intensify as the number of those affected climbs. Loss of mental faculties and being a burden on the family (two problems that are closely related) are the most important criteria underlying treatment cessation—equally important to patients and proxies. As knowledge of the multiple dilemmas associated with dying in modern institutions continues to diffuse throughout our society, more people will inevitably realize that "the only way to be reasonably certain of a good death is to plan it," if possible, while one is still in reasonably good health.[29]

Familial and societal values, expectations, and needs influence individual choices and have potential for either hastening death or delaying it. Patients seldom want to decide alone and many prefer to either share the burden with significant others or to withdraw entirely from the decision-making process. Various scenarios are possible: for example, significant others may give tacit "permission" to die to a patient tired of struggling or encourage acceptance of death too soon by elders who sense rejection. Thus professional caregivers, relatives, and friends inevitably influence individual decisions—even their refusal to talk about a topic can affect the patient's thinking. Shaping a patient's deliberations can be a very subtle process and some outcomes may not be consciously intended. The ability and willingness of significant others to comply with the patient's wishes also affect the options chosen and limit those considered. Finally, since "dying is a social process which is guided by expectations of appropriate behaviour," if expectations change, behavior will eventually follow.[30]

In summary, the average person spends a lifetime trying to avoid death, minimize personal suffering, and cure, or at least manage, chronic illness and functional limitations. He also strives to earn the respect, if not the admiration, of significant others. Although these goals sometimes conflict with other desires, they are all indications of a strong wish to control and direct life events. Those who have become accustomed to exercising freedom of choice in other areas of life may see no reason to stop at the threshold of death. And clearly, those who fail to act risk being acted upon.

All of the for going assumes that the dying patient is competent to decide her own end. But growing numbers of incapacitated elders now have decisions made for them—by relatives, medical professionals, ethics committees, or others. Such decisions should be altruistic, made with good intentions, and in the incompetent patient's best interests. But it is not safe to take this for granted—there is more danger of abuse as decision making becomes further removed from the individual, competent patient. Hence family, medical, and societal perceptions of advantages to death control also merit concern.

Perceptions of Advantage: Families

The taxi driver was interviewing me on the way from the airport—How long would I be in Chicago? Did I like the weather? What was the purpose of my trip? When I reported that I planned to speak at a professional meeting about caregiving to frail elders, he began to tell me about his mother's experiences in the nursing home where, he said, employees repeatedly stole the small personal items her family brought to cheer her up. The anger in his voice plainly indicated his belief that his fragile mother was a helpless victim of an insensitive system and he, though he had tried, equally helpless to prevent her suffering. Indeed, employee theft is a major form of crime in nursing homes, running into tens of millions of dollars each year.[31] Soon the driver's voice choked up, and the burly, middle-aged man was in tears, making no effort to disguise his emotion. When he recovered himself, he shared more details about his mother's illnesses, eventually venturing an opinion that "sometimes people just live too long." As I recalled the painful circumstances of my father's death five months earlier, I had to agree.

Like the taxi driver, family members commonly express love and concern for aged relatives, and sometimes that same love and concern make them wish for the elder's peaceful death. Health care choices affecting a frail elder, such as institutional versus home care, also have serious consequences for the family members who must participate in decision making, arrange for appropriate care, or provide it themselves. The family is typically viewed as the institution best suited to meet elders' everyday needs, physical, social, and emotional. And, indeed, families provide the bulk of care to most of the nation's frail elders. Assistance is often required for years, not just weeks or months—44 percent of caregivers to non-institutionalized disabled elders in the United States have been providing care for one to four years, and an additional 20 percent have been doing so for five years or more. Most caregivers (80 percent) provide services seven days a week, for an average of four hours a day, in addition to all their other responsibilities.[32]

Technological medicine and increased longevity have added to demands on caregivers over and above the provision of food and shelter more characteristic of the nonindustrial societies of the past, when little could be done to postpone death through medical means. Family care providers now routinely perform services at home that previously took place only in institutional settings, or at least were performed by medical professionals. The trend toward home dialysis, for example, requires a lay person "to assume an unprecedented amount of responsibility for operating a complex life-support system."[33] Other examples include giving injections, tube feeding, administering oxygen, and managing incontinence. In general, the care required is more difficult and longer in duration.

Care management is also more onerous and more time-intensive. For example, since few doctors make housecalls, a caregiver must drive, perhaps some distance, for an elder's medical appointments, an activity that now may also entail leaving work or arranging for child care in her absence; an elder who may be confused, recalcitrant, or suffer mobility limitations must be physically and psychologically prepared for the medical encounter; finally, considerable waiting time may be involved. In earlier eras, in contrast, the doctor might never be summoned, or the caregiver would have been home doing other chores while waiting for him to arrive. A recent study suggests other forms of increasing responsibilities for family caregivers since the implementation of Medicare's Prospective Payment System in 1983. For example, since the workload for nurses appears to have increased, relatives must be patient advocates even in the hospital to ensure adequate care. And since the new system contains incentives for discharging patients "quicker and sicker," necessitating that a larger portion of recuperation take place at home or elsewhere, relatives must act as mediators, supervisors, planners, and coordinators of care to a degree unprecedented before the new system was initiated.[34]

As elders become frailer over time, the intensity of assistance must increase, and caregiver involvement often extends gradually to encompass total management of the elder's affairs. Even institutionalization does not signal the termination of family care efforts, since many relatives continue to engage in "protective caregiving" aimed at remedying institutional shortcomings, as well as other forms of care. For example, they may come in at mealtime to help the patient eat. Conditions in institutions for the aged are a persistent national problem, as described earlier in this volume. Residents' quality of life is a low priority for the busy, often overworked, nurse's aides who perform most of the daily services needed by frail clients. Forced to cut corners in order to survive on the job, aides are likely to leave important tasks undone; examples are changing the wet sheets of incontinent patients, repositioning those who are immobile (important for preventing bedsores), and routine mouth care. Watchful relatives can ensure that their loved one is adequately cared for by complaining to the administration, befriending staff, or taking over some tasks themselves.[35]

Worker characteristics, characteristics of the institution itself, and the relative powerlessness of their charges help create the potential for abuse and neglect. Hence it is incumbent on relatives to select a home carefully, to monitor the care provided, and to make alternative arrangements if circumstances warrant. Since most nursing homes have waiting lists and many discourage visitors' "interference," these responsibilities may prove formidable. For example, when Frank Robinson complained that his mother was not being fed properly and that her personal hygiene was neglected, the staff threatened to discharge her; he knew and they knew that it would be difficult for him to make other arrangements. And indeed the situation was so difficult that he eventually shot her to death.[36]

Greater longevity for frail, aged relatives thus both pleases and distresses their families. While longer lives provide more time for positive family interactions, they also provide more time for negative interactions. Simultaneously, they allow the accumulation of yet more chronic conditions and the worsening of existing conditions for the care recipient and the appearance or worsening of health problems for providers, which complicates care provision on both sides. Prolonged survival of frail elders also creates greater potential for psychological distress and economic difficulties, as the psychic and financial resources of both parties are depleted. As an elderly relative's health deteriorates, the family's attitude may be radically transformed—from sympathy and concern to annoyance and feelings of burden to, finally, relief at an overdue death.[37]

Social, economic, and demographic trends contribute to constraints on family care provision. For example, the long-term movement of American women into the paid labor force limits the potential supply of caregivers for the elderly, as it does for children. Women's employment is highly correlated with a tendency to seek institutionalization for aged parents, as it is with day care for small children. Inflationary pressures that require both husband and wife to work, along with desires for personal freedom, self-fulfillment, and leisure time, affect ability and willingness to provide long-term elder care. Families are also smaller, leaving fewer siblings to share parent care. Delayed marriage and childbearing help to create competing obligations, and divorce too seems to inhibit caregiving to aged parents. Family capacity to provide hands-on care is further limited by the geographic distance that often separates parents and adult children. Meanwhile, growing numbers of elders and their escalating needs indicate that more family caregivers, not fewer, will be required in the years ahead.[38]

For families who supply direct care for elders, the psychological costs—the sense of burden, feelings of inadequacy, anger, guilt, and fears about their own present and future well-being that inevitably arise—are good examples of the human costs associated with long-term care provision. Time, energy, activities, and opportunities must be sacrificed to care for an incapacitated relative, affecting the caregiver's relationships with spouse, children, friends, and others, as well as with the recipient. Relinquished opportunities can include the caregiver's job and any psychological, monetary, and social benefits associated with it. Household routine must be rearranged and the caregiver must schedule time for the multitude of activities associated with long-term elder care. She must learn new skills, take on new roles, and coordinate them with her preexisting responsibilities.

For all this, family care providers may no longer recognize (or be recognized by) a demented yet demanding elder, however close their previous relationship. Caring for Alzheimer's patients is particularly stressful, for example, because victims are often unable to appreciate caregivers' efforts and may be hostile and uncooperative as well. Thus family members nursing frail relatives may resent unreciprocated calls for emotional support on a long-term basis; if they cannot withdraw from the relationship due to lack of alternatives or psychological bonds, they often find themselves chronically depressed or angry. A wife asks, for example, if her sacrifices in caring for her sick husband are worthwhile, because "there could be a life for me if not for this disease...my life is draining away." Thus the patient's problems have considerable ripple effects on the family, and the quality of life of both is likely to be adversely affected. A large and growing body of research documents caregiver stress and burden, and growing numbers of caregivers worry about the moral dilemmas created by their competing obligations to family, career, and personal well-being.[39]

Middle-aged adults are those most often torn by competing obligations. Many question the sacrifices entailed in providing elder care that seems to yield no appreciable benefits to the patient or anyone else, despite the effort expended. In one case, for example, a son and his wife each took weeks off from their jobs to care for his frail and confused mother, to the point that both jobs were jeopardized. Publicly funded home health care was insufficient to meet their needs, and the couple could not afford private care; hence, their 13-year-old daughter stayed home from school to look after her grandmother. This kind of dilemma is repeated daily in thousands of American homes. While no one expects families to deny themselves food, clothing, or shelter in order to provide elder care, gray areas exist regarding other choices. Should children attend the local community college in lieu of the more distant school they prefer, in order to help out at home? Should the family remain in their cramped, older home instead of moving to a better one that will require a long commute to help a frail parent? Should they forgo vacations, reduce hours on the job, or dip into their own retirement savings? What do family caregivers (or potential caregivers) who are themselves elderly (35.5 percent), poor or near poor (31.5 percent), or the one in three whose own health status is fair at best expect of themselves? What do we tell a middle-aged caregiving daughter who reports that because of her father's illness, "The rest of my family is on the verge of collapse. Our children hate to come home because of the anger and fear in our house." When are the benefits too few or the costs too great? Finally, who is to make such decisions and on what basis, and who is to enforce them?[40]

Questions of how much support the family should give to the elderly, how much families can realistically provide, and whether family caregiving is the most desirable form of long-term care are thus far from settled. Families do want to protect their elders, but they have others to protect as well. Children (and hence child care responsibilities) are usually freely chosen, their birth timed for the convenience of the parents, and an end to parental obligations can reasonably be foreseen at the start of the commitment. None of this is true for elder care, a responsibility that is typically taken on in a crisis and is highly unpredictable in both intensity and duration. Hence motivation to provide elder care may well be weaker from the start and responsibilities more easily relinquished due to competing obligations.

Family members also dread having to watch the slow, painful dying of a relative, the person they once knew often irrevocably changed by illness, or unrecognizable due to severe dementia. Those whose parents suffer from Alzheimer's disease, for example, worry that they might be glimpsing their own future and its troubling impact on their own children. The extreme pain of watching helplessly as a loved one deteriorates may be so severe that some families, for their own well-being, must be discouraged from visiting an institutionalized relative; others cease visiting voluntarily if they believe that care is adequate.[41]

Relatives also object to seeing loved ones become victims of technological medicine, their dying prolonged with no enhancement of the quality of additional days. A common public perception now is that the health care system is capable of victimizing the persons who should be its beneficiaries by prolonging their death with worthless treatment. Novelist Philip Roth, for instance, has shared his thoughts regarding his difficult decision not to prolong his unconscious father's life. After considering "what the tumor had done with him already" and "the misery that was sure to come," the loving son opted to forgo respirator treatment for his father. In another case, a daughter who experienced her father's "bad death" determined that she would not "let her mother down" and even became a social worker with a hospice unit in an effort to help others die well.[42]

Economic considerations play a role in family decision making. "Most caregivers are shocked to learn how little financial help is provided by health insurance or Medicare and how much they must pay for themselves." As early as 1970, a survey of heads of families found that three out of four agreed that there was a health care crisis in the United States, one that threatened to ruin families with overwhelming medical bills. Yet, for all the dollars poured into it, there was a growing sense that the system was inadequate for the needs it was supposed to serve. Clearly, when it had exhausted its ability to cure, the system could not even provide a good death to its "failures." It is not the financial outlay per se that people object to, but the fact that the expenditures do not seem to yield commensurate benefits, especially when spending on costly but futile care adversely affects families as well as patients.[43]

Even if community alternatives to direct care by families were widely available and affordable, which they are not, it seems doubtful that such options as institutionalization, adult day care centers, or home health services could satisfy all relatives regarding their loved one's care or, more important, their quality of life. Many relatives do not consider institutionalization a viable option because of its general low quality. Like Father Hugh McCormley, chaplain at a Pennsylvania nursing home and an eyewitness to institutional shortcomings, they might say, "I would rather bury my mother than ever put her in an institution." Family dissatisfaction with available formal care services may be exacerbated if the relative is mentally impaired. The irony of the "pleasant activities" planned by earnest social workers for dementia victims—reading to them from children's books or helping them play simple games, for example—may greatly distress those who remember a mentally vigorous person who would have been appalled at such "toddlerization."[44]

The paucity of adequate alternatives has led many to wish for the release of a gentle death for their loved one. But some relatives take a more active course, such as abandoning elders in hospital

emergency rooms when they can no longer cope with care requirements. According to the American College of Emergency
Physicians, 70,000 elderly Americans were abandoned by their
families in 1991. Other relatives have assisted in the patient's suicide, negotiated the death of one who is incompetent, or literally
killed them. For example, his mother's suffering, poor outlook,
and the "appalling care" she received in formal institutions, combined with his own fruitless search for a suitable nursing home
and the refusal of medical personnel to help her have a peaceful
death, caused considerable anguish for Frank Robinson. So he
shot his mother, at her request, in 1979. When the case came to
trial, the sympathetic judge commented that in similar circumstances he too would have ended his mother's suffering.[45]

Children who help end the life of a parent seem to examine their
motives carefully, asking themselves if they are doing it for selfish
reasons or to ease their own suffering. The answer seems to be
"yes," in part, but the primary motive is compassion. Many emotional accounts of those who kill for merciful reasons also contain
a second major theme: others should not have to suffer as they and
their loved ones did; in that cause, the perpetrators of these "compassionate crimes" are often willing to speak candidly about their
experiences. In a moving account of her father's suicide, for example, which she aided, Betty Pelletz noted her happiness about his
choice. Because "neither his body nor mind were letting him enjoy
life as he wanted," his suicide was rational and his daughter was
proud of him because he regained control over his life and served
as a role model to others.[46]

Recall from Chapter 2 that the devoted families whose filial behavior toward frail elders conforms to societal prescriptions are
largely figments of our collective imagination. Among *real* families, many are indeed conscientious and compassionate, but many
are also severely constrained by other obligations, and others are
callous or indifferent. The assumption that families are basically
close and loving and that only antagonistic outside forces prevent
their warmth and concern from manifesting itself more fully is
now being challenged. However disconcerting the thought, we are
forced to admit that families are seldom as strong, generous, and
altruistic as we would like, facts that have important consequences
for their more vulnerable members. Surveys on topics such as fam-

ily willingness to support needy elderly relatives may yield answers that reflect what people think they should say or feel rather than their true perceptions, and thus should be interpreted cautiously. In relying on such reports, many researchers have been unduly optimistic about the family's role in the care and well-being of aged members. Most research, in fact, has focused on the *fact* that care is provided or on its *quantity* rather than its quality or the willingness of the providers.[47]

The stresses of care provision may lead to physical and psychological abuse of the frail elder. Since they let elders know they are unwanted, unloved, or burdensome, such incidents are indirect forms of death hastening. Much abuse is either undetected or unreported, but we do know that those in poor health are three to four times more likely to be abused. Family members predominate as abusers of the elderly, as they do in other forms of abuse. Documented examples include screaming, threats of punishment, hitting, throwing objects, and psychological manipulation, such as threats to institutionalize. Severe physical abuse, sometimes with permanent damage, is not unknown, as in the case of a 78-year-old widow who was hospitalized with serious injuries inflicted by her son, and the 89-year-old who lost an eye under very suspicious circumstances while in the care of her grandnephew. Neglect, a more prevalent form of mistreatment than abuse, tends to be concentrated among the oldest and most impaired elderly and is closely related to caregiver stress and sense of burden, especially when the patient is demented. For all parties, the miseries of such an existence may predispose thinking of a quicker death as a way out.[48]

Another emergent trend with important implications for death control is evident in the tone of recent expert advice, which warns caregivers and potential caregivers against the dangers of overcommitment to elder care. A tendency among some professionals and lay persons to romanticize family caregiving under adverse circumstances may be pathological. Long-term care experts like Elaine Brody suggest instead that adult children accept limits to what they can or should do for their parents. The American Association of Retired Persons encourages members to consider their own abilities, needs, and limitations, as well as those of other family members, before committing themselves to in-home care for frail elders.

Ethicist Daniel Callahan, addressing the question of what children owe their elderly parents, concludes that the extent of moral obligation is ambiguous even when affectional ties are strong; moreover, "there is a pronounced distaste, on the side of both children and parents, for burdening children with financial obligations toward their parents." When time is money, especially with more women in the labor force, the boundary between financial obligations and other kinds of filial duties is a fine one. But it is noteworthy that financial hardship is not the reason most people institutionalize elderly relatives. Purely economic costs may, in fact, be greater following institutionalization than prior to it, implying that family caregivers are willing to exchange money in return for diminished social and psychological responsibility.[49]

Monetary concerns are relevant in decisions to choose death. For example, a network of professionals has developed to counsel families on how to preserve income and assets by making an infirm elder eligible for Medicaid assistance in a nursing home. This apparently occurs despite the fact that Medicaid patients receive decidedly inferior care in American institutions, possibly dying prematurely as a result, and implies that such families either don't know this, or don't care; mentally alert elders presumably care, of course, but may feel helpless to oppose their children's wishes, whereas those who are senile or confused are at risk of financial and other abuse. Any government tightening up of Medicaid rules to discourage asset transfers will threaten children's inheritance. Instead of passing to heirs as they now do, elders' assets would, with better enforcement of existing regulations, be used to pay their long-term care costs directly or to reimburse Medicaid after their death, with only the remainder of the estate going to beneficiaries. Some children are poor and some are greedy, and financial abuse of the elderly by their relatives is commonplace. Hence, prudent observers must ask what might happen to frail elders if such legislation is better enforced, especially if death control is more readily available. State efforts to pass and enforce relative responsibility laws—holding families responsible for helping disabled older relatives financially—should raise parallel concerns. This combination of circumstances might provide incentives to some relatives to safeguard their inheritance by facilitating an elder's quicker, ostensibly merciful, death—but one which may, in fact, be premature.[50]

Regardless of the initial situation, as the duration of caregiving increases there is greater potential for family conflict and strain, as well as greater distancing, both physical and psychological, between the parties. When the patient is very old, is visibly suffering, and has no expectation of improvement, the question of "Why?" must be asked repeatedly by everyone. As one caregiver put it, "She would be better off if she had a massive heart attack. I often think that. . . . Ideally, that would be the solution, because I would be free." With the advice of physicians and significant others, caregivers may turn away from their charges in desperation because of the consequences for their own lives; patients, too, aware of having become a burden, may offer an "abandonment" rationale and suggest institutionalization. But if institutionalization is not seen as a viable option, caregivers "often feel trapped because they realize that caregiving will only end when their relatives die." In one case, for example, a 71-year-old wife and her 92-year-old husband each promised never to place the other in a nursing home. The husband became bedridden with multiple illnesses; he was also deaf, suffered severe hallucinations, and was in constant pain. After eight years of caregiving, the wife, a former nurse, was on the verge of a breakdown. Rather than break her promise, she strangled him. Later, she told police that "Walter would thank me. Walter would appreciate what I did."[51]

For many, caregiving is a socially imposed "relationship of bondage" which would be avoided if choices were available. The results of one recent survey showed that morale was highest among caregivers whose elderly relative died or was institutionalized during the twelve months prior to the interview and lowest for those who were still providing care. Strikingly, only 2 percent of respondents in another survey agreed that caregiving had been an enriching experience for them. Such factors may lead families to serious consideration of negotiated death as they continually reassess the costs and benefits to themselves and the patient of prolonging his dying. A more timely death may be seen as less of an "abandonment" than institutionalization, especially since nursing homes are popularly viewed as highly undesirable by both patients and families. This choice will become more frequent too as death control becomes more accessible and role models increase among the average person's acquaintances.[52]

It seems clear that prolonged care needs, especially when accompanied by the continued deterioration and suffering of the recipient, will predispose relatives to choose death if circumstances allow. In 1990, for example, one in three respondents in a Gallup Poll answered that a person had a moral right to commit suicide if he or she was "an extremely heavy burden" on the family. "A good and acceptable death releases not only the terminally ill, but also those who have waited and watched, cared and cried, reached out and were in turn responded to, hoped and felt hope ebb." In a more cynical vein, a timely death also releases less altruistic caregivers from demands on their time, energy, and pocketbooks, concerns we would be extremely remiss to disregard. Thus we must ask three interrelated sets of questions. First, what do families have to give up in order to provide elder care? Second, what do they stand to gain that might make their sacrifices seem worthwhile? And, finally, what advantages might they see in "stopping behavior" with regard to unwanted or futile treatments?[53]

Collectively, the trends I have discussed in this chapter suggest that families will feel increasingly constrained in their ability to meet the everyday care needs of very frail, aged relatives. They will seek other options and, increasingly, may find them in deliberate death, as the mass media circulate information and provide dramatic role models, new legislation facilitates such choices, or doctors become more willing accessories to patient and family preferences, with or without legislative approval.

Finally, recall that a significant proportion of frail elders have no immediate family members and thus lack whatever protection from premature death or delayed death that concerned relatives might provide. For example, about half of female nursing home residents are either childless or have outlived their children.[54] "Strangers" in the health care professions, forced to make key life and death decisions for familyless patients, may also perceive important advantages in facilitating death.

Perceptions of Advantage: Health Care Workers

In a recent article addressed to his peers in the medical profession, Dr. Timothy Quill explained why, in defiance of the law, he assisted the suicide of a patient: his fear that an unaided suicide attempt might be unsuccessful and leave her worse off than she already was; the consequences of a violent death for her family; his concern that a relative who assisted her instead would suffer severe personal or legal repercussions. It is significant that Dr. Quill, former director of a hospice program, was well acquainted with pain control and comfort care. Yet when his patient rejected this course, he accepted and facilitated her choice to die. His concern for her family also merits comment. It bespeaks a renewed concern among professionals with the need to see the family as a whole, a unit containing several members whose various needs must be delicately balanced so that one member is not seriously disadvantaged for the sake of another. In other words, the needs of the family are more likely to be recognized nowadays than in the more recent past, when the needs of the patient took precedence over everything else.[55]

Among medical personnel, it is primarily physicians who must struggle with hard choices at the end of life and who are expected to advise patients and families about the best course of treatment. So, when a competent patient, or his representative, refuses life-prolonging treatment, the doctor must decide between "omissions" (legally acceptable) and "acts" (now illegal) for complying. Although both "acts" and "omissions" are deliberate choices that result in the same end, death, confusion reigns as some maintain that there are significant moral differences between the two, an argument that failed to impress the court even as early as the *Quinlan* case in 1976. Nonetheless, in our current legal climate doctors risk prosecution for the one but not the other, despite the fact that the very existence of a meaningful distinction has been disputed. If one turns off a respirator, for example, is she acting (literally stopping the machine) or omitting (to continue a particular form of treatment)? Is there a difference? If so, is it morally significant, especially if death is always the predictable result? Whose view of morality should prevail? If "omissions" merely prolong suffering, perhaps "acts" are preferable in some cases, but we must decide which ones. For example, if hemodialysis is discontinued, death may take up to two weeks and can be quite uncomfortable for the patient, a distressing situation that some argue could (and should) be avoided by resort to a quicker death with lethal drugs. Others maintain that "comfort care"—aimed at minimizing pain and suffering rather than curing—can ease the dying process sufficiently to avoid that kind of distress. Should a patient be permitted to decline "comfort care" and opt for the quicker death, like Dr. Quill's patient?[56]

Like people everywhere, medical professionals want to go home at the end of the day feeling good about themselves and their work, and to sleep well at night. Practitioners want what they do to make sense, to be morally as well as legally justifiable. But these goals are proving very elusive. Today, for example, doctors risk prosecution both when they try to do too much to keep a patient alive, unduly delaying death, and when they do too little, unduly hastening it. If others—patients and families—make the choices and accept the responsibility, and the law supports their right to do so, and peers and professional organizations concur, practitioners' doubts about their own helping role will be reduced. Having a "Do Not Resuscitate" order for a nursing home resident, for instance, reduces anxiety among staff concerning their responsibility if the person's heart stops; similarly, other decisions discussed in advance of a crisis, such as whether to hospitalize a patient, serve to simplify management decisions, as well as, presumably, avoiding excessive treatment and prolonged suffering for the patient.[57] Thus many medical professionals may see advantages to themselves in respecting, and promoting, patient autonomy at the end of life. Of course, they will have to sacrifice some of their enormous power in the process but, in return, they may be able to regain their credibility as patient advocates.

Economic considerations may support or impede the humanitarian goal of a peaceful death. For example, hospitals and physicians now have strong economic motives for encouraging greater selectivity in the type of treatment they provide to Medicare patients and its duration; this is especially true for patients whose cost of care threatens to exceed available payment.[58] Fewer tests and procedures may free some patients from overly aggressive, useless treatment, lessening their suffering, but others may be worse off if treatment is inadequate and causes their premature death. On the other hand, if certain treatments, tests, and procedures are economically profitable to provide, some frail elders will have their death unduly delayed.

Taking care of frail elders is also time-intensive for doctors and other medical workers. Since they have lived longer, more health problems have accumulated, so must be probed for in the medical history and accounted for in the treatment plan. Frail elders may be garrulous or uncommunicative, forgetful or confused, unable or unwilling to give a clear account of their problems and symptoms. Drug effects and drug interactions may affect their mental alertness and inhibit communication. Their reactions to medication are less predictable, suitable dosages are more difficult to ascertain, and there is greater risk of complications. Predicting outcomes is thus more hazardous and explanations of procedures and alternatives generally takes longer, creating problems for busy practitioners.

Doctors are not necessarily uncaring, but the external pressures to hurry on to the next case are often overwhelming, a point that applies equally well to other health care workers. Thus it may be appealing to many workers, and institutions, to minimize their dealings with patients who slow down their pursuit of other goals. If the worker's income depends on how many patients she is able to see, there is an economic incentive for more superficial dealings with frail elders. Unnecessary suffering and premature death for the vulnerable aged may again be the result. On the other hand, economic considerations aside, if the sickest patients are allowed or helped to die, caregivers' feelings of efficacy, self-esteem, and job satisfaction may increase. The satisfactions of facilitating a "good" death may come to replace or outweigh negative feelings about the failure to heal. Or regret about the "bad" death that might have occurred because medical heroics went too far may be avoided. Young doctors may learn from the experiences of their predecessors. One retired anesthesiologist, for example, regretted that his work had sometimes contributed to others' suffering by unduly prolonging an intolerable existence: "When I look back on some of the operations we did to prolong life, and each time I walked through a rest home and saw the misery, I always shuddered to think we would not treat animals this way. It would be inhumane." Finally, as workers focus their skills on people they *can* help, feelings of efficacy should be further enhanced and, concomitantly, provider stress and burnout should be reduced.[59]

Perceptions of Advantage: Society

The single overriding factor in the economic needs of the elderly, and the most obvious basis for societal perception of advantages to death control, is the rising cost of health and long-term care and accompanying perceptions of excessive burden on other segments of the population. The bulk of formal health care services to the elderly are publicly financed, primarily through Medicare and Medicaid.[60] This fact ensures that decisions about what and how much to provide are largely public decisions but which, in turn, shape and constrain private choices.

Sophisticated new medical equipment, drugs, and specially trained personnel are expensive. For many patients, treatment choices in the acute-care setting set the stage for chronic care and a need for continued technological support over the long term. The ongoing costs of care may far exceed the initial costs, but there has been no attempt yet to quantify their full economic impact. Very high public costs are associated with long-term care, whether provided in the client's home, the community, or an institution. The government share of these costs came to $30.4 billion in fiscal 1988, more than half of the $57.8 billion total spent on long-term care in that year. The Medicaid program paid for the bulk of these services. It should be noted, however, that the typical frail old person incurs relatively high costs in *both* acute-care and long-term chronic care settings prior to death. Projected changes in the size and composition of the elderly population (the "aging of the aged"), the likely increase in morbidity prevalence and severity as people live longer, and the growing prevalence of dementias, in combination with escalating health-care costs, are trends that pose a tremendous challenge to care provision and help make rationing concerns explicit. It is worth noting that past projections of the size of the elderly population and their health care needs and costs have typically been underestimates. The very frail, of course, require the greatest number of per capita health dollars and caregiving hours, and current trends imply that ever greater commitments of funds must be expended on their needs, producing a situation that will require our society to accommodate to new realities about life and death, to discard inappropriate solutions, and to be flexible in adopting new ones.[61]

The projected cost increases are staggering. From $387 billion in 1984, for example, health care costs rose to $604 billion in 1989 and are projected to rise to $2 trillion by the year 2000. The overall cost of Medicare tripled in the 1980s, and the Hospital Insurance Trust Fund, which pays all government reimbursements for hospital care of Medicare patients, is projected to become insolvent by the end of the century; proposed remedies, such as tax increases or delaying the age of eligibility, are politically unpopular. Even with optimistic assumptions about future trends in health, the aging trend alone points to substantial cost increases. Assuming *no* increase in per capita physician or hospital visits or the percentage of people living in long-term care facilities, costs will rise because there will be proportionally more older persons in the population.[62]

It is likely that foreseeable improvements in medical technology and personal health practices will enable us to delay the onset or severity of *fatal* diseases and enhance survival prospects for their victims. But this does not mean that a need for long-term care for those afflicted will be eliminated or even reduced. Nor is there evidence to support the belief that medical advances will affect the onset or progression of conditions like arthritis—that is, those which do not kill but which may require years of ongoing care and management. Longer survival for those suffering from "killer" conditions, combined with the intractability of many chronic, *nonfatal* diseases of aging, implies substantial growth in the disabled population. Many agree that we are unable to finance adequately the long-term care needs of today's frail elders. Our current approach shows no indication of being able to respond well to future long-term care needs either, as the population of disabled and chronically ill elderly swells. In a climate of growing disillusionment with medical technology, policy makers, along with families, are asking if the gain is worth the cost, and there is growing concern with cost containment in the Medicare and Medicaid programs. Governments at every level recognize that not all services can be provided to everyone to the extent that citizens might wish. No one who has been the victim of a crime, for instance, thinks that the amount of police protection is adequate, nor are those whose children cannot read pleased with the quality of the educational system.[63]

Health care expenditures will rise even more if pessimistic projections of morbidity rates prove accurate. Assuming that utilization of health services will remain constant at each age as our population ages, as some analysts do, may prove overly optimistic, since new and expensive medical procedures will continue to appear and other costly procedures may be performed more frequently. Some experts maintain, correctly, that the concept of costs used in many studies is too narrow: *total* costs include many that are typically omitted from discussion, such as safety monitoring of new equipment, record keeping, interdepartmental coordination of care arrangements, and continuing care at home. They anticipate a long time lag before early disease prevention strategies reduce the costs of health care.[64]

Although continued improvement is expected in the overall economic well-being of the elderly, a recent simulation model shows that long-term care costs will rise faster than the incomes of the very old. The result is that the elders most likely to need care will actually be worse off in terms of their ability to pay for it. Where will the necessary funds come from? There is little support in the United States for using legal means to force adult children to provide financially for elderly parents, despite rapidly rising public costs. This means that the public share must increase, exacerbating already-considerable pressures for cost control, or that new ways to contain costs must be devised, because measures tried to date have had little success. Rising costs have already inspired increased emphasis on alternatives to institutionalization, commonly believed to be the most expensive way to care for frail elders.[65]

The government policies that have emerged are basically cost-avoidance strategies, designed to shift costs from institutions and government to families and the private sector. To the extent that family burdens are increased, family perceptions of advantages to deliberate death will be strengthened. For example, government strategies making asset transfers to heirs under Medicaid "spend down" rules more difficult and attempts to recover public monies from the estate after the elder's death are likely to increase. One study has concluded that almost $600 million could be recovered annually by such efforts—an amount that some believe is seriously underestimated. That these kinds of strategies may have important latent effects (intensifying both individual and family desires for more timely deaths by threatening bequest motives and inheritance, for example) merits concern. It would be quite erroneous to conclude that *any* public effort to curb costs or restrict access to services will have no effect on private decisions in favor of earlier death.[66]

Real cost increases or real crises in financing health care, however, are not necessary for increased willingness to resort to deliberate death—the mere *perception* of a crisis, encouraged by the mass media, may be sufficient to influence both policy makers and the public. Further, it is not ability or willingness to pay alone, but value received for dollars expended (in terms of the patient's improved functional status, better quality of life, or enhanced ability to engage in meaningful social roles, for example) that must be considered. Heavy spending on the high-care needs of exceedingly frail, incompetent, or demented patients, especially those who require total care for years, risks leaving other critical needs unfunded and raises thorny issues of distributive justice. Unlimited costs cannot be met, and lines must be drawn because government has responsibilities to other groups and must meet other compelling social needs. One might argue that some of the $700,000 a minute spent by the Pentagon in 1986, for example—a year in which the United States was not at war—might be better diverted to the needs of frail elders, thus reducing motivation for resort to death control. But this use of part of the "peace dividend" also raises questions of limits if little seems to be gained for the additional dollars allocated. No amount of money, for example, can make the frailest well again, nor can dollars necessarily ease their suffering. Moreover, an important function of government is to protect those who need it, including protecting them from unwanted, futile, or painful treatments that only delay death. Hence altruism alone on the part of legislators is sufficient to make deliberate death easier, without regard to financial incentives. Thus economic considerations alone do not (and should not) guide decision making. Legalization of physician-assisted dying is not essential either—society may continue to tacitly support death hastening for frail elders, as it currently does, but refrain from explicitly *promoting* it. Such denial and secrecy, however, open the door to serious abuses.[67]

In the business world, companies watch and worry as health

care spending consumes a growing portion of profits, and employees juggle job responsibilities with long-term care provision to frail relatives; stress, depression, and role overload inevitably affect job performance. There are proposals for on-site elder care to help employees cope, but these have costs either directly to the business or indirectly to consumers in the form of higher prices for goods and services and thus encounter considerable resistance. Millions of American workers cannot afford health insurance for themselves, and others have had their benefits cut or copayments increased. Union members have waged bitter strikes over health care issues. And a recent report from the Manufacturers' Alliance for Productivity and Innovation urges employers to promote "informed decisions" about end-of-life care among their employees in order to use limited resources more efficiently. Since most people fill multiple roles as family members, workers, and taxpayers, role conflict is inevitable. While some demand expensive care for their own aged relatives, heedless of public costs or the small chance of benefit, the same people in their role as taxpayers may be reluctant to finance futile end-of-life care for the aged relatives of strangers. This seems most likely in the case of the very old, the very frail, and especially the mentally incapacitated, for whom life prolongation may be deemed a useless waste of resources, scarce or not.[68]

Current health care policies, such as Medicare's Prospective Payment System, also reward providers (both institutions and individual practitioners) for delivering treatment at lower cost, with quality and humane considerations often taking a back seat to financing concerns. Where more likely for cost-saving potential to be perceived than in the quicker death of frail old people who are not only expensive to care for, but whose needs extend over long periods of time and who are unable to get well regardless of the effort expended? And, despite all the money already spent on them, there are still enormous unmet needs.

No health care policy now in force ethically justifies the use of economic criteria in decisions concerning life-sustaining treatment. But ethicists at the Hastings Center suggest that coordinated policies be developed to identify treatments whose benefits do not justify large expenditures, relative to alternative uses of those resources. They have advanced the concept of "costworthy care," which assesses the value of treatments vis-à-vis the sacrifices they entail by requiring us to give up other legitimate individual and societal goods.[69]

Gradually, it seems that citizens and policy makers are coming to realize that unwarranted efforts to postpone death bring with them multiple disadvantages the nation can ill afford, and that facilitating deliberate death is a potential solution to these growing dilemmas. But are there other solutions that should be tried before resorting to death control for frail old people, even at their own request? Surely there are other, better ways to provide quality end-of-life care? Alternatives and their shortcomings are the topic of later chapters, following a discussion of the third element in the paradigm of preconditions for death control—the means—in Chapter 6.

The Means of Death Control

Just as they see an urgent need to prevent aggressive overtreatment in the last stage of life, innovators have increasingly come to recognize that a right to choose death is worthless without adequate means of communicating and implementing the decision. A case in point is Mary Severns' dying dilemma. An active member of the Delaware Euthanasia Educational Council, Mrs. Severns had indicated repeatedly that she never wanted to live on in a vegetative state, but neglected to document her wishes. When she suffered irreversible brain damage in an automobile accident in 1979, her doctor refused to withhold life-sustaining treatments because there was no legal protection for him due to her oversight. A year of litigation, accompanied by much emotional and financial distress for her family, followed before she was allowed to die.[1]

Earlier in this book, I discussed themes of responsible dying and the importance of preplanning for ensuring that one's last wishes are respected. The legal history of advance directives like living wills was summarized in Chapter 4. Can resort to these documents protect patients, keeping their wishes at the center of decision making? Will they allow us to implement our choices and avoid unwanted outcomes such as overtreatment? In short, are they a reliable means for achieving the desired end—a "good" death?

Advance Directives: A Solution?

In theory, advance directives can avoid the sort of dilemma experienced by the Severn family. They offer patients autonomy in terminal-care decisions, a chance to avoid expensive, invasive, and futile procedures, and the possibility of a more acceptable death.[2] The documents allow elders to consider and record their treatment preferences while they are still competent. Thus they can instruct proxies about their care wishes should they become unable to communicate them directly. A valuable lesson that many elders, whether currently sick or not, seem to have learned from the well-publicized tragedies of others is the importance of advance planning for self-protection from medical heroics. In fact, the absence of an advance directive can understandably be interpreted by the medical team to mean that the person wants everything possible done to maintain life, even in a vegetative state—the precise situation that many wish to avoid.

Documentation of one's wishes has been strongly encouraged by medical and legal experts and the popular media. Advance planning fits well with dominant American values, such as individualism, self-reliance, and an active as opposed to a fatalistic outlook. Relatives and doctors are relieved of the burden of making life and death decisions and of the risk of misunderstanding the elder's preferences. In the absence of direct discussion, for example, physicians often fail to predict patients' desires for resuscitation accurately, a finding that will greatly trouble all conscientious practitioners.[3] So advance directives help to reassure caregivers that, in a case of lost competency, they are doing what the elder would have wanted had she been able to express an opinion.

The cooperation of professionals, especially physicians, is essential if advance directives are to function as the signer intended. Some planning advocates are urging doctors to initiate discussions about advance planning with their patients, and nursing home staff are urged to do the same.[4] In the right combination of circumstances, advance directives can deter unwanted overtreatment, balancing the medical system's bias to treat against the values and preferences of the individual patient. But how much reliance can be placed on them? In fact, despite the extensive advice literature, relatively few Americans have signed advance directives to date, and a bias in favor of better-educated and higher-income categories seems likely. For those who do execute them, how well do they work in practice? Although advance directives are easily available and widely promoted, systematic empirical data on how well they work are just beginning to appear.

One highly publicized form of advance directive is the living will. This document, which can only be signed by an adult of sound mind, specifies that life-sustaining treatments should not be used if the signer is terminally ill and treatment will merely prolong suffering; comfort care and pain relief are to continue until death occurs, however. Many people believe that by signing a living will they can avoid "medical torment of all sorts."[5] But the facts are at variance with this common belief.

Although more than forty states had living will statutes by 1991, most have major shortcomings. First, they apply only to the "terminally ill," a determination that is notoriously difficult even for experts to make accurately and which excludes those whose condition is not terminal, even when they are suffering greatly. Further, they often limit the specific types of treatment that can be refused and, contrarily, may lead to undertreatment in some situations. They make no provision for substitute decision making if the signer becomes incompetent and contain no penalties for health care providers who fail to honor them, although a patient or his family may file suit if they are dissatisfied. Furthermore, the degree of foresight required by those who sign is quite unrealistic; no matter what contingencies are foreseen, the crisis that materializes may be far different from those that were envisioned. Or an emergency may preclude medical personnel from searching for a directive or interpreting the document in light of the particular situation at hand. There may be no time to interview surrogates about what the patient might have wanted. Concerns that may be extremely important to patients—such as their concern for the emotional, physical, or financial toll of their illness on the family— typically are not covered in a living will.[6]

In some cases, those who thought they had planned well nonetheless died in what can only be described as modern versions of a horror story. In one New York case, Brenda Hewitt, an editor and poet, understood the serious nature of her ailments very well. Anticipating the worst, she signed a living will and appointed a health care proxy, a man she trusted implicitly with her life when she could no longer decide for herself. In what turned out to be her final crisis, the proxy arrived at the hospital with her. But he was ignored, pushed aside, and threatened by staff members as he tried repeatedly to act according to the patient's instructions and prevent the aggressive medical interventions she had feared all along. The doctors, it seems, were just trying to do their job.[7]

It is all too easy for a physician to assert that a patient is suffering from "impaired mental status" and so is incompetent to request release from suffering; it is also all too easy to get consulting physicians to corroborate this judgment. Moreover, documents filed in one state may be useless in another. The Supreme Court's decision in the *Cruzan* case in 1990 leaves it up to the individual state to decide the legal requirements for discontinuing treatment for incompetent patients. This means that a state legislature may change existing rules at any time, draft new laws when it sees fit, and ignore the positions of other jurisdictions. Only twenty states allow families to refuse life-sustaining treatments for incompetent relatives, and these differ as to which patients are covered, the kinds of treatment that may be withheld or withdrawn, and which family members can make the decision. Hence those wishing to be protected by an advance directive must devise one that will be effective in multiple jurisdictions. Concern for Dying developed such a general form, which is available to the public on request, but individuals should complete their own state's form too.[8]

In short, advance directives may provide sufficient protection only to those who remain mentally competent to the end, who escape an intervening emergency, and who are lucky enough to have other key factors on their side. Physician Ronald Cranford has described the necessary confluence of circumstances: "If a patient has made her wishes very clearly known and understood, and if she has a loving, caring family ... and if there happens to be a physician in the family experienced in termination of treatment issues, and if a caring, experienced hospice nurse is involved, then the patient can be reassured that he or she will have control over the dying process and will die in the style she has chosen."[9]

But, in the words of an expert on health law, tragedies like Brenda Hewitt's are "a cruelly common occurrence." Even physicians may be unable to prevent a delayed death for their own relatives, as Norman Paradis learned in the course of his father's dying. The father, also a physician, was subjected to "endless procedures ... that could not possibly cure him or relieve his pain," that in fact worsened his condition. The tests and treatments were contrary to both the patient's wishes and his family's repeated instructions. At one point, before he deteriorated too far to complain, the old man pleaded, "They are treating me like an animal. Please get me out of here." But neither the younger Dr. Paradis nor his brother, a lawyer, could prevent their father's misery. Paradis concluded that "if a doctor and a lawyer could not get decent care for a doctor, what chance does the public have?"[10]

A serious problem is where death occurs. In sharp contrast to past eras, more than four in five deaths now occur in institutions, primarily acute-care hospitals; in a crisis, even nursing home patients are likely to be moved to a hospital. Hospital admission implies, even for those brought there involuntarily, that aggressive treatment is wanted. In an emergency, when the patient is likely to be met by on-call staff who have never seen him before, there is no time to ask about, or search for, an advance directive, and staff members risk legal liability if they fail to treat aggressively when the situation is in doubt. Part of the blame for the New York tragedy described above was the fact that the woman's primary physician, who was well acquainted with her wishes, failed to convey that information to the physician in charge at the hospital. In other cases, documents are too vague to be adequate guides to the patient's wishes. Every eventuality cannot be foreseen, so what the now incompetent signer would want in her current unique situation is frequently uncertain. Research has also shown that physicians may be unaware of the existence of advance directives signed by their own patients. They may not ask, for example, or the patient might not have volunteered the information in timely fashion.[11]

One team of researchers found that care was consistent with patients' previously expressed wishes three times out of four, but that the consistency could not be credited to the presence of written advance directives in medical records: in only 25 of 71 hospitalizations from a nursing home was the advance directive successfully delivered to the hospital, for example. This was attributed to the fact that nursing home staff, subject to frequent turnover, were unfamiliar with the document. Inconsistency was more likely for patients who were incompetent at the critical time than for others; the treatment provided was sometimes more aggressive than previous wishes, but was generally more conservative. Relatives of incompetent patients, for example, sometimes decided that the aggressive care the elder had requested (while he was still competent) was futile given his current circumstances.[12]

According to the same study, there were sometimes compelling medical reasons, not foreseen by the signers, that resulted in advance directives not being followed. For example, one patient had refused artificial ventilation in the directive, but when a seizure occurred it was clear that a brief period of such treatment would be of substantial benefit to him, so he was treated accordingly. The authors also speculate that the high rate of consistency between what patients requested and what they received in this study could be serendipitous because the interview process itself facilitated discussion about treatment wishes among staff, patients, and families. They conclude that written advance directives have limited potential for enhancing the autonomy of patients who become incapacitated—regardless of how specific and accessible the directives are, no amount of preplanning can anticipate all possible situations, or the patient's change in attitude over time.[13] In fact, then, it is unlikely that simply filing an advance directive will produce the kind of death that the signer envisions.

To counter such dilemmas, some have suggested a durable power of attorney for health care, a form of advance directive wherein a trusted other is empowered to make health care decisions for a person who has become incapacitated. This allows the doctor to discuss treatment options on the spot with a competent individual who has legal power to make a decision, and the appointer, in theory, has the security of knowing that her agent must act in good faith and make decisions consistent with her best interests. But we saw in the New York hospital case above that even this is no guarantee. As one critical care nurse put it, the agent must act as a "bodyguard," present night and day, to ensure that unwanted treatments are not forced on the patient in her absence. For example, if the patient develops breathing difficulties at 3 A.M., she may well be intubated and placed on a ventilator as doctors reason (1) that her mental status is impaired *because of* the breathing difficulties, and (2) that they risk litigation if they fail to relieve the problem. If the proxy decision maker is not on the scene or is unable to protest successfully, the die is cast. Once the patient is put on the venti-lator, it is difficult to withdraw that treatment.[14]

Other serious problems are becoming apparent as researchers investigate the dynamics of proxy decision making. For instance, individuals are often more willing to accept negative health out-comes—such as being on a respirator, confinement to bed, or in-continence—for a relative than for themselves. In other words, they seem to be more confident about their own feelings than someone else's and prefer to err on the side of caution for their rel-ative. Discrepancies between what they would accept for them-selves and what they would accept for a loved one were higher for elderly respondents. Such discrepancies suggest a greater probabil-ity that unacceptable outcomes (that delay death with aggressive interventions) will be imposed on a patient, albeit with good inten-tions, than that his death will be hastened. It is important to note that these findings do not rule out the possibility that others' deci-sions, including those in express opposition to the earlier docu-mented wishes of a now-incompetent patient, are actually better-informed and more in his best interests. Thus the evidence also suggests that in some circumstances advance directives should not be honored.[15]

The validity of substituted judgments has been called into ques-tion in other recent studies. Results of one investigation, for exam-ple, indicate that the resuscitation preferences of elderly patients often are not understood "even by their primary care physicians and spouses of long duration." Spouses tended to err in the direc-tion of "overresuscitation," while physicians tended in the other direction. Lack of discussion among the principals seemed to be only a partial explanation for the large discrepancies observed—discussions did take place in some cases, and many surrogates *be-lieved* they knew what the patient wanted.[16]

There are additional problems with proxy decision making. For one, only competent adults who take the trouble to execute a legal document appointing a surrogate are theoretically protected. Relatives and friends do not generally want this kind of power, however, and appointment of an agent does not preclude tensions and disagreements among family members, which the patient is now in no position to help resolve by clarifying his wishes. Under unanticipated circumstances, there is no guarantee that they will decide as the patient would have wanted. Proxies may not be immediately available in an emergency, either. Even if the agent arrives at the emergency room with the patient, there may not be sufficient time to consult with physicians about specific interventions. If the familyless patient has discussed her wishes only with her primary physician, the doctor may not be readily available in an emergency—she may be out of town or attending to another urgent case, for example. Will the staff on call be aware of formal documents or have time to look for them? Will the paramedics? The bottom line is that often strangers—the medical personnel who happen to be on duty at the critical time—will make the crucial choices.[17]

Furthermore, a life-threatening emergency may occur more than once to the same individual, raising all the same issues each time, with the risk that ignorance will encourage aggressive treatment. Hence the patient still has a very real chance of dying with all the horrors he tried to avoid with advance planning. To forestall such a scenario, a few members of the Hemlock Society have gone so far as to have "No Code" or similar orders tattooed on their chest, but the utility of this highly unorthodox form of communication is by no means certain. More promising, perhaps, are bracelets bearing the message "Do Not Resuscitate"; laws authorizing these as means of facilitating compliance with individual treatment preferences were recently passed in New York and Montana, and similar guidelines have been adopted in California and Connecticut. But their usefulness in practice has yet to be tested.[18]

The fact that many elders eschew formal arrangements and wish to let relatives decide their fate creates other kinds of risks. This is especially true of a "proclivity toward group decision-making" expressed by many old people. When interviewed, they make such statements as "my spouse and children will decide for me when the time comes" or "I'll leave it up to my four children."[19] This behavior bodes ill for both the timeliness of decisions and their congruence with patient wishes; since relatives may be geographically distant and must discuss and resolve their own differences of opinion, aggressive treatment to maintain the patient's life may well be required in the interim before consensus is reached. It would thus seem far less risky to appoint *one* trusted person as surrogate decision maker.

What of the potential for both *better* use and *greater* use of advance directives? Can improvement in provider sensitivity and better communication among patients, providers, and family members reduce discrepancies and enhance patient self-determination? There is undeniably scope for professional intervention in devising advance directives, and professional cooperation is essential if they are to be successfully implemented. And certainly far more people want advance directives than now have them. Most nursing home residents, for instance, prefer to be involved in decisions about resuscitation, but only a small minority have thus far been given the opportunity to do so. The fact that little agreement has been found between what residents want in terms of information and involvement in treatment decisions and what their nurses think they want suggests a strong need for better communication in advance of a medical emergency. Most professional caregivers do not understand the preferences of elderly persons regarding end-of-life health care, and since most elders have neither signed advance directives nor discussed such matters in sufficient detail with possible surrogate decision makers, there is considerable room for improvement. Of course, the worst-off patients, especially the severely demented and the most physically impaired, are no longer able to participate in decision making. And, typically, they are not cared for by a physician they have personally chosen, or one familiar with their history, personality, or preferences.[20]

Achieving better doctor-patient communication on end-of-life treatment choices may be exceedingly difficult, even for a competent elder. Discussions with patients and families to work through misunderstandings, review treatment alternatives, and resolve conflicts are all time-consuming, and busy schedules on both sides may inhibit thorough communication with professionals. There may also be a strong desire among all parties to avoid, deny, or postpone these unpleasant topics. But when a crisis occurs it is too late to initiate discussion. Doctors may also think they know what a patient wants or what is best for her, or regard the subject as beyond discussion owing to their vast differences in medical knowledge. And they may be right, because patients can be ill informed or unduly fearful. Even when their knowledge is adequate, patients and their caregiving relatives may hesitate to question, let alone challenge, the doctor's opinion because they fear his anger, rejection, or even abandonment.[21]

Moreover, many doctors continue to oppose patient empowerment, tend to distrust patient and family judgments, and are reluctant to give up any of their professional authority. These physician characteristics and proclivities, in combination with the great legal uncertainties about what may or may not be done with respect to life-sustaining treatments, conceivably lead many doctors to decide for themselves when care should be limited. Such reasoning led one physician to conclude that "the notion of informed consent...remains a fairy tale." Thus, despite "the chorus of voices urging doctors to speak frankly to their patients," the vision of the patient as the ultimate decision maker is far from being realized in practice. All this leaves doctors deciding what treatments are futile, what alternatives should even be mentioned to the patient, and what criteria are most relevant for decision making. Thus, although improvements are certainly called for, they will not be easily achieved.[22]

If preplanning is no panacea, what are the implications for death control? First, recall that advance directives are intended to avoid aggressive overtreatment. As knowledge of their considerable shortcomings in achieving their primary objective becomes more diffused in American society, we may expect individuals to search for better forms of self-protection. It follows that we may also expect greater resort to "active" means of death by choice— while the individual is still both alert and competent enough to persuade others to comply with her wishes. Prospective identification of those who will die within a specified interval is difficult or impossible for a physician to determine; predictions of remaining "quality time" may also be far from the mark. Hence choosing the time and circumstances of one's death inevitably means dying somewhat "too soon." Some will not wish to risk waiting, however much they disvalue premature death. Others will not wish to be labeled incompetent and turned into someone else's responsibility, if they can avoid it. Since elders have often been caregivers in their lifetime, and even dying patients care about others, they may well wish to avoid burdening relatives with long-term care or hard choices about terminating treatment on their behalf.

Better communication between providers and patients, greater resort to written advance directives, and establishment and enforcement of penalties for noncompliant providers, to the extent they become a reality, will result in deaths that occur earlier than they otherwise would. For example, interviews with a group of alert nursing home residents indicated that 30 percent were inclined to reject aggressive treatment unless it was necessary for comfort, pain control, or safety; rejection was especially likely in hypothetical scenarios involving dementia.[23] Presumably, under the old regime of "bias to treat," these patients would be treated more aggressively, their biological life prolonged. If patients are encouraged to think about the issues and to make their own decisions, with staff cooperation, death will occur somewhat earlier for many.

Means of Causing Death

Help, especially from medical personnel, is often necessary if the circumstances of death are to coincide with an individual's preferences for a dignified, peaceful, and timely end. Lethal drugs may be very difficult to obtain without a physician's cooperation, and their toxicity may decline if too much time elapses while a supply is stockpiled. The right dosage must be determined and the drug administered appropriately, with due consideration for the patient's debilitated condition. An insufficient dose may not kill, or it may kill too slowly or with too much discomfort. A bungled attempt may be devastating to both patient and family. Current dilemmas are illustrated by one physician's recent account of how, out of fear of the law, he failed to aid a death despite his explicit promise to the patient. In the face of a serious, protracted, and clearly terminal illness, the man was determined to die on his own terms. He planned to take a fatal overdose of pain medication but was worried lest his extreme physical weakness and severe diarrhea inhibit absorption of the barbiturates, causing the attempt to fail and very possibly worsening his situation in the process. Hence he consulted a physician, who agreed to check on him after he swallowed the pills and to administer a lethal injection of morphine if he happened to be still alive. Without informing the man, however, the doctor did not appear as promised. When the sick man's live-in companion, who had deliberately absented himself to facilitate the suicide attempt, returned, the patient was still alive. Not knowing what else to do, the companion called an ambulance, and the patient was "saved."[24]

This account of a well-considered, yet nonetheless frustrated, suicide effort illuminates why Americans are coming to see a need for, and advantages to, removing remaining barriers to physician-assisted dying. The ironies of the situation are compounded by the doctor's admission that each year he renews his license to prescribe narcotics, because "someday I might have need of them...to kill myself easily should the occasion arise." Surely many other physicians think along the same lines. Indeed, physicians have substantially higher rates of suicide than either the general population or comparable professionals. Thus it seems that doctors can readily help themselves but are prohibited from helping others.[25]

An analogous situation occurred when birth control was still controversial, as many physicians limited the size of their own families but refrained from helping their patients do the same; although they may have cautioned an unhealthy woman not to get pregnant, few would tell her how this could be accomplished. Others occasionally helped a woman in "exceptional" cases where they deemed that assistance was called for. Compared to birth control, however, the means for achieving death control are simple and straightforward. Anyone can end a life, if sufficiently motivated, and do it successfully (that is, quickly and relatively painlessly for the recipient), although at some legal risk to the perpetrator. As Chapter 2 explains, in all times and places there has been scope for providing a merciful death when circumstances seemed to warrant. Methods of ending life in the past may have been crude, and were typically violent—stabbing, strangling, or pushing off a cliff, for example. Those who killed seem to have had little choice about employing violent means because, although pain-relieving drugs have long been known and used, dosages could not be accurately calculated until quite recently in medical history. Nor could drugs be administered efficiently enough to ensure that death was quick and painless. For example, the hypodermic syringe was not developed until the 1850s. Nonetheless, the wish to end useless suffering is timeless and universal.[26]

Today, guns and knives, bridges and tall buildings are accessible to anyone with enough physical stamina and determination to use them, but a natural human repugnance about resorting to pain and violence to achieve a merciful goal inhibits their use. Means that are unpleasant, if not actually violent, are also understandably rejected by those who see an alternative. Highly motivated people, for example, have drowned themselves in a toilet bowl, set themselves afire, or deliberately starved to death.[27] Although such gruesome methods are effective, no one can claim that these are "good" deaths, and few are anxious to imitate them. Further, such means are often impractical or impossible for persons who are aged, ill, and weak, or who live in an institution under more or less constant surveillance.

For compassion to become action, communication (among family members, between patient and doctor, or doctor and family) and sufficient will to act are indispensable. If deliberate death is unthinkable, communication will not occur, sufficient resolve to challenge laws or prevailing social norms will be difficult to muster, advance directives will be ignored, and empathy will rarely be translated into action. Thus, although means of death control are always readily available, cultural, legal, or religious prohibitions have often made their use inconceivable. As with the concept and practice of birth control, however, sooner or later innovators such as Dr. Timothy Quill and Derek Humphry emerge as new conditions demand appropriate responses. Their ideas may be embraced and their actions imitated by others, helping diffuse them throughout the society, or they may be rejected and punished, thus effectively discouraging innovation. Tellingly, Dr. Quill's actions have been generally praised, not condemned, and he was not indicted, and *Final Exit*, Humphry's "suicide manual," has enjoyed brisk sales.

Another lesson from our experience with the history of birth control is a gradual shift from less reliable, highly obtrusive, or dangerous methods to safer, more efficient, and less obtrusive means. No one today, for example, would think of resorting to ancient Egyptian recipes for vaginal plugs to prevent conception, which called for crocodile dung, gum, and acacia, among other ingredients. (These worked, by the way.) Relatively high failure rates, the need for constant vigilance, and the interference with pleasure and spontaneity characteristic of many early birth control methods fueled the public's demand for improvements, demands that research institutions and medical practitioners were quick to respond to. Because of these improvements, couples today have higher expectations of their birth control methods—why shouldn't they be easy to obtain, easy to use, and virtually foolproof? One consequence of higher expectations is dramatic increases in the United States in the popularity of contraceptive sterilization, despite the finality of the method, as word of its advantages spread and fears related to ignorance and misinformation were dispelled. Certainly there are risks attached to the sterilization choice, as well as to every other method, but couples have freely accepted them in light of the greater advantages.[28]

In advanced industrial nations, scientific medicine provides the capability to keep people biologically alive almost indefinitely, regardless of the social quality of their life. The same expertise, however, has produced more humane ways of ending life painlessly for the incurably ill. Practices in the Netherlands—the nation in the forefront of public and medical support for death by choice—are instructive. The Dutch Society for Voluntary Euthanasia has published and distributed a tract advising physicians about the most suitable drugs for euthanasia, their proper administration and dosage. One means of ending life quickly and painlessly is to administer a series of injections to first induce sleep, then a comatose state, and finally respiratory arrest.[29] This method of death control, where "appointments" may be made by the dying person or the family, is obviously more humane than pushing an elder off a cliff or burying him alive, methods used in some premodern societies.

But the most effective and most humane means are not necessarily used, as the account of the unkept promise reveals. In analogous situations, defective newborns and incurably ill adults are allowed to starve to death in modern American hospitals and long-term care institutions owing to legal and ethical proscriptions surrounding the use of lethal injections. Even though the decision to let die has been made in such cases, the appropriate means (how the decision is implemented) remain controversial. In one court case, for example, a wife's request to have her husband's feeding tube removed was granted on the grounds that if he could speak, he would have wanted it removed. Death was not imminent, however, as perhaps many people envision. Nor does death follow quickly (or easily) when a respirator is disconnected or hemodialysis stopped. In this case, it took eight days for a "natural" death to occur—days of watching and waiting, of decision makers hoping they did the right thing and simultaneously realizing that the choice is irrevocable and, of course, mounting costs for survivors. Whether this too is what the dying man would have wanted if he could speak must, I think, be considered open to question. Further, we have little idea how those who participate in these death watches are affected by the experience. But Richard Besdine, a physician who has observed such situations firsthand, notes that once the decision to limit treatment has been made, family and staff have an increased need for counseling and support. And both hospice workers and relatives report considerable stress from protracted death watches.[30]

Further, "Do Not Treat" orders do not preclude medical interventions to "alleviate suffering" in the interval between the decision to let die and the occurrence of "natural" death. This is true of hospice care also. Invasive procedures (including amputations and other surgeries), radiation, and chemotherapy may be used to alleviate symptoms or to prevent their development. An effort is made to weigh benefits and costs, but this is always difficult; for the patient, of course, these measures may themselves cause discomfort or pain. I suspect that many patients and families now learn these things by sad experience; if so, this too suggests that greater knowledge will lead to decisions favoring quicker deaths with lethal drugs. Significant attitudinal changes in this direction have already occurred in the United States, as shown in Chapter 4. For example, volunteers in Washington were able to collect over 212,000 signatures of registered voters to qualify Initiative 119, the Initiative for Death with Dignity, for the ballot. The bill would have allowed just the sort of physician assistance that would forestall the protracted deaths and frustrated suicide attempts I have described. Although grassroots lobbying by volunteers was sufficient to prevent substitution of a weaker bill by opponents, the initiative failed to pass by a margin of 54 to 46 percent. A similar bill in California in 1992 failed by the same margin. The close votes are indicative of enormous changes over time in public tolerance for aid-in-dying, however, and further efforts at legislative change are sure to follow.[31]

If death is to be allowed at all, many would argue, on humanitarian grounds, that it should come quickly, out of consideration for the dying patient, the family, and caregivers. On looking back at her husband's death, for example, one wife wished she had known more about drugs, so he could have died more quickly. "I don't think he suffered," she said, "but it was a long, terrible night for us. I wrongly assumed that the morphine would work faster." Nursing home patients often express a wish to be done with the waiting and the suffering. Hospice patients become weary with lingering and the uncertainty surrounding the actual time of death. In the words of one, "The worst thing is not knowing the when. I know that it's going to happen, but I don't know when and I don't like this. There is no control. No way of being able to say I have this amount of time and then I'll die. I lie here and think about it all." Long death watches (five days or more) are hard on families and hospice staff too, and all hope the ordeal will end soon. As a patient lingers, family exhaustion and staff stress inevitably heighten, creating discomfort over the patient's inability to let go and grief over a "hard" death.[32]

Although it may not be protracted, a hospice death is not necessarily peaceful. Even with an experienced terminal care team, for example, some patients suffer such unendurable symptoms that they must be heavily sedated for their last days; according to one recent study, sedation was needed for 16 percent of patients in their last week of life. Most hospice workers, dedicated to relieving suffering and providing compassionate care to the dying when successful treatment is not deemed possible, are nonetheless opposed to "active" euthanasia and assisted suicide; they maintain that hospice care makes such means unnecessary. Yet if assisted suicide were decriminalized and reasonable safeguards devised, 38 percent would support it, according to a recent survey of hospice groups; another 18 percent were unsure, whereas 45 percent would remain opposed.[33] Support for patient autonomy and recognition of hospice's inability to provide a "good" death to every patient underlie the supportive stance of the first group.

Comparisons are often made between the "easy" deaths that are not only acceptable but obligatory for animals, such as family pets, yet not acceptable for human beings. As a practicing clinician in Massachusetts put it, "My dog died last year with more love and dignity than my mother did in 1972." Statements by nurses involved in caring for Nancy Cruzan, whose body survived twelve more days after her feeding tube was removed, are also telling: "The Humane Society won't let you starve your dog," said one. From another, "They don't starve death row inmates." (The prisoners, by the way, are always killed quickly, for "humanitarian" reasons.) Although these nurses were objecting to the removal of the tube per se, their repugnance at the method is apparent. One nurse specifically noted that a quick death by lethal injection would be more humane and easier for the staff to deal with. Others believe that the "agonizing battle to breathe" endured in a "12-hour ordeal" by a dying man, after the decision to forgo life-prolonging treatments had been made by his son, constitutes pointless suffering that a lethal injection could have prevented. It is abundantly clear from an examination of human history that avoidance of suffering is a strong motivator behind many behaviors. The *manner* chosen for a deliberate death would also seem a likely candidate for efforts to avoid suffering.[34]

The presence of close friends and family members for a final farewell to a loved one would also seem desirable. Since the law in many states currently prohibits assisting a suicide (although suicide itself is not illegal), one is forced to die alone in order to protect from prosecution the survivors who assist him. In describing how he aided the death of a patient, Dr. Timothy Quill queried whether leaving a patient in this "final aloneness" is either necessary or humane.[35] Clearly there is room for improvement if our already-conceded right to choose death is to have real meaning and, as the existence of efforts such as Washington's Initiative 119 demonstrates, innovators are already demanding it.

Improvements to the Informal Care System as Alternatives to Deliberate Death

As Alzheimer's disease slowly destroyed his wife's mind, 79-year-old Hans Florian cared for her at home, with the help of his son. Together, they "bathed Johanna, pried open her mouth at feeding time, woke to her screams, picked her up when she stumbled and changed her clothes five or six times a day as she wet and soiled them." For nearly two years, unless she was heavily drugged, Johanna screamed almost constantly, using only two words: the German words for "fire" and "pain." Finally, for all their sakes, Hans moved her to a nursing home. There the screaming grew worse, terrifying other patients, and he was asked to remove her. Ten days later, he shot her to death. A grand jury refused to indict.[1]

Collectively, the demographic, social, and economic trends reviewed to this point suggest greater demand for and resort to death control in years to come, especially "active" forms of assistance, such as lethal injections. Are there no alternative solutions to the formidable problems of extreme frailty and prolonged dying in old age? Perhaps more and better family caregivers are the answer to long-term care dilemmas, up to and including the dying process itself. A related notion is that more and better formal support services can help families help their frail relatives. Consider the tragic story above, for example. How could the community help the Florians to care for Johanna? What more should the nursing home have done both for Johanna and for her family? What should Hans have done when the home refused to keep her?

The "if only" school of thought has many adherents, and most professionals in the aging field believe that improvements to the informal care system are possible and highly desirable. Financing issues affect the probability, nature, and extent of improvements, of course. While there is no doubt that more and better caregivers, supportive services, and additional money will help improve care in the last stage of life, the more important question is whether improvements will be sufficiently great to deter increased resort to deliberate death.

The ideal caring scenario would ensure that both premature death and delayed death are avoided; that personal, medical, and social services are sufficient in both quantity and quality to meet the needs of frail elders; that symptom management and pain control are adequate for those who need them; that nonphysical suffering is ameliorated to the point where it is bearable; and that no one is seriously hurt by the treatment choices of others. Thus "caring" should be defined broadly, to encompass not only its physical element but solicitude, concern, and empathy for another's suffering. This chapter explores possible alternatives to the expansion of death control and examines their disadvantages for reducing or eliminating choices for deliberate death. By definition, the chapter precludes discussion of familyless elders—a significant minority of frail elders. For example, one-third of female nursing home residents have outlived their children, and most have outlived their spouse. Informal care by more distant relatives or friends is relatively rare, more narrowly defined, more perfunctory when it does occur, more open to abuse and neglect, and more easily relinquished to the formal system when it becomes burdensome. Grandchildren seldom provide care to grandparents, and assistance from siblings, cousins, nieces, or nephews is exceedingly rare. Lacking concerned relatives, some elders are more dependent from the beginning on publicly provided care, possible improvements to which are the topic of Chapter 8.[2]

Informal, unpaid caregiving by relatives is by far the dominant mode of meeting the long-term care needs of frail elders, and cost containment is by far the chief concern of policy makers, a duality that implies little public incentive for mitigating family burdens and, concurrently, considerable incentive for maintaining or increasing them. Yet the impediments to long-term family support are substantial and are likely to contribute to family perceptions of advantages to deliberate death for frail aged relatives. Moreover, as age and dependency increase for frail elders, obstacles to continuing family care are more difficult to overcome. We begin with the relevant characteristics of family care providers and potential providers.

Obstacles to Quality Care: Caregiver Characteristics

Claire Quinton was in very poor health for her age. Five spinal fusions had necessitated her early retirement from the workforce; she also suffered from high blood pressure, was overweight, walked with a cane, and had difficulty lifting. Her doctor believed she had a drinking problem, and for six years she had been receiving professional help (medication and psychotherapy) for depression. Finally, she had just learned that she might need yet another operation for the back problem. Her plight would seem to constitute a compelling case for health care and supportive services. Yet, in this true story, Claire was a *provider*, not a recipient, of long-term care: the recipient was her 80-year-old mother, who also suffered from a variety of serious chronic conditions, including severe osteoarthritis. Moreover, the mother often seemed not to appreciate her daughter's efforts and openly preferred Claire's sister, who offered little concrete help.[3] Sadly, Claire's story is not unique, and illustrates the difficult family situations in which elder care may be embedded.

The public resources allocated to long-term elder care are directly related to the family resources expended on providing it, since public support is intended to supplement, rather than replace, family efforts. Currently, little is known but much is assumed about the supply of informal (unpaid) caregivers for frail elders, despite renewed policy emphasis in recent years on family care.[4] Love, concern, altruism, and considerable willingness for self-sacrifice are often taken for granted. But data on the quality of family care or the real ability of relatives to accommodate elders' needs are generally lacking. Thus it is important to assess not only the numbers of potential family care providers, but their characteristics as they affect their capacity to provide adequate long-term care.

More than the presence or absence of kin must be considered. Geographic proximity, competing obligations, health status, social and economic well-being, and many other factors impinge on the ability and willingness of relatives to provide elder care. The possibility of rapid changes in circumstances on both sides of the caregiving equation is also relevant; in particular, the trend toward caregiving responsibilities at older ages will tend to increase the prevalence of morbidity among potential carers and thus constrain their caregiving capacities. Family caregivers typically cannot self-select into the role as readily as formal providers, especially if an emergency precipitates the need for care, leaving no time for calm reflection about one's capabilities or for exploration of other options. Few have a realistic idea of the demands of long-term care. Alternatively, a potential caregiver may misjudge her capabilities, the elder's needs, or the changes that might occur over time in either or both. Often social expectations that relatives will provide care preclude any real choice about doing so. Hence many relatives undertake home care out of a sense of family responsibility, not out of affection or a desire to reciprocate for past help, and despite a troubled relationship with the frail elder. In such circumstances, caregivers tend to be less steadfast in their resolve and burnout occurs more rapidly.[5]

That social expectations force many families to provide care unwillingly and perhaps against their better judgment is supported by data on decisions to institutionalize a frail relative. For example, a study of family involvement in nursing homes revealed that bed availability and geography, not staffing quality, quality of physical care, or the patient's preferences, largely guided the selection of a home; half the families did not even visit the facility prior to the placement. The families did not seek out or utilize community alternatives that would have prevented or postponed their relative's institutionalization, even though the majority were aware of the existence of such services. The authors conclude that "no alternatives would have been acceptable at that late date." Families had apparently had enough. Although they usually continued to visit their frail relatives, few looked forward to visiting, and visits were often unenjoyable, especially if the patient was cognitively impaired. "Many families felt that they just sat and stared at their relative for an hour twice a week."[6]

These findings strongly suggest disengagement or a desire for disengagement on the part of relatives; families seemed to want to remove their burden entirely, not just mitigate or lessen it with community support services. Other investigators have also concluded that "regardless of the type of support service that was offered to a caregiver, the data suggest that the best way to relieve the caregiver of burden and to increase morale is to relieve the family of the responsibility for care."[7]

Even if we assume that family caregivers freely volunteer for the role, can we also assume sufficient capability to carry out the necessary tasks? Do they self-select wisely, in other words? Caregivers are more likely to be poor and to report worse health than their age peers in the overall U.S. population; they are also less likely to be employed. These characteristics all suggest either poor judgment or lack of alternatives to taking on responsibility for elder care, not an eagerness to add one more demanding dimension to already-strained lives. Moreover, some caregivers who make a good decision in the first place ultimately overextend themselves because the needs of the care recipient increase over time, presenting ever-greater challenges to the provider. The increasing duration of care provision itself may exhaust the provider and cause her own health to deteriorate. Over an eight-month interval, for example, 17 percent of the spouse caregivers in one survey reported declines in their own health. And a recent national survey showed that one in three caregivers to noninstitutionalized elderly persons reported that their general health was fair or poor; yet they were still providing care, presumably at some risk to both themselves and the care recipient.[8]

Maintaining multiple roles may help in mitigating the stress and burdens of caregiving. For instance, going to work may have buffering effects for care providers if they enjoy the work and get emotional support from co-workers. But such benefits seem to accrue disproportionately to caregivers of less impaired elders, especially those who are cognitively intact. For example, the authors of one study were careful to note that their finding of positive impacts applied to caregivers of elders who seldom required assistance with personal care and did not suffer from severe mental impairment. In other words, these elders were largely independent, requiring only occasional help with transportation or heavy chores rather than more time-consuming and onerous forms of care, such as those involving body contact. Although helpers who report a positive relationship with the care recipient are less likely to say they feel burdened, regardless of the level of care provided, the progressive mental deterioration that often occurs with advancing age makes continuation of an initially positive relationship much more difficult.[9]

"Excessive caregiving may represent not emotional health or heroism or love, but pathology," according to one expert. Adult children may intensify parent care as a substitute for a failed marriage, the death of a spouse, or problems holding down a job, for example, or use care provision as an excuse to delay independence from parents. "Enmeshing techniques," wherein the care dyad withdraws and becomes increasingly isolated from social contacts, or the caregiver becomes so entrenched in her role that it supersedes all other social roles, are also unhealthy responses. There is even a possibility of delayed death if caregivers become so bound up in their role that they lose sight of the suffering of the patient in their desire to maintain the caring role.[10]

Discussions of caregiver stress and burden must distinguish between family strains that precede caregiving and those that result from it. Some preexisting characteristics of potential caregivers, for example, are serious enough to endanger their charges through abuse and neglect. Abuse may take various forms, ranging from beating an elder, to threats to institutionalize her, to stealing her money or possessions. Neglect may encompass such actions as ignoring the person or refusing to purchase needed medicine or special equipment. In 1988, gerontologist Jordan Kosberg identified fifteen categories of high-risk caregivers: (1) problem drinkers; (2) medication or drug abusers; (3) persons suffering from senile dementia or confusion; (4) victims of mental or emotional illness; (5) those inexperienced with caregiving; (6) persons who are economically troubled; (7) those who were abused as children; (8) those who are stressed emotionally, socially, professionally, or economically; (9) persons who are unengaged outside the home; (10) those who are blamers; (11) individuals who are unsympathetic or callous or (12) lack understanding (of the elder's condition, prognosis, or the care needed); (13) those with unrealistic expectations; (14) persons who are economically dependent on their frail relative; and, finally, (15) those who are hypercritical.[11]

These health and personality problems, Kosberg convincingly maintains, are sufficiently serious to result in elder neglect and abuse. Using both qualitative and quantitative data, for instance, Suzanne Steinmetz has confirmed that "like mother, like daughter" patterns of abuse are transmitted intergenerationally, and much of the abuse carries the potential of grave harm to the frail elder. In one case, a social worker became concerned about entrusting a debilitated elderly woman to the care of her sons, with whom she was living prior to hospitalization. The first son, Sam, is "loud, hot-tempered, threatening, and often speaks nonsensically." Ike, the second, "appears to be actively hallucinating and delusional." Both are slovenly chain-smokers, both have long psychiatric histories, and their apartment is "unsafe and unfit." Their brother Jack often promises to visit but never shows up. Yet the men insist that their mother continue to live with Sam and Ike.[12]

If caregivers or potential caregivers are already severely stressed, their attempts to care for another may predictably result in a worse situation for them as well as endanger the welfare of the dependent. It follows that persons who fall into one or more high-risk categories should be screened out of the caregiver population or counseling, support, and supervision should be provided before they are entrusted with the care of a frail relative. How many people might this be? Although Kosberg performed a valuable service by compiling his list of high-risk categories, he stopped short of estimating the numbers or proportions of Americans who, for their own well-being and that of others, should not be asked or expected to provide care. How many should be subtracted from the population of potential care providers? How many more stable individuals are left to share the duties of elder care in our society? What are the implications for long-term care provision and death control?

As an experiment, I tried reading Kosberg's list to a variety of audiences, mainly colleagues and students. Invariably, I got no further than halfway down before some (usually incredulous) voice in the group ventured, "Who's left?" Follow-up discussions indicated that virtually everyone placed himself or herself in at least one of the high-risk groups. We were led to conclude either that some of the categories are too broad, encompassing some individuals who would be perfectly adequate caregivers, or that many people are providing care despite strong indications that they should not be doing so. The latter may account for a large share of reported elder abuse and neglect. Admittedly, respondent self-reports—from which much of our empirical evidence on American attitudes and behavior are derived—may be imperfect indicators of unsuitability for caregiving tasks. But, given the frequent human tendency to deny problems and present a socially acceptable persona to interviewers, survey data are more likely to *underestimate* than *overestimate* the respective numbers in high-risk categories. In other words, the respondent who is asked if he is "unsympathetic," "callous," or "hypercritical" may well be inclined to deny it, regardless of what he really thinks; likewise, those who are substance abusers or merely "confused" are not reliable respondents either. Since interviewers may avoid questioning some people entirely because they seem incapable of responding or because their answers are erratic, respondents in the average survey are probably more emotionally stable than persons not selected for the sample. Again, the effect would be to *underestimate* the prevalence of high-risk characteristics in the population.

There is plenty of evidence indicative of the extent of problematical attitudes, behaviors, and circumstances among potential caregivers. Unemployment data and poverty statistics are suggestive of financial stress (and its concomitant psychological stress), data from the National Center for Health Statistics indicate the prevalence of substance abuse, and attitude surveys and opinion polls suggest the extent of lack of compassion, "blaming the victim" tendencies, and social isolation. Data from the 1985 National Health Interview Survey, for example, show that almost one in five persons aged 45 to 64 (the ages when potential elder care responsibility is most likely) reported being under a lot of stress, and 14 percent said that stress had a strong deleterious effect on their health. Nine percent of respondents in the same age category considered their stress-related problems sufficiently serious to warrant seeking help from professionals or other sources. Among persons already providing elder care, caregivers of dementia patients use more psychotropic drugs, average more stress symptoms, and have lower levels of life satisfaction than comparison groups. At least some of these problems may *result* from caregiving rather than predate it. In either case, care provision in such circumstances endangers both provider and recipient.[13]

Marital disruption is another kind of stress which, especially for women, often results in financial difficulties and hence a greater need to be in the paid workforce. Adult children who have experienced a marital disruption provide less help to parents than those in intact marriages; the majority cite job responsibilities as the main reason limiting help.[14] For those lacking alternatives, who must provide care regardless of their own circumstances, we are ignorant of the quality of care that results or the consequences for the carer.

Finally, while no single characteristic on Kosberg's list is necessarily predictive of elder mistreatment, *combinations* of characteristics, other things being equal, should increase the risk of abuse and neglect. These are forms of death hastening that may cause death directly or indirectly, through physical trauma or the effects of psychological abuse on the will to live, for example. Similarly, relatives who are "unsympathetic," "blamers," or "hypercritical" may be predisposed to forgo life-sustaining treatments for frail elders when this is unwarranted. Others, out of guilt, confusion, or a desire to keep the elder's pension checks coming, may insist on continued treatment against the advice of professionals, thus unduly delaying death and increasing the patient's suffering. Substance abusers or those who are extremely stressed economically may have incentives for financial abuse of the elder, up to and including facilitating premature death in anticipation of an inheritance.

The risk for elders is especially great if they are cognitively impaired and an unsuitable relative obtains guardianship powers or has durable power of attorney for health care. Our judicial system assumes that family members are the most appropriate guardians for frail elders—that their knowledge of the elder's values and preferences and their concern for his welfare will override their interest in preserving the estate. This assumption is invalid in some cases. For instance, the youngest son of a 79-year-old woman was appointed her legal guardian. But her social worker had to plead with him to purchase necessities, let alone small luxuries, for his mother; the son's attitude led the case worker to believe he was more concerned with preserving the estate than in enhancing his mother's well-being. In another case, a son acting as conservator instructed the operator of the home where his father lived not to allow visits from church members. Because he feared that his father would revise his will in favor of the church, the son was willing to deny him the comfort and companionship he might derive from the visits.[15]

Both physical and mental impairments may hinder an elder's self-defense when she is mistreated, and dependence on the perpetrator may well prevent her from reporting problems even if the opportunity presents itself. Social workers and other professionals may be aware of the family's problems, but may be unable to do anything because of budget limitations, long waiting lists at the better nursing homes, or the old person's refusal to move. On the other hand, gerontologists who serve family caregivers have been cautioned to be aware of their conflicting goals, especially when cost containment points to continued at-home care but the care provider's needs are best served by the residential placement of her charge.[16]

Greater recognition of negative family interactions and more realistic assessments of family caregiving potential are long overdue. Identification of incompetent or inappropriate caregivers is essential if compassionate care is to be delivered to those in need and mistreatment avoided. But problem areas extend well beyond the characteristics of individual caregivers. Kosberg has provided two additional important lists: of high-risk *elders* and high-risk *family systems*. Frail elders have a combination of the high-risk characteristics Kosberg identifies: advanced age, and a population that is disproportionately female, dependent, isolated, and highly impaired; their dependence and functional impairments, of course, increase caregiver stress and may induce negative changes in caregiver well-being that, in turn, exacerbate the risk of elder maltreatment. Since, by definition, nothing can be done to change most of the high-risk characteristics of frail elders (their age, sex, degree of impairment and dependency), interventions must focus on changing the negative characteristics of caregivers or transferring the elder to some other care arrangement.

However, even when a competent caregiver exists, there are high-risk family systems to be concerned about. These are systems that are isolated, overcrowded, contain a substance abuser, or suffer from unemployment, marital conflicts, or other serious stressors. All may endanger frail elders despite the exemplary behavior of the primary caregiver. Others in the household may abuse the elder, for example, and the primary caregiver may be unaware of or unable to change that person's behavior. The depressing reality is that an adequate caregiving individual is not enough if the family system in which she is embedded is dysfunctional. In fact, the caregiver herself may be dependent on a family member who mistreats her as well as her charge.

Given Kosberg's warnings and considerable evidence of elder abuse and neglect, great skepticism is required in interpreting surveys of caregiver burden. Many seem to downplay the risks to both parties. For instance, I think we would do well to mistrust such statements as this, from a recent study: "A common theme expressed by these women was the desire to continue with the diverse activities they were pursuing, but in a more organized and efficient manner. In fact, the notion of relinquishing any caregiving responsibilities to accommodate their own interests seemed intolerable to them." There is an aura of unreality here, and of denial. In contrast, research such as Suzanne Steinmetz's should give us pause: although in most respects the female caregivers she studied "probably represented model caregivers," they engaged in an "astonishing" amount of psychological, verbal, and physical abuse, and the behavior of nearly one in four carried the potential of severe physical harm to the elder. With her, we may well wonder "about the treatment being provided by caregivers with less noble intentions." We may wonder as well about the psychological abuse (for example, the threat of abandonment) that is hard to measure but may be just as devastating to elder well-being—if it leads to severe depression and thoughts of suicide, for instance. We know that bad things happen in families, but is it only a tiny, deviant minority that does them? Has the family's potential for providing for the needs of the elderly been greatly exaggerated? To believe otherwise, and to design public policies based on false, overconfident assumptions, is unrealistic and dangerous. We must continue to challenge our collective complacency regarding family caregiving potential.[17]

Families frequently exchange visits, telephone calls, and a wide variety of goods and services. But, as we have seen, there is no justification for assuming that because these kinship relationships exist they are inherently supportive for either party. In fact, studies of social support are quite consistent in finding no positive effect of contact with adult children on the well-being of parents; in sharp contrast, frequent interaction with friends is positively related to elder morale and life satisfaction. So there is little rationale for concluding that either generation wants or is capable of handling extensive care for indefinitely long intervals. Yet, despite contrary evidence, study after study has concluded that "informal networks are doing such a fine job of supporting older persons . . . that formal agencies should take pains not to interfere with or disrupt their operations." This assumption fits so conveniently with cherished images of traditional family values and policy makers' efforts to contain public health care costs that it is rarely challenged. Thus policies remain in force that disregard "the possibility that, while many older people may be in no position to refuse assistance from kin, they may not *want* it"—and would prefer formal, paid services. This suggests that if informal networks are replaced by formal agencies, life satisfaction and quality of life of elders (and their families) would increase. But such reasoning does not take adequate account of the shortcomings of formal services (see Chapter 8) and the unlikely scenario that policy makers will soon deemphasize family care at the risk of substantially increasing public costs.[18]

Time constraints, heavy caseloads, and financial considerations may preclude recommendations by social workers to institutionalize frail elders for their own protection, as may the elder's own reluctance and the long waiting lists characteristic of many nursing homes. So there may be literally nowhere else for the elder in a dangerous care situation to go. Social supports for caregivers are also severely limited, as we will see, and are insufficient to prevent elder mistreatment. Interventions with caregivers and their families to reduce or remove the strains that make them high-risk providers, rather than moving the care recipient, are also costly. Moreover, we have little idea of what to do or how to do it, and families may well resist such intrusion into their private affairs. Mistreatment by relatives, elders' anticipation of mistreatment, and their dread of institutionalization may, in turn, reinforce the individual motives for deliberate death discussed in Chapter 5. For families, professional care providers, and society generally, facilitating a quicker death helps resolve these troublesome issues, particularly if it seems in the frail elder's best interests. A good illustration is Frank Robinson's story. When his mother was critically ill, "he discovered that people would make vague sympathetic noises about [her] condition but never actually volunteer to do anything or even to visit her." Eventually he killed her, as she had repeatedly asked him to do. At that juncture, the same people—about 300 of them—signed a petition declaring that he was a good son who loved his mother and asking the courts to show him mercy.[19]

Formal Supports: Does "Help" Help Enough?

Can community supports help families to help their frail relatives? Can they help high-risk caregivers change in appropriate directions—to become better carers? Can they help enough? Insofar as formal support services screen potential caregivers for high-risk attitudes and behaviors and are able to ameliorate them, the quality of family care should improve. And insofar as formal support services actually reduce stress and burden, both caregiving relatives and their charges should benefit. There is no doubt that needy elders are drastically underserved in the present service environment. Data from the 1982 Long-Term Care Survey indicate that only one in four community-based frail elders uses any home-care services, for example. Even more underserved are their caregiving relatives. Ironically, some are unable even to take advantage of the few existing services because of their caregiving activities. For example, they cannot leave the elder long enough to attend a support group meeting. This section describes the shortcomings of the "helps" that are available.[20]

The thrust of public policy initiatives currently being discussed is on how to promote in-home care by relatives for impaired elders. Tax incentives to encourage coresidence, public monies for support services such as respite care, and cash grants to caregiving relatives are among the items that have been discussed (but seldom produced). Expansion of community-provided home care services is predicated on the formidable arguments that this is conducive to both elders' welfare and their preferences to remain at home, while simultaneously helping to keep down public costs by preventing or postponing institutionalization. But home care services are nonexistent in many communities and sorely inadequate in others, assuming that elders or their families can afford the out-of-pocket costs in the first place.[21] Elders may also find fault with home care attendants, flatly refuse their help, or be so demanding that aides quit in frustration—all of which puts more pressure on family caregivers to remain in that role.

For elderly patients who are technology-dependent, such as those who require tube feeding or hemodialysis, home care requirements are often too complex to make it feasible; at the same time, however, institutions are reluctant to accept or keep technology-dependent individuals, lacking both the staff and financial incentives to do so; the same is true of other patients who have high care needs that are nonmedical, such as those suffering with dementias or those with a history of violence. Adult day care centers, for example, are often reluctant to admit patients who are demented; wandering, incontinence, and disruptive behavior are also common reasons for rejection. Cognitively intact clients as well as staff may resist the inclusion of such elders in their programs, despite mounting social pressures to include them (because their numbers are increasing and their care onerous). Both costs and access can be problematical too. There are now about 2,000 centers in the country, with an average capacity of twenty participants. Costs averaged $30 per day in 1986. Today, providers believe that a charge of $40 per day is needed to maintain cost-effectiveness. Although the number of such facilities is growing, the total remains far fewer than the number of communities.[22]

Financial support for family caregivers is exceedingly rare, and stringent eligibility criteria exclude most from receiving even minimal reimbursement, despite the fact that a significant proportion desperately need financial assistance. Pamela Doty, an expert on health care financing, examined the possible impact of government supports and incentives on family caregiving. She concluded that nothing thus far proposed would induce families to provide more informal care to impaired relatives than they now do. Cash grants or tax incentives, for example, would do little to prevent institutionalization, because decisions to institutionalize are seldom financially motivated. Hence researchers believe it is highly unlikely that financial inducements will prompt American families to provide more care; but if they do succeed, family members who are ill-equipped to provide elder care may be tempted to take on the role and this would not be conducive to high-quality care.[23]

Financial compensation seems to have no effect on the emotional and physical strains that constitute the most oppressive aspects of elder care. That money does not remove all the burdens is well illustrated by this statement from an affluent daughter-in-law: "Money doesn't seem to solve the problem of my 89-year-old mother-in-law. She has three shifts of nurses, but we can't even get away for a vacation. If a nurse doesn't turn up, I have to fill in and spend hours trying to get another." A teacher was forced to quit her job for similar reasons. She could afford to hire round-the-clock help, but the arrangements "constantly came unravelled," some attendants were incompetent, and others quit on short notice.[24]

Some people see the private sector as "an untapped source of potential support for family caregivers," though few companies have initiated programs to aid employees who care for old people, and most of those are token efforts. Information provision and referrals to service agencies, allowing pretax dollars to be set aside for elder care, flextime, and personal leave policies allowing several weeks of unpaid leave per year are examples of what some companies, such as Travelers, have offered their employees; family leave insurance and low interest loans to help cover the costs of expensive medical equipment have also been mentioned. But employees seldom use whatever services are available, in part because they fear bosses' reactions to their family commitments. There have been no organized efforts by employees aimed at ameliorating their problems with elder care.[25]

The nature and duration of care needed by frail elders typically call for *large*, enduring commitments, not short-term, emergency-oriented accommodations, so employer-provided services may be completely inadequate. A few weeks of unpaid leave are not nearly enough to cope with the long-term needs of the chronically ill. More important, representatives of the private sector, such as the U.S. Chamber of Commerce, are prominent among the *opponents* of family leave bills. Business leaders fear that their costs will increase and eventually be passed on to consumers and that small businesses will be especially hard-hit if compliance is mandatory rather than voluntary. If the private sector continues to resist, some suggest that the public sector will need to offer incentives, such as tax breaks, to induce businesses to assist their employees, a move that will do nothing to curb public costs.[26]

According to a recent review, no federal or state family leave bills were passed prior to 1987; of 28 states that introduced such legislation in 1987, only six included elder care. The four bills eventually enacted did not result from the efforts of grass-roots movements, however, but were placed on the agenda by party leaders. Lobbying efforts by advocates for the elderly or by caregivers simply did not occur. An examination of hearing transcripts for nine states showed no signs of involvement by the American Association of Retired Persons, the Gray Panthers, home care organizations, regional gerontological associations, or family caregivers or their representatives. Lobbying efforts for the inclusion of elder care in a national family leave policy have also been sparse at the federal level. Bills passed by Congress in 1990, and again in 1992, which would have applied only to employers with fifty or more workers, were vigorously opposed by business groups and vetoed by President Bush. In any case, none of the family leave bills thus far proposed are adequate to meet the need.[27]

Allowances for family caregivers are common in Western Europe, but very rare in the United States. A new elder care policy in Sweden has been recommended as a model program for other nations. Like many suggestions in the United States, Swedish policy reflects a renewed interest in family caregiving. The new care leave policy entitles workers to time off with pay for up to 30 days in the lifetime of the care recipient, making it inadequate for the long-term chronic-care needs of many frail elders. If care exceeds 20 hours per week, however, the provider receives a salary from the government that is equivalent to the pay of a municipal home health aide, along with benefits, pension rights, and vacations. Despite the fact that Sweden's initiatives have been proclaimed "the most farsighted and innovative approach to caregiver support found anywhere in the world," they are seriously flawed in other respects. The skills used in elder care are not easily transferred to other jobs, for instance, and such experience may not impress prospective employers once caregiving obligations have ceased. Because pay and benefits are offered, however, potential caregivers (primarily women in Sweden, as elsewhere) are less free to refuse care. But neither the monetary compensation nor the psychic rewards of caregiving may approach those which could be obtained in other work that the caregiver might be qualified for, prefers, or, indeed, already has. Finally, even one episode of extended caregiving may limit work experience to such an extent that future episodes of caregiving become more likely, with cumulative negative effects on the provider's well-being. That is, if a woman forgoes other work for caregiving, her "experience" may make it seem logical to family members (and to her) that she continue in the role when other relatives fall ill. Hence choices, especially for women, may be limited by public policies aimed at encouraging family caregiving.[28]

Providers' responsibilities also typically extend beyond services they personally provide, and the stresses and burdens of caring do not cease when formal services are initiated. For example, assuming that community-supported home help is available and affordable, relatives must still evaluate, select, and supervise it; hidden costs include taking up the slack for "no shows." In *Kate Quinton's Days*, journalist Susan Sheehan chronicles how a search for in-home services that would allow a middle-aged disabled daughter to keep her frail mother at home involved tremendous coordination efforts, misunderstandings, and gaps in service as they worked with fifteen different home health aides over a five-month period. A partial chronology of the Quintons' experiences, as shown in Table 7-1, helps illuminate the sorts of problems families may encounter.

Were the Quintons problem clients? "No," according to the case coordinator, they were merely unlucky. Are their experiences typical? It is hard to say because few accounts of clients' experiences with the home care industry have been published, none as detailed as this one. I believe that experience will show that the Quintons are not unusual, that home care aides generally will exhibit levels of absenteeism, job turnover, and attitudinal/behavioral problems similar to those of their counterparts in the nursing home industry.

A variety of counseling, training, and education services have also been proposed to buttress family continuance in caregiving roles. Although reports indicate that these are enthusiastically received by caregivers and are indeed beneficial in some respects, they also serve to shift responsibilities from formal organizations

TABLE 7-1

A Chronology of One Family's Home Care Experiences

March 3	Mercedes Robbins, the first home-care attendant assigned to 80-year-old Kate Quinton, fails to show up.
March 4	Ms. Robbins does show. She is wearing designer jeans and high-heeled boots and carries a number of textbooks. She performs her tasks "capably and grudgingly," and then reads her books or watches television. She does not provide the companionship the old woman craves.
March 6	Ms. Robbins begins a pattern of arriving late and leaving early. Claire Quinton is afraid to leave the house while she is there because the aide might not hear her mother's calls for assistance. Ms. Robbins remains on the job until March 19.
March 20	Margaret Clayton is pleasant and proficient, but annoys the client with loud religious music and wants to hold a faith healing session in her living room. The aide asks if she can send her Aunt Nellie to help the Quintons while she attends church services.
March 22	Alice Kuster does not appear as scheduled. She had been given inadequate directions and was unable to locate the correct address.
March 23	Tina Ortiz appears on the scene. Pleasant and efficient, she is well liked by the family.
March 24	Ms. Ortiz calls to say she cannot work due to her son's hospitalization following an automobile accident. A week later, she takes another job.
March 25	Felicity Sanchez, inexperienced and with no aptitude for cooking (part of her assigned duties), begins to work for the Quintons. She also falls into a habit of arriving late and leaving early.
May 30	Belinda Fernandez, the weekend substitute, does not inform anyone that this is her last day on the job. She thought the Quintons were too "picky" and that being a home attendant was too stressful, so she returned to work in a garment factory.
June 5–6	Cecille DuFief is described as slovenly and inefficient, and spends too much time sleeping on the job.
June 12–13	Jeanne DuFief, Cecille's sister, brings her needlework and tells the old woman to "wait a minute" each time she asks for something, such as assistance in getting to the bathroom. Some of the "minutes" are very long. Like Cecille, Jeanne is studying nursing.

TABLE 7-1 (CONTINUED))

June 19	Dominique Jaqua gets lost on the way to work. When she finally arrives, she is wearing four-inch-high stiletto heels and a party dress. She doesn't want to stay.
June 20–21	Zenobia Nelson, an aide with "wonderful experience," is unable to work. Martine Latour is called to substitute. It turns out that Martine is working on another case, so her roommate, Elise Gentil, impersonates her and takes the job. At the Quinton home, it becomes clear that Elise knows nothing about caregiving.
July 6	Anita LaLuz, a far more skillful aide, comes to substitute for Felicity Sanchez, who is on vacation (one of many conflicting stories she told the Quintons).
July 10	Yolanda Encalada seems less than promising. She "cast[s] a cold eye on the commode" and has to be reminded that it is part of her job. Her humming and crude manners annoy the client considerably.
July 19	Felicity Sanchez does not show up. When the agency tracks her down, she reports that her son is sick and she cannot work.
July 20	Eugenia Warren, sent to substitute for Ms. Sanchez, proves herself a very accomplished home attendant. The family is sorry to see her go on July 23.
August 9	Jasmine Pagano arrives. The Quintons are well pleased, but Jasmine has many family problems that affect her work—an unemployed husband who is often drunk and abusive, for example. Claire Quinton gives Jasmine time off to go to the food stamp center and sometimes drives her there herself.
September	Suzanne Blanc is shy and sickly. She spends hours in the bathroom or sitting with her head in her hands.

Source: Susan Sheehan, *Kate Quinton's Days* (New York: Mentor, 1984), passim.

to families and hinder social reform in the direction of more equitable distribution of caregiving burdens. Refusing to accept help in the forms offered by society also penalizes the caregiver (and possibly her charge as well), and she may well realize that any help is better than none. Such programs are of doubtful utility for another reason: since those who are highly motivated either already provide good care or actively seek out the help they need, the programs may not attract the more marginally committed caregivers who conceivably need them most. Other forms of help, such as expert advice about better time management, may have limited usefulness in helping carers to cope with the real problems of their situation. If physicians and clinics have more evening hours, for example, as some have recommended, this alone cannot reduce caregivers' exhaustion, though ostensibly employers gain because appointments are shifted into the employee's "leisure" time and elders gain because they get the medical attention they need.[29]

Some experts may exaggerate the benefits of care provision to relatives, in part because they are affected by strong institutional pressures to contain costs. In describing a model respite care program, for example, one group of investigators maintained that respite care (an average of four weeks a year when caregivers were relieved of primary responsibility) could transform "a dreary, exhausting job" to "a rewarding and life-enriching experience." However, they provided no evidence of such a transformation among participants.[30] Recipients of such services may hesitate to complain because they fear that, if they are not suitably grateful, the services, however meager, may be withdrawn.

Evidence from a recent study shows that although formal services may alleviate *objective* burdens, they can do little to relieve caregivers' *subjective* burdens—their lives remain severely constrained. Home attendants can help with housework and the patient's personal hygiene, for example, but the burden of "having one's social world shrink through the long-term responsibility of caring for a dependent relative ... cannot be relieved by formal service provision." Even institutionalization may not relieve the caregiver's sense of burden, since the relative's mental and physical condition often continues to worsen and considerable time may be spent in visiting the patient, worrying about her, and monitoring care; new problems and concerns thus replace the old ones, and financial worries may be heightened, particularly for spouses. Despite the considerable burdens families already bear, some studies even view them as neglected resources that should be further exploited to the mutual advantage of patients and institutions.[31]

Hence we return to the question with which we began: how many formal "helps" really help? How many just exacerbate psychological pressures on relatives to continue in the caregiving role and forestall their complaints about the paucity of public services because ostensibly some are provided? Gerontologist Elaine Brody has studied family caregiving issues for many years. In her view, social policies that "cheer the family on" and call for relative responsibility at any cost mask social irresponsibility, disadvantaging everyone and adding to the problems rather than resolving them.[32] In short, while needs proliferate and proposals for change are abundant, formal services to help families remain meager and the real changes necessary in the long-term care arena are nowhere in sight. Families are caught in the squeeze, left to cope as best they can within a manifestly unhelpful system.

Carers as Victims

Caregiving has consequences, both short-run and long-run. It is not uniformly deleterious, however, since some withstand its rigors well and others adapt over time to the additional demands without ill effect.[33] Many professionals have assumed that because frail elders prefer home care over institutional care, home care should be provided, or at least managed, by relatives. Many policy makers have further assumed that efforts to save public monies, even more than elders' needs or preferences, should take priority over the needs and preferences of family members. But gains to frail elders are sometimes achieved only by the considerable sacrifices of others. Families may be more than temporarily "stressed" or "burdened" in our current system—they may be victimized. Up to now, we have taken a rather narrow view of victimization—as if only frail elders were hurt by the inadequacies of current long-term care arrangements. This section goes beyond two indisputable conclusions—that many families need more formal help than is now available and that others should not provide care at all—to argue that even willing caregivers need *protection* from overcare, that this too is a social obligation, and that it too suggests greater tolerance for deliberate death in years to come, as more caregivers recognize limits to their obligations to frail relatives.

A conclusion that relatives are victimized over and above any temporary feelings of stress and burden seems indisputable. First, the evidence suggests that caregiving roles are not assumed freely and willingly, due to personal values, but instead are assumed "as a consequence of values imposed by public policy"; given a choice, few families would opt to provide personal care.[34] But that choice is rarely available. Further, caregiving obligations are unevenly distributed within families. There is an implicit preference structure underlying caregiving arrangements, with primary responsibility assigned first to the spouse, then to children, other kin, and non-relatives, in that order. When there are several siblings in the family, one of them assumes a disproportionate share of responsibility or is involuntarily selected into the role of primary caregiver because the others live too far away, are estranged from the parent, or decline the responsibility for some other reason; moreover, daughters are more likely to serve as caregivers than sons are.

Compared to nonspousal caregivers, spouses spend more time in care provision—a minimum of 35 hours per week. Caregiving is more burdensome for them because they tend to be older, to have poorer health and lower incomes, and to provide more intensive care for longer periods. The marital bond should not be interpreted to mean that spouses are more willing to provide care, however. In fact, they have the least choice about doing so, given the "universal expectation" that they will—regardless of their own health, competing obligations, the state of the marriage, or the effects on their own well-being.[35]

Nonspousal caregivers are usually better able to distance themselves from the patient, physically and psychologically. In the case of adult children, feelings of obligation to elderly parents may grow weaker if there are role conflicts, if they live far away, or if family disagreements interfere with a positive relationship. Compared to spouses, adult children and other relatives can more easily decline the caregiving role and can withdraw from it more readily when it becomes too demanding. Significantly, researchers have found that spouses were caring for more disabled elders than were adult children, leading them to conclude that children are less willing to care for highly impaired elders.[36]

Caregiving relatives may suffer a variety of mental and physical health problems related to long-term care provision, symptoms that go well beyond temporary stress or inconvenience to threaten future well-being and even life itself. The burdens of care provision, combined with lack of sufficient supportive services, sometimes have tragic results. At the extreme, some providers have committed suicide, or simply killed their charges, risking trial and imprisonment. But most negative effects are less dramatic, less visible, and less easily measured. The extent of premature illness and death for caregivers that is brought on or made worse by the stresses of care provision, for example, has not been systematically investigated. Problems include severe depression, anxiety, a sense of helplessness, sleep interruptions and sleepless nights, and physical and emotional exhaustion. In one study of caregivers of Alzheimer's victims, for instance, 42 percent of those under 65 and over half of those over 65 showed signs of clinically significant depression. Moreover, many dementia patients exhibit aggressive behavior toward family caregivers, including severe violence (kicking, hitting, or biting, for example) or threatening them with a weapon. According to a recent study, significant violence occurred in 17.4 percent of patient-caregiver dyads in which the patient was diagnosed with Alzheimer's disease; in contrast, the prevalence of violence in the other direction—from caregiver to patient—was 5.4 percent.[37]

Serious family conflicts may arise over care provision and its toll. As one caregiver explained: "My husband thinks it's time for a nursing home. My son said when she began to go downhill to put her in a nursing home. My daughter says I can't put her in a nursing home. She said it would be better if she fell over dead at home." Elder care may also interfere with the family's life-style, privacy, future plans, and income, as well as divert the caregiver's time from other family members who also need attention. Are there long-term deleterious impacts to these forms of interference? If caring for a frail elder necessitates that less time be spent with a child, for example, there may be lasting consequences for the child. They may be good or bad, or not even measurable. Similar reasoning applies to the net effects on the family system. Should we continue to disregard these impacts?[38]

Adult children seldom make direct financial contributions for care provided to frail relatives by others, whether in the parent's own home or in an institution. But the opportunity costs of caregiving daughters and sons who sacrifice work time and experience to provide parent care may be substantial. As our population ages, growing numbers of midlife and older workers are called on to serve as caregivers for aged relatives. The call is likely to come at a time when they are also deciding whether to remain in the workforce. At issue is the fact that workers who retire too soon may shortchange themselves in terms of the resources they will need for retirement.[39]

There has been little attention to the impact of class and race on caregiving demands or caregiver well-being either, despite the fact that low-income people—often members of disadvantaged minority groups as well—face additional obstacles in providing care, such as less flexible work schedules, less access to formal services, and aged relatives who are, on average, sicker and more in need of assistance than the white middle class.[40] To assume that families encounter only short-term inconveniences in the course of providing elder care, with no negative long-term effects, or to suppose that any negative impacts will cease with the institutionalization of the frail relative is to expose both informal caregivers and their families to unknown, but potentially very grave, risks.

None of this is to deny that caregiving can be ennobling to providers—a chance to return the love and care received in the past or to express willingness for self-sacrifice, perhaps in anticipation of their own future needs. Caregiving may also be a challenge and an opportunity for closer relationships between spouses or between generations. It may, at the least, serve as a means of avoiding guilt or gaining the good opinion of others. Different individuals may evaluate the caregiving relationship differently, even when objective conditions are similar, and find meaning in the most demanding of circumstances. But all this implies that the inevitable sacrifices seem worthwhile to the provider. Even willing relatives may still be victims in some circumstances—for example, if their health deteriorates owing to their caregiving efforts. Moreover, public costs may swell if caregiving demands are so onerous that they create two disabled and needy patients where there was one. Since the risks of long-term care provision are often objectively measurable, whereas the rewards are intangible, and perhaps fleeting, a minimally adequate long-term care system should fully inform potential family caregivers of both the risks and the benefits and allow them the freedom to say "no"—an option not now available to most. As the next section shows, it is primarily women who are disadvantaged by our present system.

Women Disproportionately Victimized

Assignment to caregiving roles on the basis of gender reflects long-standing cultural values and has important social, psychological, and economic implications for women as the primary providers of informal care to frail elders. Within each class and ethnic group, women are the primary victims of the "compassion trap"—the social manipulation of an individual's psychological resources for the benefit of others, to her own detriment. A reading of the growing literature on caregiving demonstrates how deeply American women have succumbed to the compassion trap and how difficult it is for them to refuse care, given the paucity of alternatives. As care provision has become more demanding of providers and longer in duration, women carers are increasingly victimized by the inadequacies of our long-term care system. The resurgence of interest in family responsibility for elder care also affects women disproportionately. For example, the recent trend within the hospice movement to contain costs by shifting caregiving tasks back to the family, if successful, will succeed largely at women's expense.[41]

Seven in ten informal caregivers for the elderly are women. They not only provide hands-on care themselves, but have primary responsibility for selecting, coordinating, and monitoring care provided by others, both within and outside the family. Generally speaking, "the most difficult and emotionally draining level of assistance"—personal care and health maintenance—has been socially defined as "women's work." Moreover, women carers are often "on call" for caregiving activities whereas men are usually more peripheral carers and can more freely choose what they will do and when they will do it. Owing to differential socialization, men in general seem more willing to delegate caregiving tasks to female relatives or pay outsiders for services rather than perform them themselves. Finally, women carers typically receive less assistance from either formal or informal helpers. These gender differences in caregiving experiences help explain why the adverse consequences of elder care affect women more than men.[42]

That elder care is basically women's work is documented in Table 7-2. These data—the first national estimates of informal caregivers to noninstitutionalized disabled elders—provide important insights on the costs of informal care to providers.

Identification as the primary caregiver, for example, indicates a high level of responsibility for patient welfare; this group is predominantly female. Shared living arrangements probably reflect severe impairments among care recipients, and hence greater call on caregivers' time and energy; women also predominate in this category, as well as among those who have provided care for five years or more. A higher proportion of nonwhite than white caregivers are female, suggesting greater commitment, or fewer choices, among women of color. Sociodemographic trends, such as higher morbidity among minority elders, a lower rate of nursing home utilization, and more competing responsibilities, combine to place minority women at relatively greater risk as caregivers.[43]

Table 7-2 suggests other hardships experienced by caregiving women. Three in four caregivers living near or below the poverty line are women, for example. Women are also disproportionately represented among care providers reporting their own health as fair or poor. They are "more apt to become submerged in caregiving" and more likely to experience it as a "boundless, all-encompassing activity." Some researchers assert that women are more likely to assume responsibility for improving the overall quality of life for elderly care recipients, even when this is difficult or impossible. In contrast, men are more likely to take a task-oriented approach and to remain more distant and detached.[44]

Clearly, women are providing an enormous amount of care to frail elders despite both current hardships (poverty, ill health, and competing obligations, for example) and predictable future hardships as their ability to accumulate resources for their own old age is constrained. Moreover, caregivers' health problems may be caused or exacerbated by the emotional stress and physical requirements of care provision (sleep disruption and role conflict, for example). A caregiver who has quit her job to provide care and then becomes disabled herself is doubly disadvantaged because she is not eligible for Social Security disability benefits unless she worked outside the home for five of the ten years prior to the onset of her disability.[45]

Women's assignment to "serial caregiving" roles for relatives— first children, then elderly parents and parents-in-law, and finally their spouse—contributes to the more serious consequences they suffer. In one analysis, for example, nearly half the caregiving

TABLE 7-2
Caregivers to Noninstitutionalized Elders: Selected Characteristics and Percent Female, 1982 National Long-Term Care Survey/Informal Caregivers Survey

Characteristic	Number	Percent Female
All caregivers	2,201	71.6
Primary caregivers*	1,565	74.1
Age		
45–64	911	74.3
65+	781	71.6
Race		
White	1,750	70.6
Other	451	75.2
Lives with disabled person	1,627	68.8
Poor/near poor	693	74.6
Health fair or poor	735	70.5
Provided care for 5 years or more	445	70.1
Quit work to provide care	196	79.1
Employed caregivers who:		
Worked fewer hours	215	70.7
Rearranged schedule	301	72.8
Took time off without pay	190	75.8

* Includes those with and without formal or informal help.
SOURCE: Calculated from data presented by Robyn Stone, Gail Lee Cafferata, and Judith Sangl, in "Caregivers of the Frail Elderly: A National Profile," *The Gerontologist* 27 (1987): 616-626, esp. Tables 2-4.

daughters had helped care for their father before assuming responsibility for their widowed mother; one in three had already helped other elderly relatives. Women in American society continue to have major responsibility for child care. Hence those who care for frail parents or in-laws often do so *after* spending years out of the workforce or as marginal workers owing to child care responsibilities. Finally, since women are statistically more likely to be widowed than men are, husband care in his final illness may demand similar sacrifices of labor force experience and postponement of personal interests and goals. Caregiving requirements by the different generations may overlap, of course, but this seems to hold for only a small minority of women.[46]

More than opportunity costs may be involved in elder care. The types of personal assistance needed by many frail elders—feeding, bathing, toileting—are similar to the needs of young children. But children's functional capacities improve with age, and an end to intimate forms of care can typically be foreseen, whereas the functional capacity of frail elders continues to decline, their needs increase, and the duration of caregiving is far less predictable. In effect, many women are faced with "parenting" their own parents, in-laws, or spouse, and may well spend a larger portion of their lives at it than in parenting small children. Home care services and other proposed "solutions" to elder-care dilemmas—training programs in patient care, hospice, job sharing and flextime, for example—rest on unstated assumptions about women's availability and altruism, and about the gender division of labor. Insofar as serial caregiving duties confine women to the home, they limit earning power and access to other valued social roles. Hence they operate to reinforce existing gender inequities, maintain a patriarchal society, and threaten the substantial social and economic gains women have made in recent decades. But the problems of serial caregiving have yet to attract the attention of policy makers.

The dilemmas of caregiving wives are somewhat different from those of caregiving daughters or daughters-in-law. In their research on family caregiving, Baila Miller and Andrew Montgomery point out that "for elderly married couples, caring for an impaired spouse is a normative stage of life and an inherent part of the marriage contract." But because women generally marry older men and because men die sooner, it is much more likely that the average woman will provide care for her husband than vice versa. In two out of three couples, the wife is the caregiver and the husband the recipient. These demographic facts have important implications for women's well-being in widowhood and old age. Relatively little is known about husband-wife caregiving experiences, but caregiving wives seem to feel more depressed and burdened. In one such investigation, many women reported feeling "trapped during a time in their life when finally, they thought, there would be time for themselves," and resenting the situation because they had hoped to leave the caregiver role behind. Some women are troubled by the need to assert control over a now-incompetent husband if he was previously the authority figure in the marriage, and a few fear violent reactions when they attempt to do so.[47]

The prevalence of stress and burden may be underreported by wives (and women carers generally) because of widespread social assumptions about appropriate roles for women. Women may hesitate to tell an interviewer, for example, that a traditional role they are "supposed" to fill lovingly and purposively is instead one they would gladly forgo if options were available. Others may be ambivalent about their feelings or deny their legitimacy because they fear being labeled "selfish" or "ungrateful" or because they anticipate criticism for deviating from the ideal of the "good" wife or "good" daughter. Male caregivers, in contrast, may be more willing to complain because care provision is not a traditional male role.

Women's frustration and resentment may have a strong negative impact on their quality of life and hopes for the future. Elder care is very demanding of the provider, and there are no guarantees about how long care will be needed or what its ultimate effects on her health and economic well-being will be. A woman cannot know at the outset of her commitment how much time, if any, will be left for self-fulfillment after everybody else in the family has been taken care of. This kind of uncertainty may play a large role in the depression and resentment that many women caregivers report. In a recent survey, for instance, investigators found an *increased* sense of burden among caregivers despite their receipt of formal help and their positive evaluation of the support program. They attributed this anomalous result to the fact that most of the caregivers were "powerless individuals with few alternatives to those offered by the bureaucracy":

> The bureaucracy certainly provided them with an incentive, that of marginal support, to care for a dependent family member at home, but it also forced them to continue to assume a large burden. Some of their increased sense of burden may have stemmed from a feeling of helplessness that there was no longer any chance that their life situations could be improved.[48]

Objective measures also suggest the deleterious impact of long-term care provision on women's welfare. First, higher male death rates and age differences between spouses mean that wives are not only more likely to provide care to husbands than vice versa, but that they are more likely to become impoverished by doing so. By the time they are widowed, women may have spent down the couple's joint assets on expenses associated with the husband's final illness. "Since the income and financial resources of a spouse are tied to those of the dependent individual, their choice is to pay for tasks, perform the caregiving tasks, or share the poverty that is required to obtain assistance."[49]

Spousal impoverishment resulting from current Medicaid policies threatens women more than it threatens men. Since Medicaid policies require that spouses be economically responsible for one another, the surviving spouse (typically the wife) is virtually assured to be on the Medicaid rolls, particularly if her institutionalization eventually becomes necessary. American nursing homes are filled with aged widows, many of whom presumably cared for their husband before he died, paying for it with the couple's joint assets or "spending down" to qualify for public aid. Women are thus more likely to be Medicaid patients at admission or to run through their remaining assets more quickly once admitted, because there is less to spend down. The longer the stay, the greater chance of reliance on Medicaid as a payment source, and the proportion staying in a nursing home for five years or more is far higher for women than men. Class distinctions and downward mobility exist even within the nation's nursing homes; as people outlive their resources, they are moved from private to public-aid wings, the latter characterized by noticeably inferior care. Medicaid conversion in the community is an even greater risk for disabled elders; again, women's longer lives and the fact that husbands predecease them put them disproportionately at risk. Thus a widow's last years are much more likely to be spent in poverty than were her husband's.[50]

Substantial numbers of adult children, especially daughters, also provide care to frail elders, often at considerable sacrifice to themselves. Sons tend to become primary caregivers only when a daughter is not available, and their caregiving experiences are significantly less stressful than those of daughters. That caregiving is primarily a female role is also demonstrated by the involvement of many daughters-in-law.[51] And, of course, caregiving daughters and daughters-in-law are likely to eventually become caregiving wives.

Since elder care is typically a long-term responsibility, many women face hard choices about whether to discontinue or cut back on paid work in order to become caregivers, whether to combine caregiving with a job, or whether to stay out of the workforce if they are already out. These are tradeoffs that most men are never required to make. As Table 7-2 shows, women comprise 74 percent of care providers aged 45 to 64—the most likely ages for elder care responsibilities to occur. *Continuous* work, especially at those same ages, is crucial for accumulating assets and ensuring pension availability to avoid impoverishment during retirement.

Women are gravely disadvantaged relative to men on several counts. First, they are likely to have spent other years out of the workforce or as more marginal workers because of childrearing responsibilities, paying the penalty in terms of reduced occupational status, lower income, and fewer benefits.[52] Caring or having cared for children may, in fact, provide a rationale for continuing care provision into middle age or beyond because of the lower opportunity costs associated with less intense or less continuous paid work. Thus women may seem more "logical" candidates for elder care than their husbands or brothers.

The data in Table 7-2 also indicate that women are disproportionately likely to quit a job to provide elder care (four in five who did so were women); since in such cases all taxpayers in the household are not working, federal regulations prohibit them from claiming a Dependent Care Tax Credit, clearly a form of double jeopardy. In one survey, 22 percent of the daughters who were not currently working had quit a job to provide care. Twenty-eight percent of another sample of nonworking women had quit jobs because of the need to provide elder care; a similar proportion of working women were sufficiently conflicted to consider quitting, and some had already reduced the number of hours worked. Women predominate among caregivers who work fewer hours or take time off without pay. Finally, women wishing to enter the labor force may find that caregiving constitutes a serious obstacle.[53]

If caregiving requires quitting a job or cutting back on hours, there are important repercussions for women's future well-being.

"Early departure from the workforce often means sacrificing accrued pension benefits if the required vestment period is not achieved prior to leaving. Group health benefits, life insurance, and wage benefits tied to longevity are also sacrificed." Thus care provision is likely to compromise women's welfare in their own old age and helps explain why women constitute 58.7 percent of the elderly population, but a full 72.4 percent of the elderly poor.[54]

Compared to their male counterparts, women working full time are four times more likely to be primary caregivers. For women who combine the two roles, caregiving interferes significantly with work performance. Absenteeism may increase and worrying about elder care may reduce her ability to concentrate on the job. Her own health may suffer due to the strains of care provision. Work interruptions for care-related phone calls or doctors' appointments are additional distractions. For example, Jean Tyler's husband, a victim of Alzheimer's disease, phoned her frequently at work—he needed reassurance and, later, forgot that he had just called ten minutes earlier and dialed again. By one count, he called her office fourteen times between 8 A.M. and noon. She, in turn, called him often too, because she worried that, home alone, he would hurt himself, forget to eat, or wander off. Jean's morning routine also affected her job performance. She rose at 5 A.M. to prepare her husband for the day, so that she could be at work by 8. She needed extra time to bathe, dress, and feed him because he "played and dawdled," resisted her efforts, undid what she tried to do. Understandably, she was often exhausted and depressed, but they desperately needed the money she earned.[55]

Most studies show that employed caregivers provide as many hours of care as the nonemployed. This implies that rest and leisure are forgone, as in Jean Tyler's case, and that job performance suffers in consequence. Statistics are lacking on the numbers of women who turn down training, promotion, or travel opportunities because of caregiving demands, or are not considered for them because of employers' knowledge of their family responsibilities. Nor do we know how many postpone a job search or job change due to caregiving constraints, or forgo the additional schooling that could lead to a better job. What we do know, however, is that women predominate among the elderly poor and that even women with substantial work histories may find themselves in a precarious financial situation in old age. While some may resist withdrawing from the labor force for caregiving, the current lack of affordable alternatives "may raise the opportunity costs of labor-force participation to the point where the material and psychic rewards it affords cannot compensate for tensions generated by a needy or untended elderly patient." Those who quit involuntarily, however, may face greater personal tensions as a result.[56]

By limiting labor force opportunities, elder care reinforces women's dependence on male earnings and on the institution of marriage itself. The woman who forgoes work experience to provide care to a parent, for example, may be disempowered in her marriage owing to her loss of earnings. "Sons-in-law may question the imbalance in emotional and material resources committed to their wives' families [and] may resent the interruption in plans for the future and the effect of caregiving on the marital relationship."[57] Or the widow who devoted her life to her family is forced to rely on a fraction of her dead husband's pension benefits for her financial needs in old age because she has no resources of her own to fall back on. A woman is also less able to leave an unsatisfactory relationship if she is not financially independent because she is tied down by caregiving obligations. If elder care has economic costs in addition to those associated with more limited labor force participation, the husband's earnings must be stretched further and her dependent status is reinforced. Increasing family financial stress may also cause marital strain. Without the woman's earnings, children's plans for college may have to be modified, a move to better housing reconsidered, vacations and other leisure activities forgone, for instance. Finally, since the duration of elder care is often unpredictable, the average provider cannot plan for an expeditious return to paid work.

As part of a series of caregiving episodes, elder care promises to compound women's current disadvantages in the labor force. Valuable work experience, pension rights, job advancement, and self-fulfillment continue to be sacrificed as caregiving duties extend into middle age and beyond. Women's workforce participation may thus be constrained over most of the life cycle. Like child-rearing obligations, their commitment to elder care is likely to strengthen existing notions that they are intermittent workers and so serve as a rationale for employment practices that maintain the already substantial gender gap in status and pay.[58] For example, employers may hesitate to hire, train, or promote women because they will leave the workforce for caregiving not once but several times during the working ages. Thus women's second-class status in the labor market may be reinforced.

The very limited efforts of private employers to help workers fulfill family care responsibilities do nothing to make long-term care burdens more equitable between the sexes—it is still mainly women who are expected to adjust their schedules and sacrifice pay and benefits. Although flexible scheduling may reduce strains for some, the time spent on paid work versus caregiving is merely rearranged rather than reduced, so there is no real lessening of fatigue or role conflict. Such policies merely encourage women to do more and, since ostensibly they are being "helped" (and may be expected to be grateful), it becomes more difficult to protest inequities. This is especially true of any hidden costs—promotions or training opportunities not offered, for example, are extremely difficult to document.

Employer policies that "allow" workers to combine child care responsibilities with paid work at home may not be truly helpful either. Women may find themselves still confined to the home sphere as children's needs give way first to the long-term care needs of impaired elderly parents and parents-in-law and then husbands. Viewed this way, home work is much more convenient to employers and the public purse than to women's long-term welfare, as it allows both child care and elder care to remain firmly among women's responsibilities.

In short, while gratifications undeniably attach to caregiving, they are largely subjective, transitory, and intangible, whereas many of the costs can be measured objectively (forgone income, loss of pension eligibility, for example) and are substantial. When "helping" means maintaining the *status quo* in the gender division of labor while containing public costs and "family" means primarily women, one sex is still disproportionately burdened. Men and male-dominated institutions in the United States seem justifiably confident that women will not let their children go unfed or unwashed if they do nothing; hence the lack of any substantial shifts in child-rearing burdens. Similarly, the implicit belief that women will take up the slack for needy elders makes social change in this area extremely difficult as well. To date, women's groups have been generally silent on elder-care issues. While individuals are encouraged to adapt and endure, the need for broader social transformations toward more equitable caring arrangements is overlooked even by those most directly affected.[59] Thus the solutions proposed for today's long-term care dilemmas tend to solidify women's disadvantaged position in American society.

In pressing for women's rights to birth control, feminists assumed that freedom from unwanted childbearing would loosen the traditional role expectations that subordinated women in other areas of life. Gains in the educational, political, and work spheres were viewed as impossible without the ability to control their reproductive capacity.[60] Now policies designed to maintain (and reinforce) elder care as a family (that is, primarily women's) responsibility threaten hard-won gains in other spheres. Because women bear the brunt of negative outcomes associated with long-term care and because formal "helps" have serious limitations, policies that move toward more equitable distribution of caregiving burdens (and satisfactions) demand, but are not receiving, close attention from policy makers. The fact that both the public and many professionals talk about caregiver stress and burden in gender-neutral terms has helped to obscure differential impacts on well-being by sex. Elder care continues to be enshrined as women's work, despite its changing nature, duration, and impact, and women continue to be disproportionately stuck in the "compassion trap." Hence it seems that preventing greater resort to death control by enlisting yet more services from families risks grave injustices to caregivers in general and to women caregivers in particular.

Implications for Death Control

Death control issues are salient for family caregivers in their roles as the primary providers of long-term care to disabled relatives, as proxy decision makers for incapacitated elders, and as decision influencers for others. The growth and aging of the elderly population are expected to result in a large increase in the number of incompetents, especially dementia victims, and medical interventions may themselves diminish competence in the last stage of life.

Hence many frail elders who have living relatives will need to have decisions made on their behalf; the assumptions are that spouses are able to speak for one another and that children speak for widowed parents. The most difficult choices for relatives involve incapacitated persons without advance directives. To date, comparatively few Americans have signed living wills; depending on the survey, the proportion ranges from 4.0 percent to 17.5 percent. Even fewer have arranged for a durable power of attorney for health care. This general lack of preplanning makes the responsibilities of caregivers more onerous, since they must make life-and-death decisions with little to go on.[61]

Relatives must also resolve ethical dilemmas involving conflicts between elder care and other important commitments, such as those to minor children. Consider, for example, the complexities of resolving this situation faced by a 41-year-old caregiving daughter: "Being a caregiver and trying to work and raise a family is a tremendous physical and emotional strain. I can never think at work and am always tired. Is it fair to me and my family and my job to do this? Is it fair to my mother not to?" As the duration of care and its associated burdens increase, caregivers often look for alternatives to establish greater distance, physical or psychological or both, from the patient, including institutionalization. Aware of the negative publicity accorded institutionalization, knowing that elders strongly prefer to remain in familiar surroundings, yet unable to cope with the daily demands of caregiving, adult children may feel tremendous guilt when a parent enters a nursing home. They may feel that somehow they should have done more, and repress their feelings of anger, resentment, and burden, making the admission process an emotionally wrenching experience for everyone. But relief may be at least as important an emotion as guilt. In either case, allowing or helping a seriously ill relative to die may be perceived as an alternative to the problems of institutionalization and thus influence family decisions to terminate treatment; patients themselves may suggest it.[62]

Relatives play a major role in determinations to initiate or withdraw life-sustaining technologies. First, in discussions with the patient, the doctor, and one another, they help shape the patient's assessment of the best course of treatment.[63] They must seek information and advice from medical professionals, reconcile conflicting expert opinions, convey information to the patient, if possible, and try to ascertain their relative's best interests if he or she is not competent. For growing numbers of dementia victims especially, they must often make life-and-death decisions without knowing what the patient might have wanted if he could choose for himself. When all is said and done, they have to live with the consequences. Caregivers must be altruistic enough, knowledgeable enough, and strong enough to decide wisely.

It is especially incumbent on women, as the primary caregiver in most caregiving relationships and as the surviving spouse in most marital dyads, to become familiar with new options, discuss them in advance with loved ones if possible, as well as with professionals, and act responsibly in making very difficult decisions about life and death. It is important to realize that men seem to be more favorable to both suicide and euthanasia than women are. One important implication of this sex differential is that women caregivers may hesitate to act on a loved one's wishes even when the patient asks to be allowed to die. Thus the patient's suffering may be prolonged as death is delayed. Or the greater passivity associated with female socialization may cause some women to defer overmuch to male decision makers—doctors, lawyers, ethicists, or relatives, for example. Despite their greater familiarity with their frail relative's preferences, they may hesitate to question, let alone challenge, expert opinions. Since many professionals continue to be influenced by negative stereotypes of women, women's concerns as caregivers to aged relatives may be given short shrift, thus risking a death that is either premature or delayed for the patient.[64]

Inevitably, long-term care provision entails following through to the elder's death. Whether death occurs in an acute-care setting, a long-term care institution, a hospice, or at home, family carers, good or bad, loving or spiteful, generous or selfish, will typically make or influence decisions about its timing and circumstances. So we must ask what happens when new choices are presented, temptingly labeled "death with dignity"? On the other side of the coin, decisions to initiate or continue life-sustaining treatments, when otherwise the patient would die, prolong the caregiving relationship without circumventing the need for further life-and-death decisions down the line. In other words, decisions about terminating treatment may be postponed, but not eluded altogether, and postponement itself has repercussions for both patient and family.

Family carers have little to guide them. The difficult goal is to protect a loved one against decisions that make death premature as well as from those that delay it too long and cause too much suffering in the process. Fifty-one percent of the general public in one recent study reported personal experience with either a friend or relative who needed end-of-life treatment decisions made on his or her behalf. As more families deal with elder care firsthand, caregivers will learn specific coping strategies from more experienced friends and acquaintances; they will share their feelings of anger, resentment, guilt, and helplessness. It seems likely that the death option will be among the coping strategies that are shared, that a growing number of role models will help further legitimatize deliberate death. Eventually support groups for "death with dignity" may take their place alongside those offering help to families of Alzheimer's patients and cancer victims.[65]

How well life-and-death decisions are now being made is unknown, but the evidence cited above suggests serious problems. Especially in light of the existence of dysfunctional families; of caregivers with little or no real caregiving potential; of the burdens and constraints facing many whose intentions, at least, are good; of the likely victimization of many others; of the general failure of social supports to provide sufficient help; of the lack of guidance from courts and legislatures, we would be quite remiss to ignore the considerable potential for poor decision making—that is, not in the best interests of the elder.

This chapter began by asking if more and better informal caregivers could be found, or created, in American society. The conclusion must be a very cautious "yes," but clearly the process will be exceedingly difficult, as many social, economic, demographic, and psychological factors militate against success. But assume for a moment that, against all the odds I have discussed, America does succeed in producing enough willing and dedicated family caregivers to meet the needs of frail elders, and that no one is unduly victimized in the process. We are still left with elders who reject the care and sacrifices of others, no matter how willing the providers. And we are still left with elders who are appalled by the possibility of extreme frailty, dependency, or loss of self to dementia, who prefer to forgo even "comfortable" suffering or "pleasant" senility. Finally, since the purpose of caring is to demonstrate a strong commitment to the well-being of others, to empathize with them in their suffering, and to do one's best to alleviate it, there is nothing in the definition that is incompatible with merciful aid-in-dying. Indeed, there is much that would suggest such aid as the most appropriate form of care in some circumstances. In other words, "caring" may require "letting go." And "letting go," to produce a compassionate, dignified, "good" death, not a lingering "bad" death, may well require help. More and better family caregivers, then, may be conducive to *increased* resort to death control, including "active" means, the same outcome predicted if there are too few providers, if they are ill-suited to the job, if they are too burdened, too poorly motivated, or too selfish to provide adequate care.

Improvements to the Formal Care System as Alternatives to Deliberate Death

Patients may choose active euthanasia primarily because they lack access to effective supportive care....Caring for the terminally ill through the widespread availability of supportive care must be a high priority. This our society has yet to do. Abandoning the effort without even having tried cannot be justified.

Thus the American Geriatrics Society, in a 1990 policy statement, called for more supportive care in order to avoid resort to deliberate death. Although the Society concedes that some might benefit from "active" euthanasia, the risk that others may be abused is too great to press for its legalization. According to Dame Cicely Saunders, a pioneer in the hospice movement, hospice care "is the alternative to the negative and socially dangerous suggestion that a patient with an incurable disease likely to cause suffering should have the legal option of actively hastened death."[1]

The inability of the medical profession to cure the chronic ailments that prolong dying necessitates a transformation of health care priorities from "curing" to "caring," according to prominent ethicist Daniel Callahan, who also opposes "active" euthanasia. A panel of Jewish and Christian theologians, philosophers, and legal scholars recently made the same point. With effort, they maintain, we can return to the traditional wisdom on which the human community and civilization itself are based—an "understanding . . . of the imperative to embrace compassionately those who suffer" at the end of life, "always to care, never to kill." Reflected in all these views is the belief that the patient's desire to die or the family's wish for a quick release if their loved one is too ill to speak is unreliable—too distorted by pain, anxiety, or fear to be credible. Sufficient supportive services would, "care" proponents maintain, calm the fear and ease the pain, so that no one need ever voluntarily choose death.[2]

But although these writers stress the need for reordering national priorities, they do not discuss precisely how a new emphasis on caring can be achieved or, indeed, if it is achievable at all. The importance of good end-of-life care is undeniable. Its requirements include concern, sympathy, and relief of pain and suffering, as well as sufficient personal, medical, psychological, and social support to allow a gentle, dignified, "good" death for everyone. Because it is now well established that families cannot do all of the needed caring work, despite good intentions, most activists call for a mix of private and public efforts to meet the growing challenges. Some of the manifold difficulties of achieving caring objectives in the informal care system, along with the shortcomings of social supports that would allow caregiving relatives to continue in that role, were reviewed in earlier chapters.

Among the "mores and betters" called for from the formal sector are home care and home health care, adult day care and other forms of respite for caregivers, hospice services, and improvements to long-term care institutions such as nursing homes. Simultaneous progress in the recruitment, training, supervision, and backup support of the people who perform these services—home care aides, nurses, physicians, and hospice volunteers, for example—is also crucial. Since many frail elders need but do not receive formal long-term care services, or are underserved, enough "mores and betters" must be provided to cover them too. The efforts of the women's movement to humanize the American health care system by deemphasizing its cold, technological approach and replacing it with a warm, empathic one may facilitate a shift to caring over curing, so they merit comment as well. Finally, a "compression of morbidity," postulated by a number of researchers in recent years, can conceivably avoid or mitigate the problems of long-term care for future generations of aged, so it must also be accounted for in predictions about the prevalence of death control in years to come. This chapter will consider the potential for significant social change in each of these sectors and the implications for death control.

More and Better Formal Services

To a large extent, where one is cared for is irrelevant, since a supportive environment can be found almost anywhere—at home, or in a hospital, skilled nursing facility, institutional hospice, or other formal setting. Appropriate, affordable public services, however, can facilitate choice, respect individual preferences, reduce search time, and lessen burdens on informal providers. The ability of formal services to meet elder-care requirements in American society, and thus limit resort to deliberate death, is explored below.

Home Care and Home Health Care

With a combination of the right "helps" from relatives and the community, many frail elders can remain in their own homes almost indefinitely. Substitution of home care for institutional care is a primary goal of Medicare, Medicaid, and privately managed care plans throughout the United States. Both population aging and reimbursement incentives have encouraged the industry's growth; the earlier discharge of sicker patients from acute-care facilities under Medicare's Prospective Payment System has also increased demand for in-home services. Services delivered in their home are also more congruent with elders' wishes. Since 1980, home health care has become the most rapidly growing segment of the Medicare budget. Can more home care services ease family caregiving burdens, deter deliberate death, and eliminate or reduce indirect forms of death hastening, such as abuse, neglect, and unwanted or premature institutionalization?[3]

Unfortunately, the potential benefits of home care have probably been overstated relative to their true cost. Home health agencies are now providing a variety of more sophisticated services—respiratory therapy, intravenous infusion therapy, and intravenous feeding, for example—to patients with more complex problems. The work thus requires considerable skill and involves highly disabled patients. Yet it is often performed by aides with limited training, and we have little systematic knowledge of its quality. Training requirements vary by state and funding source, but few agencies provide the sixty hours that the National Home Caring Council considers minimal; aides are given little information about the specific case, and direct supervision on the job ranges from negligible to nonexistent.[4]

Nationally, the most frequent complaint about home care services is their unreliability.[5] Late-shows or no-shows are a serious problem for old people who depend on home care workers for meals, medication, and personal care, and can be life-threatening. It is hard to wait for dry sheets and clean clothing, for example, when one has not made it to the bathroom in time. Serious health complications may arise if medication is not administered on schedule, or frail clients may fall and injure themselves trying to attend to their own needs. The uncertainty of not knowing when, or if, an attendant will arrive also causes considerable anxiety for both aged clients and family members.

Other drawbacks in the system include physical injury to clients by aides (intentional or accidental), inadequate performance of duties, attitudinal problems, and theft or financial exploitation of clients. "The potential for fraud and abuse is staggering," according to the president of the Community Health Accreditation Program. Yet monitoring what happens behind the closed doors of thousands of private homes is a challenge currently far from being met by regulatory agencies. Government regulations have had limited scope and effectiveness, mainly because inadequate funding makes regulatory activities a low priority in many states. Hence quality assurance for noninstitutional long-term care is in its infancy, and compliance mechanisms and remedies for inadequate care are generally lacking.[6]

Barriers to effective regulation include the fact that patients are dependent and vulnerable and may be afraid to complain lest they lose desperately needed services. Tremendous problems of coordination also arise, as illustrated, for example, in Susan Sheehan's dramatic account of the efforts, eccentricities, and shortcomings of a New York City home care agency in its encounters with the Quinton family. Recall from Chapter 7 that fifteen different aides were assigned to Mrs. Quinton over a five-month period. Few worked out as hoped: they came late, left early, got lost in transit, or failed to show up; they took other jobs without notifying either the agency or the client; they had personal and family problems that interfered with work; they were slovenly or neglectful; they annoyed the patient with loud music, crude manners, or religious

218 . *Last Rights*

proselytizing. For one reason or another, even the best ones seemed unable to stay on the job for long. Such problems were agency-wide, not specific to the Quintons, and "the case coordinators' Cardexes were rarely the same two days in a row." Consequently, someone "was constantly on the telephone, assigning and reassigning" them.[7] (Note that although Sheehan does not discuss the aides' point of view, it is certainly possible, in the general case, that clients and their relatives may severely try a worker's patience with excessive demands and poor treatment, contributing to the rapid turnover.)

For patients who depend on medical technology, such as intravenous feeding, home care is often not feasible, certainly not without substantial inputs from both family and community services and sufficient private resources to pay for them. These conditions are very difficult for any patient to meet and are likely to preclude home care for most frail elders. At the same time, however, many nursing homes are reluctant to accept technology-dependent individuals, or keep them if they become so dependent, since most homes are chronically understaffed, most employees minimally trained, and financial inducements lacking. Unless state laws prohibit such discrimination, homes are also averse to Medicaid beneficiaries and heavy-care patients, such as those with severe dementia, even when they do not require complex medical services. Hence frail elders and concerned relatives are often caught in the squeeze, forced to resort to in-home care despite its great stresses and possible contraindications because there are no alternatives. Yet even home care does not always work. For example, when his mother became verbally abusive to attendants, physician Charles Jannings reported that the agency refused to send others to help her. A fiercely independent woman, she had vowed never to enter a nursing home. Her way out of this dilemma—suicide.[8]

Respite

In addition to a pool of capable primary caregivers, a backup pool of persons to provide respite for them is needed for adequate long-term care. This is especially true if elders' preferences to remain in the community are to be respected and the institutional alternative—generally (but erroneously) thought to be more expensive—

avoided or postponed. In theory, for example, adult day care provides needed respite to allow family caregivers to continue in that role. Users of adult day care services, however, are typically less incapacitated individuals; their caregivers are those better able to cope with the strenuous demands of getting an impaired relative ready for, and transported to, the facility. Centers tend to reject elders who are severely demented or who suffer from serious physical or behavioral problems. They may be ill-equipped to cope with such clients, staff may resist working with them, or other clients, especially those who are cognitively intact, may be depressed by their presence and drop out of the program. Program coordinators must walk a fine line in devising activities that will both hold the interest of nondemented clients and stimulate the demented, without frustrating either.[9]

Users of respite services are usually middle- and upper-income; since the services are not reimbursed by third-party payers, many low-income families cannot afford them, even with a sliding-fee scale. In order to be cost-effective, for example, adult day care programs must now charge $40 per day. Hence many who desperately need them have limited access to the services. On the other hand, "It is not uncommon...for caregivers to be reluctant to accept respite because the patient becomes (or might become) upset by a respite worker providing in-home care or by the environmental change involved in nursing home respite." Caregivers who do receive services often want, and need, more than is usually available. In one demonstration program, for example, caregivers received in-home respite for an average of only 10.7 days over a one-year period.[10]

Despite the fact that all respite services are rated very positively by recipients, they do not improve caregiver well-being or mental health: they are a welcome temporary relief, but caregivers must then return to an arduous role that becomes more demanding as the elder's condition deteriorates. Recent evidence has also shown that respite services prolonged the elder's stay in the community by only 22 days on average before he or she was institutionalized. When elders are highly impaired and family caregivers exhausted, "continued community care is often simply not possible unless services can actually substitute for the bulk of the sustained care needed on an ongoing daily and nightly basis. Such a plan requires virtually unlimited funds with which to employ three shifts of paid caregivers plus substitutes for staff vacation time, time off, and illness." Moreover, hands-on respite services are typically provided by home care attendants whose high turnover, unreliability, limited skills, and inappropriate attitudes have already been noted. Increasing staff quality has difficulties of its own, including the infusion of funds required, as shown below. Thus it is very unlikely that formal respite services will either save money or deter institutionalization.[11]

Long-Term Care Facilities

In theory, nursing homes and other long-term care institutions relieve family stress and burden by allowing the transfer of care to professionals when it becomes too onerous for relatives to manage themselves. In an ideal world, residential placement would allow frail elders to live out their remaining days comfortably, under the watchful eye of caring specialists while relatives continue to maintain a warm relationship through frequent visits. But finding a suitable, affordable institution with an available bed is often a discouraging and time-consuming effort for families, since occupancy rates for most homes approach 95 percent and many have long waiting lists. The supply of beds has been growing, but has not kept pace with the increasing numbers of potential users, and it is unlikely that enough new beds will be forthcoming to meet demand. Institutions also prefer private-pay patients or, if that is not always possible, those with the least difficult physical, behavioral, and social problems.[12] In other words, the patients most onerous for caregivers, formal or informal, to care for at home are those whom institutions also tend to reject.

Moreover, conditions in many institutions for the aged are a continuing national disgrace, as shoddy care and a variety of abuses persist. Problems range from lack of privacy, dignity, and autonomy for residents to neglect and injury, and, in some cases, premature death. Research suggests that healthier patients receive more humane treatment and that the cognitively impaired are more liable to maltreatment from staff members. For example, two elderly sisters, both severely demented, starved to death in a facility supervised by the state's Department of Human Services.

Weak, confused, and locked in a room by the home's operator, how could they complain effectively? It is worth noting that in this particular case the facility in question was under the supervision of the Adult Protective Services division, which apparently saw nothing amiss.[13]

Many writers have commented on the multitude of resources needed to rectify institutional shortcomings—more money, more staff, more training, more compassion. In 1987, under pressure from Congress, the Department of Health and Human Services proposed sweeping revisions of federal rules for nursing homes. The dual goals are to improve the caliber of care and to protect patients' rights, and represent an effort to cope with the 1986 finding of "shockingly deficient" care in many nursing homes that receive federal funds. But government regulatory approaches for improving nursing home quality are an acknowledged failure, and many marginal or substandard homes continue in operation.[14]

Because the threat of negative sanctions has been largely ineffectual, there is growing interest in positive incentives—rewards, monetary and nonmonetary—for superior performance. Scott Geron, an expert on nursing home incentive schemes, provides an excellent overview of such efforts and their inherent difficulties in over 800 nursing homes in Illinois. For example, some professional raters deliberately manipulated the scoring system to help (or hinder) a home's rating and some operators temporarily rented equipment on the day an inspection was scheduled in order to gain points for a "homelike atmosphere." Most important, however, it was impossible to determine whether the standards used in the rating system really had anything to do with quality of care or whether residents' lives improved as a result of the considerable cost and effort expended.[15] Incentives like those Geron describes may even induce administrators to become more discriminatory in their admission policies, in favor of patients who are less sick, since resident participation in "meaningful" activities, clients' satisfaction with care received, and high levels of resident involvement in the community are among the "quality" indices that are rewarded. These criteria, however compelling, are hardly applicable to the frailest. Indeed, it would seem that the sickest, most recalcitrant, or confused patients would *threaten* the reward structure in such incentive plans and reinforce operators' predisposition to reject those with the most intensive care needs. Hence policy makers who devise incentive schemes must take care to avoid unwanted outcomes.

Another proposal for enhancing the quality of long-term care seems more promising. Sections of the 1987 amendments to the Older Americans Act call for increased community involvement in nursing home life. Omsbudsmen—resident advocates who have a "watchdog" effect and help foster greater accountability among institutional staff—are an integral part of such involvement. Ralph Cherry used a composite index of poor nursing care to show that omsbudsman programs are frequently associated with better care. It follows that if every nursing home had an omsbudsman (not now the case since enactment of the legislative mandate has been uneven), care improvements would be forthcoming. But Cherry's index incorporated only *nursing* care—as measured by risk rates for decubitus ulcers, catheterizations, or antibiotic use, for example—and nursing care is only one component of quality of life, albeit an important one. Thus improving nursing care is not equivalent to improving quality of life, as Cherry correctly notes, because other serious problems, such as loneliness and psychic pain, remain untouched.[16]

Nursing homes, not without justification, continue to be viewed very negatively by the elderly, their relatives, the public at large, and even the professionals who work in them. General-purpose organizations of the elderly have been relatively indifferent to nursing home issues, whereas those who presumably do care (the relatives of residents) are still a small, unorganized, and essentially powerless group, and many residents have no surviving relatives. As one expert put it, "the problem is not that nursing home residents are old or poor or without family or intrinsically hard to provide for, but that they are old *and* poor *and* without family *and* hard to care for."[17]

Little is known about resort to death control, such as decisions not to treat, in long-term care institutions, and efforts to encourage good decision-making practices have been negligible. More important, nursing homes rarely have either the personnel or the equipment required for successful resuscitation of a patient in crisis, when there is no time for discussions of patient preferences, let alone removal to a facility with the proper equipment. Some patients who would have wished to be resuscitated, if they had been asked, may be let die. In such an environment, only the most optimistic could conclude that industry interests, especially in for-profit facilities, will necessarily coincide with the interests of patients, their families, or society. What is the potential for overall improvements?[18]

In his compelling book *Why Survive?*, published in 1975, Robert Butler noted that the deplorable conditions he witnessed in American nursing homes had hardly changed since Edith Stern's 1947 exposé, appropriately titled "Buried Alive." In the last decade of the twentieth century, nearly twenty years after Butler's book, and almost fifty years since Stern's essay, nursing homes are still seriously deficient. In fact, new problems have emerged since 1975, such as a patient population that is both older and sicker. Is there reason to expect that the scholar-researchers of 2015 will no longer have to lament nursing home shortcomings? On paper, these institutions have long been regulated, but in practice the industry has been quite successful in lobbying to develop favorable legislation and block potentially threatening regulations.[19]

In 1980, Bruce Vladeck, an authority on nursing homes and their problems, envisioned a continuation of incremental changes in nursing home policy, but concluded that prospects for radical innovation were meager. Reforms and infusions of money can help, but "will never make nursing homes places where anyone, given a real choice, would ever *want* to live"—the typical home would remain "pretty awful," even when it was clean and well staffed, "because the circumstances, medical and social, of the people living there are extremely difficult to do much about." His conclusions are equally valid today. A case in point is a recent special education program intended to minimize problems of urinary incontinence in nursing home patients. This is important because urinary incontinence is associated with serious health complications, such as infections and falls. Nursing assistants were instructed to follow a particular protocol that would minimize patients' toileting accidents. But little change occurred because other problems remained unaddressed—aides were too busy, did not want to wake the patient, or thought she was too sick, for example.[20]

More generally, *any* change in institutional routine is likely to be resisted, because workers value regularity and wish to maintain "normal" work routines; thus they resent attempts at innovation, especially if they seem to add more tasks to an already hectic schedule. Floor staff may *appear* to comply, but real change is often minimal. Such resistance seems to be patient-neutral, in that workers have no real wish to harm them by resisting change or to help them by enthusiastic compliance. More perniciously, however, powerless clients are liable to abuse that "appears to be a patterned response of the aides and orderlies to their recurring problems of controlling the patients." Again, these problems are largely intractable—they are, after all, the reason many frail elders are institutionalized in the first place. Because aide-patient interactions are typically invisible to supervisory personnel, they may deny that abuse occurs. Patients who complain are labeled as troublemakers, senile, or simply crazy, whereas employees who allege abuse are disbelieved or accused of having ulterior motives, such as a grudge against a co-worker. These forms of denial help perpetuate problems, and some workers continue to slap, hit, kick, throw food and water on their charges, and verbally terrorize them without being detected or punished. Hence improvements in these areas present an enormous challenge to our society.[21]

If conditions are poor, abuses rampant, and circumstances difficult to alleviate, while a desire to avoid institutionalization is apparently universal, why are there waiting lists and very high occupancy rates? The answer is that, bad as many undoubtedly are, nursing homes fill a crucial societal need for housing highly impaired elders who have no place else to go. The nursing home has often been the best of the *available* choices to individuals and families, with patients driven there by lack of alternatives. In the words of one expert, "it is very hard to close an inferior home when there is literally nowhere to place the patients."[22] It is also very hard to fire incompetent or abusive staff when demand is high and few want to do such work. If it is very difficult or impossible to change the clients, the workers, or the institution itself, what do we do next? The great unknown is what happens when another choice—"death with dignity"—is added to the list.

Hospice

Hospice care, whether institutional or home-based, is often promoted as the best way for the terminally ill to end their days without unwanted or futile medical intervention; its palliative emphasis is promoted as the best way to avoid "active" euthanasia decisions. The hospice concept has also been suggested as a viable model for long-term care generally. But can hospice "comfort care" services preclude desire for a quicker death, as the movement's leaders and the Roman Catholic Church, among others, argue? A large part of the debate centers on whether pain control in a supportive environment provides sufficient rationale for dying patients and their families to await a "natural" death.[23]

Sixty percent of all patients are pain-free the day before their death, according to a survey by the National Institute on Aging. For those who do experience significant physical pain in the course of dying, it is commonly believed that the pain can be managed by medical means. However, adequate pain control is exceedingly difficult and requires constant monitoring. Medical training programs devote little attention to methods of pain control. Physicians may be slow or uncooperative or hesitate to prescribe enough drugs to achieve the goal, owing to unrealistic fears that patients may become addicted. Or pharmacies may be slow in filling prescriptions, especially at night or on weekends. In fact, such problems cause considerable tension for many hospice nurses. A good illustration is the actions of Montana's "Hospice Six"—six nurses accused of illegally dispensing narcotics to suffering patients, such as the one heard screaming in pain as the nurse drove up to his home and another found in a fetal position, soiled with feces, after waiting five hours for help.[24]

No individual, looking ahead, can be sure that he or she will remain pain-free or have pain that can (or will) be medically managed, or managed without undue complications. Far more important, however, is that physical pain is not the only consideration, or invariably the primary one. Other elements enter into patient and family judgments about the quality versus the length of life: the unpleasant side effects of pain-killing medications; the symptoms and side effects of the underlying diseases and conditions, ranging from physical weakness to incontinence; the psychic pain accompanying dependency and loss of control of one's body; and the suffering that one's dying causes for significant others. Virtually everyone who is alert to the end will experience these problems to some extent, and they may well be impossible for caregivers, however dedicated, to remedy. Daniel Callahan, a vehement opponent of "active" euthanasia in his books on health care issues, recognizes the difficulties. He believes that "we must persuade people . . . to endure illness and death" rather than escaping it with a technological fix or death by choice. But human history, like the death control movement itself, suggests that convincing Americans to endure rather than escape will be an uphill struggle.[25]

Assuming for the moment that pain can be managed and that only physical pain is relevant, there are other serious drawbacks to hospice. For example, hospice facilities are in very short supply relative to the national need, and waiting lists are common. There were nearly 2.2 million deaths in the United States in 1991; most of the decedents were over 65. Hospice programs serve about 200,000 patients per year.[26] Hence, the great majority of those who die do so without the benefit of hospice care. Although some may not need or want hospice services, others are denied them. While many of us have had to deal with the frustrations of being wait-listed to get into college, or standing in long lines to gain admission to a football game or a rock concert, an entirely different level of fortitude is required for the frail or dying to wait patiently for the possibility of better end-of-life care with hospice. Nonetheless, this is exactly what the current system asks.

Shortages of money, volunteers, and family help are additional problems. Hospice has been criticized for being a white, middle-class movement that primarily serves clients with the same characteristics, and effectively closes out minorities and the poor. Programs also tend to admit those who share the hospice philosophy of life and death, as described below, and this selectivity forecloses the hospice option to those who never considered the issues or can no longer communicate their beliefs. Finally, due to funding considerations and because their terminal condition is more predictable, hospices cater much more to cancer patients than to victims of other devastating illnesses. Hence, for one reason or another, the majority of frail elders are excluded.[27]

What is the hospice philosophy and how is it related to death control? First, hospice workers see patients as informed and active consumers, not passive recipients of services. Great weight is given to the patient's personal definition of quality of life and freedom of choice regarding treatment. But this emphasis on autonomy and activism militates against successful hospice care for frail elders, many of whom cannot or will not decide for themselves. Hospice philosophy defines the dying experience as "a final opportunity for the dying person's personal growth and development" and a chance to serve as a good example to others.[28] These notions are inapplicable to growing numbers of incompetent elders. For example, by the time a dementia victim is admitted to hospice, if he is admitted at all, it is too late for the spiritual growth and human development that the hospice concept envisions. In contrast, the glowing case descriptions of "good" deaths in the hospice literature focus on cognitively intact, often relatively young, patients—those who can be helped to live as fully as possible during the time they have left and to work through their feelings of denial and anger to accept their impending death. Think back to Johanna Florian's last years, described in Chapter 7. How could the hospice philosophy help her find meaning in her dying? To live more fully? To help others?

Other changes within the hospice movement impinge on vulnerable elders' already limited access to services. For example, hospice services have opened up to younger clients (AIDS victims and children, for example), making for longer waiting lists and more aggressive treatment; because the patients are relatively young, they, their relatives, and hospice workers are inclined to fight harder against the disease. More aggressive treatment helps blur the line between hospice care and conventional care, of course. It also raises the cost of hospice care and so will tend to further limit access for frail elders, especially those who are poor or who lack family members to help keep costs down with their "free" services. Finally, in their formative period, many hospices were staffed by volunteers committed to a particular unconventional philosophy. The tendency now is for hospices to hire outsiders to fill critical staff positions and to recruit people with professional degrees or formalized management skills. This too makes it increasingly difficult to distinguish end-of-life care with hospice from conventional care. In any case, indications are that the former may not be appreciably better. Such a finding casts doubt on whether hospice programs are achieving their special mission of facilitating good terminal care and to what extent they can do so for frail elders in particular, given the unique characteristics of both.[29]

More and Better Caregivers

Caregivers are more important than institutions and equipment, especially when it comes to the nonmedical aspects of caring—personal, social, and counseling services, for example—that frail elders need most. Hence the supply of potential caregivers in the formal system is important for predicting the future course of death control in America.

Supply Side Considerations

A wide range of well-trained health care workers will be required to respond to the diverse needs of older people in decades to come. According to the National Institute on Aging, the demand, under any foreseeable conditions, will far exceed the current supply.[30] Those who can afford and are capable of the advanced training needed for better jobs will presumably opt for them. But there are important differences in the outlook for different job categories within the health care sector.

In a recent report, the Office of Technology Assessment was pessimistic about the possibility of substantial improvements to the supply of health professionals with expertise in geriatrics. Barriers to recruitment include ageism, negative stereotyping of both the work and the workers, and relatively low financial rewards. Others present a rosier picture, maintaining that views of professionals who work with the elderly have been improving since about 1970: they are no longer seen as second-class citizens by peers, and working with older people is now seen as a desirable career.[31] Yet we must ask whether these attractions are specific to "curing" occupations, where one works mainly with the comparatively healthy young old, or to the "caring" ones more appropriate to the needs of frail elders. Do they apply equally well to services provided to incompetent clients who cannot get better as they do to competent and appreciative ones who show definite improvement in response to effort expended?

It may well be that many potential workers are far more willing to serve "the old" (envisioning the healthy, competent, young old so newly visible in our society) than frail elders specifically. Or young workers just entering the aging field may simply be unaware of the vast differences within the older population. For example, in a recent book aimed at helping potential professionals in the aging field to understand the field they are entering, there is no mention of job-related stress or burnout, or even of key differences between well elders and frail elders, information that might influence a young person's career choice.[32] Ease of recruitment may vary depending on which subgroup of "the old" is the target for services. When frail elders are the referent, recruitment, retention, recognition, and rewards may continue to differ sharply from those characteristic of work with other segments of the older population.

The health care industry is highly gender-segregated: four of five workers are women, and one in seven of all working women works in the health care field. Within medicine, women are seriously underrepresented in the six highest income occupations and earn less than their male counterparts in virtually all medical occupations. Such inequities must be addressed if the necessary personnel are to be forthcoming. Care work in the formal sector also involves a sexual division of labor in which technological, curative work, which is heavily male-dominated, takes precedence over care work, which is done almost exclusively by women. Nursing work (caring) has long been viewed as inferior to medicine (curing). Geriatric nursing, characterized by the most caring and the least curing activities, is the worst regarded. Moreover, working with demented or incontinent old people is particularly trying. One observer of nursing home life, for example, noted that he "witnessed quite a few cases of aides who left aghast after their first day and never came back."[33]

It is easy to understand why curative work is seen as more prestigious than caring: it is more "scientific," it is usually done by highly trained professionals (primarily men), and it is far more likely to yield quick and often dramatic results. A quadruple bypass operation, for example, may literally pull a very sick person back from the brink of death. Friends and relatives will marvel at the "miracle" and the great skill of the surgical team; they will be suitably appreciative. But the repetitive daily round of "bed and body work" done by nonprofessionals (mostly women) is largely invisible. Much like doing the laundry or washing dishes, these tasks do not *stay* done. The patient's condition does not improve dramatically either, although she will certainly be more comfortable if she is clean and well fed. The most important generalization about the lower valuation attached to "caring" vis-à-vis "curing" is that the former, in its broader sense, has no definable end for workers. When has one "cared" for a patient? When has one cared *enough*? How much warmth, empathy, and comfort must be dispensed before the worker has put in a good day's effort? Can we set standards for the number of hugs and kind words that separate good care from that which is inadequate?

This inability to set explicit limits on caring activities is a source of great distress for care workers. In sharp contrast, curative efforts are far more readily quantified, and one knows when the day's tasks have been completed, the goals attained. Hence their greater attractions are readily understandable.[34] These fundamental differences will have to be dealt with before the medical industry can reorient itself to emphasize care over cure and the growing demand for care workers can be filled. But, as we will see below, current trends within medicine are in quite the opposite direction.

Some attempts are being made to increase the supply and quality of health care workers. For example, new federal regulations since 1987 are aimed at improving training for nurses' aides, in the belief that this will improve resident care and perhaps reduce worker attrition. Yet if the results of recent efforts are any guide, success may prove elusive. The results of the urinary incontinence program cited above, for instance, indicated that the impact of training on aides' prior beliefs and knowledge was limited and, despite their proven effectiveness, the new protocols met with staff resistance. Compliance was low and the analysts speculated that constant surveillance was the largest contributor to the compliance that was achieved, since compliance declined once surveillance ceased. Low compliance has been observed in other studies too, and experts are pessimistic about prospects for significant improvements in nursing homes through mandated education programs. Part of the problem is that efforts to improve the quality of life for residents may increase the workload for already over-worked aides, thus decreasing workers' job satisfaction, increasing their stress level, and exacerbating attrition problems.[35]

There is currently no evidence that improvements have occurred in the caliber of workers entering the lowest levels of the health care system. They continue to be the least educated and most marginal workers, those with the least choice about where to work. Their ranks do include wonderful people who are literally life-savers for frail elders. Yet, due to its combination of high demands and few rewards, such work also attracts the kinds of people that an investigator saw in one home: a staff that "included former mental patients, several men who had criminal records (one was on probation while working at the home),...several people whose bizarre behavior seemed to indicate mental illness, and several men who appeared to be drifters in need of temporary employment."[36]

Nursing home employment now seems more attractive to professional nurses, and salaries have improved. There has also been substantial federal investment in enhancing job skills for these nurses. But what do these better-trained and better-paid nurses do on the job? Unfortunately, much of their time is spent on paper-work and little is devoted to direct patient care. Further, if recently published findings in Pennsylvania are generalizable nationwide, as seems likely, Medicare patients discharged from hospitals to nursing homes are sicker now than prior to the implementation of the Prospective Payment System in 1983. In combination with public policy efforts to prevent institutionalization for those who can be helped to remain in the community, this means that those in institutions are increasingly the oldest and worst off: both the median age of nursing home residents and their degree of dependency have increased since 1960. These dual trends toward residents who are both sicker and older imply a need for more registered nurses, yet staffing ratios (already poor) have failed to improve. This means an increased workload for existing staff and greater difficulties in recruitment and retention.[37]

What about jobs requiring personal, hands-on care—the kinds of help most needed by frail elders? Will they flourish or flounder? The movement of workers into long-term care seems to have lagged behind that into other industries, owing to the undesirable nature of the work.[38] Forms of reimbursement and attempts to control costs, such as "quicker and sicker" releases from acute-care hospitals, will increase the demand for workers, but may well discourage the supply because the work will be more onerous than it already is. So although jobs will certainly open up, they are not likely to be the kinds of jobs that people with choices will want.

On the other hand, those unable to qualify for better jobs will continue to constitute the pool of disadvantaged workers, chiefly women and minorities, who now provide the great bulk of daily care to frail elders. Considerations of quality of care aside, several factors suggest that increases of the size required for this labor pool will not be forthcoming. If more women are expected to stay home to care for frail relatives, owing to traditional expectations emphasizing family care, policy initiatives aimed at increasing the family's caregiving role, and the growth of the frail elderly population, the formal care system will lose some potential workers. But if better pay, benefits, and working conditions attract them into non-care-related jobs in the paid work force, their own frail relatives will need care from formal sources too, further swelling demand for care workers. The alternative is increased pressures on midlife women in particular to hold down two jobs—elder care and paid work. Later marriage and childbearing will constrain some women from both formal and informal caregiving, again limiting the supply of potential workers. On the other hand, economic necessity and such factors as a high divorce rate will impel women to search out the best-paying jobs, regardless of sector. This implies that jobs in the health care field will have to expand pay and benefits in order to compete.

Care jobs at the bottom of the health care hierarchy are very unattractive, as indicated by rapid turnover of personnel such as aides in nursing homes. Such jobs are also characterized by high absenteeism (which increases the daily workload for those who do show up), poor pay, and arduous working conditions for the marginal workers who do them. "Care" is defined minimally in terms of patients' basic bodily needs, cleanliness, and order, and cynicism and disillusionment about helping people under such circumstances often lead workers to insulate themselves—to withdraw emotionally in self-defense. In effect, they stop caring.[39] Aides are generally overworked and face increasing workloads for the same reasons discussed in connection with professional nurses.

Home care work is also done primarily by aides, and it too "illustrates some of the worst features of jobs in the secondary labor market," as it combines low pay, poor working conditions, and little opportunity for advancement with highly demanding work for severely impaired clients.[40] In the present system of long-term care, whether provided in institutions or in the community, the worst-off workers—the least skilled, least educated, and most vulnerable—thus tend the neediest clients.

The list of "mores" that are required for improving the system is formidable, especially for the aides who do most of the hands-on patient care: better training and more selectivity in recruitment to weed out those too troubled to provide care of acceptable quality; more money; more opportunity to move up the job ladder; better benefits, hours and conditions; and, last but not least, more social status and recognition. Making elder-care jobs sufficiently attractive to potential applicants will call for massive additional funding, but this is very unlikely to be forthcoming given the current cost-containment mentality of policy makers and the profit motives of many institutions. It also calls for somehow overcoming the "never done" aspects of care work discussed earlier.

Health care workers may exhibit any of the variety of danger signals detailed in Chapter 7 for high-risk family caregivers, such as substance abuse and mental illness, and some clearly should not be providing care to very vulnerable clients. The neglect that resulted in the deaths of the two sisters mentioned earlier, for example, was perpetrated by an operator who was apparently angry over her recent divorce from the women's nephew, since care had been adequate prior to that point. As this case shows, the oldest and most helpless patients, especially if mentally impaired, are those most likely to be victimized in institutions as well as at home.[41]

But workers include more victims than villains. One observer, for example, refers to those who care for geriatric patients in an American mental institution as "the living pinched and hardened by caring for the dying." Health care personnel at all levels struggle with anxieties about dependency, suffering, and death as they work with the old. Added to the bleak facts of their working lives, the personal lives of aides in particular are filled with a variety of stressors. According to a recent study, 96 percent of home care workers in New York City are black or Hispanic, almost half are immigrants, and two-thirds did not finish high school; on meager salaries, 76 percent are the primary breadwinner for their family, and they average 3.5 children. In another sample, one in five had no health insurance. The result is a situation where "two parties, both powerless, little respected, and hardly recognized by society are made to face each other in a difficult setting not of their own making." Findings from a three-year research and demonstration project that surveyed home health aides in five cities suggest a very discouraging outlook for a home care service market that can provide quality, cost-effective assistance to a growing elderly population.[42]

Yet other serious obstacles to change must be mentioned. These include the negative attitudes and stereotypes of elderly patients that are common among health care workers, including the highest-paid professionals, and the tendency of many workers to shun those who are dying. These attitudes may be a product of their experiences in dealing with highly-impaired aged, on a day-to-day basis, as well as the ageism prevalent in our society. But they too must change if caring is to supersede curing and deter resort to deliberate death. This will be an extremely challenging task. Those who become physicians, for example, tend to decide on a medical career quite early in life, compared to those who choose other professions, and their educational experiences are very different from those of other students—they are more isolated, more segregated with others like themselves, and must cope with more demanding courses and schedules; the practice of medicine is also very isolating and practitioners are largely divorced from mainstream culture. These characteristics of medical recruitment and training suggest that persons with particular characteristics are attracted to the field and that interventions to produce more caring physicians must take account of those characteristics and must begin early. In fact, doctors who demonstrate a humanistic orientation to medical care appear to be people who developed this orientation before attending medical school. They maintain this outlook in spite of, not because of, their medical training, which militates against humanistic doctoring. For example, in the first two years of medical school, students are presented with far more material than they can possibly learn; in order to survive they must be very selective about what topics they focus on. In these circumstances, the first material to be discarded is information on the "soft," social aspects of medicine.[43]

Descriptions of humane and caring encounters between physicians and patients are very rare in accounts of medical training. Although doctors talk about caring, training experiences themselves often prevent or discourage it. Compassionate doctors exist, of course, but are seen so infrequently that they become medical heroes. In general, technical skills are far more likely to be recognized and rewarded than caring skills. Medical training is part of the problem, as physician Frederic Hafferty relates:

> Traditionally, medicine has sought to establish lines of demarcation between the "art" and the "science" of medicine and therefore between science and caring. Such distinctions attempt to favor an impersonal over a personal approach to knowing. One need not journey far into medical school to hear students rhetorically asking each other whether, when seriously ill, they would prefer to be attended by a knowledgeable (technically skilled) or a caring (and therefore presumably less skilled) physician. The question, very much a part of the oral culture of medical training, frames the dimensions of skill and caring as exclusive or incompatible.[44]

After reviewing several studies of medical students, Jerome Avorn (a physician himself), concluded that "for many, the processes of bedside medical education and the socialization that is part of medical training seem to bring with them a transformation from idealism to cynicism or, at best, apathy." If their role models view elder care as frustrating, students are likely to pick up the same attitude. Part of the problem is that, within medicine, teaching is disvalued. In a report on medical education, for example, the American Association of Medical Colleges concluded that teaching medical students "often occupies last place in the competition for faculty time and attention." Medical education in the care of the dying has long been inadequate, and continues to be despite our aging population. A recent survey of schools for medical, nursing, and social work students found "no evidence of a consensus on the need for death education for health professionals, no evidence of systematic development of course content or approach, and no evidence of any attempt to integrate training and facilitate collaborative team care in this area." There is also a national shortage of geriatrics faculty, which translates into few role models for medical students. Finally, since medical training focuses largely on techno-logical, instrumental interventions in any case, there is little hope for major substantive change toward greater humanitarianism on the part of American physicians in the foreseeable future.[45]

Like other professionals, physicians learn to be emotionally detached from the people they serve. They are not taught how to talk to patients and sometimes make fun of them with crude jokes and gallows humor. At times, the pressures of work make patients seem like the enemy. Care that is time-consuming or emotionally draining, for example, may deprive doctors of sleep, slow down their progress to other patients, whose needs are also compelling, and result in stress, frustration, and depression; understandably, individuals strive to protect themselves by minimizing their involvement. Since many doctors carry prejudices about the treat-ment of old people, geriatric patients are particularly disadvan-taged by those who see little reason to dedicate great time and effort to people whose problems seem to resist all efforts at solu-tion.[46]

The history of reforms in medical education shows that changes occur very slowly. In fact, there have been frequent efforts at cur-ricular reform in the last fifty years but, in the words of one critic, they represent a "history of reform without change." Further, there is no evidence that teaching physicians the humanistic, psy-chosocial, or cultural aspects of patient care actually does make them more sensitive doctors. Educational interventions to produce doctors who are better attuned to the needs of patients also do nothing to eliminate the structural barriers that inhibit change. These include a continuing emphasis on the scientific aspects of medicine and a medical system that virtually guarantees that in an emergency patients will be treated by strangers ignorant of their values, history, preferences, or family situation. Efforts to control costs and maximize profits also help to ensure that patients are handled as speedily as possible, so these too militate against more time-intensive caring activities.[47]

There are indications that not only are professional workers not entering "caring" fields in sufficient numbers to meet the demand, but also that these areas are becoming less attractive over time.

Despite predicted shortages of primary-care physicians, for example, medical students' interest in such careers has been eroding in favor of better-paid "high-tech" specialties, which also offer greater prestige and more regular hours. High-tech fields are also attracting the better students, as measured by class rank. The main reason for this marked shift is that caring specialties such as internal medicine involve "talking to patients, listening to patients, and in general thinking about the patient's problems," activities that "represent extremely hard work with much emotional involvement" and relatively few rewards. In addition, limits on payments to physicians under the Medicare and Medicaid programs may inhibit recruitment to geriatrics in particular.[48]

For professional nurses in today's complex medical organizations, a dedication to "Tender Loving Care" is highly disvalued. Registered nurses are seldom involved with direct patient care, spending their time instead on medical treatments, dispensing medication, supervision, and paperwork. "The ambitions of nursing leaders for the elevation and 'professionalization' of nursing" are partly responsible for the trend away from caring activities. Salary structures, prestige, and authority within nursing accrue to technological expertise and administrative roles, not hands-on patient care. To move up in this hierarchy means to move *away* from patients. As one nurse put it, "the mystification of knowledge" associated with technological medicine is very seductive to nurses, and the ability to use complex equipment is highly rewarded in comparison to "comforting" activities. In her words, "we like the awe we inspire by manipulating the tubes and wires and numbers; it is another distancing maneuver, putting us closer to physicians and farther from patients and families."[49]

It is commonly thought that time and task pressures are to blame for the lack of true caring on the part of medical personnel, and that additional staff or a smaller workload will fix the problem. But this conclusion is untenable. Complaints about inadequate staffing among nurses, for example, seem to be merely an excuse for avoiding closer relationships with patients. Studies show no significant relationship between the number of nurses on duty at a given time and patient ratings of quality of interaction, for example. Nurses use the increased time for personal activities and are more bored and restless as time and task pressures are reduced. One idealistic young nurse explains how even peer pressure works to distance nurses from patients. When she tried to sit with a dying patient, other nurses thought her actions "peculiar," and the charge nurse assigned her another patient because she did not seem "busy." After several months, she too began distancing herself from patients. Even death itself did not elicit "caring": "We showed little feeling about the patients who died, and if the relatives required much time consoling, we called the chaplain." Again, the desire to distance themselves from too-close involvement with patients reflects, in part, the absence of clear end points for caring work and confirms how difficult a shift to caring over curing may prove in practical terms.[50]

All this leaves the "caring" work, by default, to the lowliest workers—the aides, orderlies, and subprofessional nurses—and suggests that a reordering of priorities toward caring activities will necessitate fundamental changes in the organization of professional nursing and its reward structure. As with physicians, there is considerable prescriptive, idealistic talk among nurses about the importance of caring. But when it comes to actual practice, there is little caring to be seen.[51] If even those at the highest levels of the health care industry, who stand to gain high pay and prestige for their efforts, are demoralized, cynical, or apathetic, what should we expect of the poorly trained and minimum-wage workers at the bottom?

In short, if the desirability of working with older people is indeed changing in a positive direction, this does not automatically translate into a preference for caring over curing, nor to an enhanced desire to work with the frailest elders. There is no evidence that antipathies to the intimate, personal dimensions of health care work with frail, demented, or dying patients have changed over time. In fact, the literature on stress and burnout in the medical profession strongly suggests that both are closely associated with working with the least "curable" clients. While there can be little doubt that improvements in wages, benefits, and working conditions will attract workers to the health care sector, there is little likelihood that we will soon see a transformation substantial enough to attract and retain the numbers needed. Further, there is no guarantee that caring will improve as a result, since we also need to convince health care workers that maintaining the lives of the frailest at great cost and with great human effort is important, especially when patients too are obviously suffering. Unless additional workers can sufficiently alleviate nonmedical forms of suffering, there is no guarantee of gains in quality of life for frail elders either. Thus even in the unlikely event that all the other "mores" are achieved, frail elders would still suffer because many of their problems are not amenable to either a medical or a social "fix."

Volunteer Potential

Volunteers are included in the formal care system because they must be recruited, trained, and supervised by representatives of that system. The notion that volunteers from the private sector can provide many badly needed services to frail elders is appealing. Little systematic research has been done on volunteer work, but many researchers and planners advocate their use in the belief that a large body of citizens, especially retired people with time on their hands, can be encouraged to perform important services for others and keep costs down at the same time.[52] And the concerned layperson may not be inhibited from truly caring by the professional biases and institutional shortcomings we have discussed.

In fact, most older volunteers spend very little time at it. In 1989, for example, more than half of all volunteers aged 65 or older worked less than five hours a week, and 77.4 percent worked less than ten hours; only about one-third worked year-round. Professionals are often wary of volunteers, with good reason. Because they are unpaid, there is no way to assure their dependability, their availability when needed, or their continuance in service following expensive training. Volunteer work is likely to be low priority when a volunteer must choose between it and some competing activity, for example. Whatever their value in other important social endeavors, volunteers constitute an inadequate pool of workers for very dependent elders whose well-being, and life itself, require that care be highly reliable rather than sporadic or intermittent.[53]

Perhaps volunteers can relieve the primary caregiver rather than assume major responsibilities themselves? Indeed, volunteer respite care has been widely recommended for its potential in supporting family caregiving and thus reducing pressures on the public purse. Few researchers have studied the feasibility of using volunteers specifically to provide occasional respite to families with highly demanding elder-care responsibilities. Two who did found that costs and staff time both exceeded expectations, whereas recruitment, matching volunteers with an appropriate family, and scheduling all proved very troublesome. Moreover, although duties for the volunteer were extremely demanding, the possibility of reward was very limited. Volunteers were expected to act mainly as companions to frail elders, rather than hands-on caregivers, and to derive their reward from the "companion" relationship, while freeing the primary caregiver for other activities. But almost half (45.6 percent) of the elders in the survey could not even be interviewed due to their extreme frailty, and many were mentally impaired, making it difficult or impossible for volunteers to provide companionship. Some patients and caregivers also tended to resist the "outsider" or were reluctant to ask for help with certain tasks.[54]

As a consequence of the various problems, only a small minority of eligible families received volunteer services. At best, respite was provided for four hours every two weeks; it was almost impossible to arrange respite for evenings, weekends, or emergencies, since volunteers were typically available only at certain days and times. Finally, many caregivers were performing complex care routines for severely disabled elders, tasks volunteers could not do without "close supervision and extensive training." There is also the personal discomfort (on both sides) that is likely to arise when laypersons attempt to perform intimate services for strangers—dealing with incontinence, for example. These factors help make volunteer respite of doubtful utility for caregivers as well as their charges. The experiences of programs in Ohio to aid caregivers of Alzheimer's patients had similar outcomes: expectations of using volunteer companions to provide in-home respite proved unworkable. Home health aides—the costlier but still problematic alternative—had to be used because care recipients were so highly impaired. So although families need and want the help, it is prohibitively difficult for volunteers to deliver because many elders are too disabled.[55]

Volunteers are a critical part of hospice because they expand the availability of services to more people and help to contain costs;

but researchers have found that keeping volunteers is an uphill struggle—up to 80 percent can be lost after training, and more leave after a few months on the job. Volunteers also report numerous work-related stressors, and some feel a need for a support group to help them deal with their grief after a patient dies. Burnout among volunteers is a serious issue. Moreover, recent dropoffs in volunteers threaten the viability of hospice care as a cost-saving alternative—its justification for reimbursement under Medicare and other third-party insurance plans. Thus the kind and duration of care needed, the degree of responsibility for very impaired clients, the risk of stress and burnout, and the difficulties of recruitment, supervision, and coordination of volunteers all diminish the potential of volunteer assistance for frail elders.[56]

Job Satisfaction, Stress, and Burnout

Are caregivers in the formal sector also *victims* of the system's inability to draw the line as to when continuing care is futile? Since they freely choose their jobs for the most part, this might seem paradoxical. But a growing literature on stress and burnout among medical workers, including professionals at the top of the hierarchy, suggests otherwise. Despite the fact that health care workers voluntarily self-select into their various fields, no group—aides, nurses, physicians, or hospice volunteers—seems immune from risk. Experts disagree about whether burnout is inevitable; some believe that it is simply a matter of time on the job, but others think it can be prevented or at least controlled.[57]

If caregiving is intrinsically satisfying, as many have claimed, why is so much stress and burnout reported by people who chose' it as their life work? According to one specialist, it is precisely *because* professional health care workers are more sensitive to the suffering of others that they are attracted to such work in the first place. Since they are dedicated to helping people in trouble and want to make a positive difference in clients' lives, they are frustrated when this proves difficult or impossible. Moreover, others have very high expectations of them—as more knowledgeable, caring, and altruistic than the rest of us, for example. Since workers often internalize these high expectations, the risk of stress and burnout increases when, as inevitably happens sooner or later, expectations are not met. They may end up deliberately distancing themselves from the very people they set out to help. Ironically, however, it is hard for workers to admit their frustrations and seek help: "People with careers based on helping the less fortunate are not supposed to become weary of their clients, dislike some of them and their coworkers, or wish not to be bothered with them, let alone express such feelings." Instead, they withdraw, become cynical, and ever more frustrated with their caring role.[58]

Those working with the terminally ill are particularly vulnerable. But attempts to manage chronic, but not life-threatening, illnesses such as dementia can also be enormously frustrating for practitioners; trained to cure, they are confronted with an incurable disease of long duration that requires a wide variety of supportive services that produce no measurable improvement in the quality of life of the recipient. Burnout is "a reaction to chronic, job-related stress...characterized by physical, emotional, and mental exhaustion," and having a wide variety of deleterious effects—sleeplessness, depression, substance abuse, family and marital conflict, feelings of powerlessness, and so on; victims may lose all sense of commitment and caring. The consequences of stress and burnout are serious and extend beyond providers to their families and care recipients as well. "Most standard medical textbooks attribute anywhere from 50 to 80 percent of all diseases to stress-related origins," and medical evidence links stress to changes in the body's ability to fight disease. Significantly, burnout involves workers who question their effectiveness on the job and the value of the job itself; intervention, such as counseling sessions, may or may not help them regain their enthusiasm, depending on how, and whether, these questions are resolved.[59]

To understand stress and burnout, we must consider what elements of care provision to the old, the frail, and the dying contribute to workers' job satisfaction and what elements are stressful. In a recent survey, for example, long-term care nurses reported that appreciation and recognition from patients was their prime source of satisfaction. Home health workers talk of "feeling needed and useful" and a "sense of accomplishment in making a critical difference" to someone's life. There are many such reports, but a major shortcoming in their interpretation is that respondents were not asked to distinguish among different categories of clients.

Which elders are they referring to? Are reactions the same for elders who are mentally competent, friendly, and appreciative, versus those who are "pleasantly senile," versus those who are severely demented or hostile? What of elders who differ greatly in background from the aide or those who treat her like a servant, or whose relatives do?[60]

Staff members at adult day care centers feel stressed by the declining health of their clients and by how much needs to be done to improve their quality of life. In nurses' reports of sources of job stress, 64 percent indicated that patients were a source of stress. Patients whose condition is visibly deteriorating, who do not respond to treatment or have no desire to get better, who do not recognize or appreciate the nurse's work, or who seem to be suffering needlessly because of inappropriate use of medical technology are prominent among the stressors listed. By definition, frail elders exhibit many of these stress-inducing characteristics.[61]

Heavy caseloads also challenge workers' coping skills, and we have seen that workloads are increasing for many. Health personnel must deal with all this in addition to the numerous stresses all of us encounter in daily life, and many are poorly compensated to boot. Women are especially disadvantaged because they comprise the vast majority of caregivers in both the private and the public sphere, a combination that can give rise to "contagion stress." Women experience significant negative effects of caring on their health, but women facing high care demands both at home and at work are at greater risk of mental and physical health problems. Contagion stress may include worrying about the problems of others and feeling helpless to assist them. A woman who is a social worker all day *and* then goes home to a handicapped child or a disabled parent is, on average, at greater risk of health problems than a woman who does one *or* the other.[62]

For nurses' aides, job satisfaction is associated with feelings of being needed, positive reinforcements, and good relationships with residents and their relatives. Aides "tend to be acutely aware of how little they are doing for each patient, and of how inadequate the services are," with demoralization frequently following. According to a recent study, aides who were highly motivated to provide high-quality care were also very likely to quit "because they just couldn't live with the contradiction between what they wanted to do and what they were able to do."[63]

The distress to nursing home staff arising from residents' disruptive behavior (verbal and physical abuse inflicted on aides, for instance) has hardly been studied. For aides, as for other health care workers, the potential for good interpersonal relationships with frail elders is limited, since many, especially those who are severely demented or otherwise highly impaired, are unable to express appreciation for services rendered, are uncooperative, or hostile. Gerontologist Jaber Gubrium's vivid descriptions of "bed and body work" at Murray Manor attest to the difficulties such patients entail for caregivers, particularly when they slow down an already rushed aide's busy schedule by "dilly dallying," false alarms (about the need to use the bathroom, for example, which sometimes serves as a way to get attention), and other "excesses" that seem to deliberately disrupt her work. Hence it is hardly surprising that both staff burnout and patient aggression are good predictors of patient maltreatment. In one recent survey, for example, one in ten staff members admitted that they had personally committed at least one physically abusive act—deliberately intended to cause physical pain or injury to a patient; four in ten admitted to psychological abuse, such as threats or insults intended to cause emotional upset. Further, many institutional patients are unable to get better and may have little desire to go on living. The oldest and worst off are also the least likely to have family members, grateful or not. Hence the trying aspects of their care may seem both futile and thankless. This is not to suggest that no satisfaction is possible from work with the frailest, but that it is generally more difficult to attain, and sustain, than with other kinds of patients. If satisfactions are limited, recruitment of workers is more difficult and stress, burnout, and job turnover more likely.[64]

The fact that health workers in many different job categories experience stress and burnout suggests that improvements in pay and benefits will not necessarily enhance job satisfaction or reduce negative outcomes for themselves or clients. Our knowledge of caregiving satisfactions is far too limited to allow us to conclude that caring work is *uniformly* satisfying to those who perform it, regardless of the recipient's characteristics. If the characteristics of frail elders have a major negative impact on providers' job satisfaction, even substantial improvements in pay and benefits will fall short of eliminating worker stress and burnout.

At first glance, hospice burnout is more puzzling than burnout in other health care sectors. Why does severe burnout exist among care providers who made a deliberate choice to work with the dying, among patients who are often selected because their end-of-life treatment choices correspond well to hospice goals? Stress and burnout among hospice workers are positively correlated with time on the job. But other important factors about hospice care encourage negative outcomes for some workers. For example, the hospice concept stresses patient autonomy and "death with dignity," viewing the last stage of life as a meaningful time for further personal growth and for living life to the fullest while learning to accept death. But there are serious discrepancies between worker expectations about helping patients achieve a good death and the realities of extreme frailty and prolonged dying. Hospice caregivers want to help patients die well and want to be present when death occurs. The timing and circumstances of death are highly uncertain, however, even in the relatively controlled environment of an institutional hospice. The worker cannot know whether she will be there when the death occurs, whether it will be peaceful or painful, or how helpful her own role actually was. These uncertainties contribute to stress and burnout. Other primary stressors include feelings of helplessness and anger over inadequate symptom control and pain management that may inhibit the good death that workers envision. Dealing with families and unresolved family conflicts can also prove stressful, as when grieving relatives push the worker away or when they argue about money or property in the patient's presence. Frail elders, especially those who are severely demented or whose dying is very prolonged, are seldom the kinds of patients whose dying, given current hospice ideology, can make workers feel good about their work: they have little or no remaining potential for the kind of closure that hospice ideals envisage.[65]

The psychological impact of spending one's working life inside the nation's long-term care institutions is a topic deserving of more attention than it has yet received. How are providers affected by high proportions of elderly patients requiring services that are transient in time and produce no tangible product that others can see or evaluate, often provided to people who are unresponsive or uncooperative? Obviously workers need support services to enhance their coping skills and keep them on the job. In recognition of these facts, caring for the caregivers has become an important new field within the health care sector. Adult day care staff need respite, "appreciation days," and "staff recognition events." Hospice workers need support groups and grief counseling. Physician stress and burnout are probably underreported, and doctors need to be trained to recognize their stress and admit that they too need care; their families need to learn to provide support to the physicians. Health care team members, in hospice or elsewhere, need to support and encourage one another. And finally, of course, family caregivers need counseling, understanding, and respite from the formal system, so they too must be included in the target population for supportive services. For some services, in fact, it is unclear to professionals whether their client is the patient or the caregiver. All this implies, ironically, that those who care for the caregivers may themselves become victims of stress and burnout in the course of their helping activities and, in turn, require care—a phenomenon I call "caregiving involution." We have not yet begun to consider the dimensions of this problem, let alone its consequences.[66]

If overwork and other job stressors cause staff to long for the death of "troublesome" patients, as anthropologist Maria Vesperi discovered from her work in nursing homes, this suggests that some deaths may be unduly hastened or that nothing might be done to avert a life-threatening incident for some vulnerable elders. On the other hand, those who work most closely with frail elders may be more willing now than in the past to terminate treatment because medical technology has gone too far and they have seen too much. An intensive survey of nursing personnel suggests that this is indeed the case, citing "too much exposure to inept medical performance" and "a certain reserve concerning medical heroics," especially for elderly patients.[67]

Interviews with physicians suggest that, with experience, most intervene less aggressively with their elderly patients; they also become more concerned with ethical issues and undue prolongation of life. Similarly, a nurse reports that "technology began to lose its rosy glow as I saw more patients being kept alive on machines when it was apparent to me that they were dying." Because the technology is typically applied without due regard to patient values, some medical workers are coming to reject its indiscriminate use. If these lessons are passed on to students in training, greater resort to death control—a tilt in the direction of letting/helping go—is a foreseeable result of the production of more humane, holistic doctors and health care workers generally. Already, individual physicians are coming forward to admit that they help patients end their lives. Nurses engage in "daring acts of guerrilla nursing," such as turning down the percentage of oxygen pumped through a breathing machine, in efforts to reduce a patient's suffering. Hospice staff sometimes administer lethal injections at the patient's request, and there seems to be considerable overlap between hospice staff and membership in the Hemlock Society, with its goal of legalizing physician-assisted dying; the two groups sometimes exchange speakers and refer patients to one another. Finally, the question of how workforce experiences influence caregivers' personal and family choices about death and dying has yet to be investigated, but carryover effects from work to family (and vice versa) are likely.[68]

More Money

In our current long-term care system, better care in institutions or in the community is available mainly to those able to finance it out of private funds. The growth of a marketing mentality apparent in the trend toward corporate medicine and for-profit institutions is not encouraging for those who need long-term care, especially nonmedical services, or for the poor. Likewise, continuing efforts at cost containment are not encouraging. Due to Medicare's Prospective Payment System, hospitals and physicians now have powerful economic incentives to be more selective in the treatment they provide to Medicare patients, especially when the cost of care may exceed available payment. Some doctors are refusing Medicare patients because of recent reductions in the payments they receive from the program. On Medicare-covered home care services, cost concerns are likely to increase and, in the interest of cost containment, a shift to paying for more complex medical services at home for the *acutely* ill is predictable because this is seen as cheaper than hospital care. Consequently, experts expect that the problems of *chronically* ill old people whose needs are mainly for custodial and supportive services (usually not covered by Medicare or other insurance) will continue to be pushed aside until an acute episode makes them eligible for services or they become poor enough for Medicaid assistance. But whereas ten years ago, almost all of Medicaid's long-term care spending was on elderly nursing home residents, today they must compete with younger recipients, such as AIDS victims and disabled children, for increasingly scarce dollars. Like the frail aged, these people too are living longer despite their infirmities, and the number of AIDS patients in particular is escalating rapidly. The near-poor unable to qualify for Medicaid find no long-term care options in the public sector.[69]

Although surveys show that the public supports increased spending for long-term care, opinion polls seldom ask respondents to make tradeoffs with education, law enforcement, or other compelling programs in order to finance them, so their results should be interpreted with caution. The market for custodial home care services is financially unattractive to the business community because the potential for profit is low. In addition, "policymakers are appalled at the budgetary implications of any expansion [of home care] that would even begin to approach the extent of 'need' they believe exists," fearing that demand will become uncontrollable as informal caregivers relinquish their unpaid services to the new programs. Finally, experience with home care has now thoroughly dispelled early hopes that nursing home costs would be reduced. Efforts to attract (and keep) workers in the long-term care industry will inevitably push costs up too. For example, a recent demonstration project aimed at recruiting nonpracticing older nurses back to work in long-term care facilities, where staff shortages are endemic, suggests that such efforts would cause costs to rise through several avenues. Before they would consider returning to work, the nurses wanted guarantees of shorter work days, flexible hours, adequate professional staff, and sufficient orientation and training. All reasonable requests, but unlikely to help curb rising costs.[70]

Nursing home expenditures are also expected to rise dramatically in decades to come, since the number of residents aged 85 and above—the most functionally incapacitated group and those least likely to have family help—is projected to increase fivefold from 1980 to 2040; the proportion of all nursing home residents 85 or older will rise to 56 percent by 2040, from 37 percent in 1980.[71] Of course, these calculations assume that the average nursing home, with a waiting list, will accept heavy-care patients if it has a choice. Those who cannot afford to pay for services themselves may also be rejected in favor of private payers as, indeed, they already are. For patients who are both poor and have heavy-care needs, the outlook is undeniably grim.

A new concern with costs has emerged within the hospice movement, a concern not contemplated by the pioneers of the movement and "symptomatic of the enormous change in attitude that hospice care professionals have gone through in a relatively brief period." Cost concerns were instrumental in forging recent new federal regulations allowing terminally ill patients to use their Medicare benefits for hospice services; the arguments for coverage emphasized cost-effectiveness as well as the view that hospice care is a humane alternative to traditional terminal care. Other aspects of the new legislation seem to favor quicker deaths, or at least do not discourage them. For example, Medicare reimbursement is limited to 210 days of hospice care per recipient, and a hospice cannot discharge a Medicare patient once he has been accepted—regulations that encourage hospices to accept patients likely to die relatively quickly (as they have historically) and deny access to others who need benefits for longer periods. These factors promise to facilitate the growing tolerance for euthanasia already apparent within the hospice movement. It is thus unlikely that hospice services for frail elders considered eligible for them will deter deliberate death, and they may actually encourage that option.[72]

The same legislation contains incentives favoring home-based hospice, again with cost containment in mind, but serving to limit access for familyless elders, on the one hand, and contain costs at the expense of relatives or workers, on the other. The cost reductions anticipated by those who drafted the new rules will be achieved largely by shifting the burden of care to families, who may be ill-prepared to accept it. Paid workers in free-standing hospices seem to experience significantly less burnout and a greater sense of accomplishment than workers in either hospital-based or home health agency-based hospices. But since free-standing hospices and paid workers are the most costly forms of hospice care, more stress and burnout among workers are predictable if the cheaper alternatives are chosen.[73]

Finally, experts are now questioning whether hospice care either provides superior terminal care or saves money. A recent study found no significant differences in such objective measures as survival time, hospital days, pain, or the number of invasive diagnostic or curative treatments that were performed; hospice costs were the same as or higher than those for conventional care. If patients are not carefully selected to screen out those likely to incur heavy costs, hospice care costs can exceed those for conventional care. The most functionally disabled patients and those whose prognosis (time to death) is less certain are unlikely to become eligible for hospice care. Very old patients are also the least likely to have the strong family support or financial resources that hospice requires in order to remain cost-effective. Thus, however attractive hospice may be in theory, access for frail elders is severely limited whereas, for those admitted, a "good" death in the absence of deliberate control is very uncertain.[74]

Reliance on the private sector to provide services and especially to hold down the public costs of long-term care is widely touted. Policy analyst Alice Rivlin and her colleagues investigated the feasibility of various private-sector options for long-term care. These included private long-term care insurance, continuing-care retirement communities, social/health maintenance organizations, and home equity conversions. Each potential solution had serious obstacles to its widespread acceptance or use, leading the researchers to conclude that even with optimistic assumptions about the extent of participation, "private sector approaches are unlikely to be affordable by a majority of elderly, to finance more than a modest proportion of total nursing home and home care expenditures, or to have more than a small effect on medicaid expenditures"; *public* spending for long-term care will still grow substantially in coming decades.[75]

Other researchers have also studied the potential of long-term care insurance. Now in its infancy, the increased use of such insurance may greatly enhance demand for services, either home care or nursing home care. And it may do so at an earlier stage of disability. That is, people who have the insurance will be inclined to use it. Those who live long enough to deplete their income and assets and live past the benefit period covered by the insurance will become Medicaid-eligible. Hence if efforts to promote long-term care insurance do not control utilization to limit insurance-induced demand, Medicaid expenditures are likely to increase, threatening the cost-containment efforts that motivate promotion of such policies in the first place.[76]

Rivlin and her colleagues also investigated a number of public sector options for financing long-term care, such as family responsibility laws, support for family caregivers, and expanded home care. Their conclusion is to advocate coverage of long-term care under a general social insurance program like Medicare. Significantly, however, this will necessitate both substantial tax increases and costsharing by beneficiaries; very strict definitions of disability would be required in the case of home care, both to keep down public costs and to control increases in service use.[77] Thus even this "best option" plan would allow substantial numbers of frail elders to fall through the cracks.

Other funding schemes include plans to control Medicaid costs by stricter enforcement of existing regulations regarding asset transfers—that is, preventing those who can afford to pay their own long-term care bills from transferring their assets to others, such as their children, in order to qualify for public monies. A New York woman, for example, transferred assets large enough to earn $168,000 in interest annually; by thus "impoverishing" herself, she was able to qualify for Medicaid-financed home health services. Like her, many of those who transfer their assets—usually to a relative—are middle- or upper-income. One expert has proposed that more diligent enforcement of the Medicaid rules will force middle-class elders to choose between public funding for their long-term care or the preservation of their estate. This will presumably encourage frail elders, and their adult children, to buy long-term care insurance or seek home equity conversion because both generations have a strong interest in preserving the estate. But both alternatives do work to reduce the size of the estate. For instance, the insurance may have a large deductible, limit what is covered, and fail to take account of the impact of inflation. All of these will increase the elder's out-of-pocket expenses over and above the cost of the premium. Home equity conversion allows elders to exchange equity in their homes for cash payments, which they can use for other expenses such as long-term care, so it too reduces what is left for heirs. Thus an unintended effect of such attempts may be to encourage a quicker death—both for individuals who do not wish to dissipate their estate in the course of "preserving" it (out of concern for survivors, for example) and from relatives anxious not to jeopardize their inheritance, especially if a frail relative is suffering and claims to want to die.[78]

The Women's Movement

Historically, caregiving has been women's work, especially with respect to the hands-on, intimate forms of care needed by both young children and frail elders. Women generally are believed to be nurturing and empathic toward those who are suffering. Thus one might ask if the women's movement will expedite a shift in national health care priorities from curing to caring. Feminists have been outspoken critics of the biomedical model, which has emphasized the technological medicine and curative approach whose shortcomings helped inspire the death control movement. They claim that medical excesses are the result of a male-dominated system of medicine deficient in the feminine values of care and concern for the whole person.[79]

The women's movement has also championed individual rights with regard to medical care and freedom of choice in reproductive matters. And it was women who founded the hospice movement as an alternative to serious inadequacies in conventional care of the dying and as a reflection of feminine values. But to date the women's movement has devoted little attention to elder-care issues, focusing instead on reproduction and parenthood.

Our national experience with child care, however, suggests that the power of the feminist movement to induce social change within a reluctant system may be very limited. Despite the continuing emphasis within the movement on the importance of adequate child care, especially for mothers in the paid workforce, little has changed. Elder-care and child-care services in the formal sector often compete for the same marginal workers; conditions of work, pay, benefits, and promotional opportunities are limited for both sets of providers, and both suffer high turnover rates. Salaries and benefits have failed to improve fast enough to draw workers to the child-care field, and many more attractive jobs are available to workers who might otherwise provide child care; parking lot attendants earn more than most full-time child-care workers, for instance. How well will frail elders fare in comparison with the nation's children? The conspicuous failure of reformers' efforts to produce adequate child care in this country belies optimistic assertions that a substantial constituency for long-term care reform, consisting of disabled elders, their caregivers, and potential caregivers, will soon mobilize to demand social change. Experience also casts grave doubt on hopes that working baby boomers, now entering the peak elder-care ages, will campaign aggressively for employee caregiving benefits. This did not happen with child care as millions of baby boomers passed through the prime child-rearing ages. Is there any reason, then, to expect a stronger mass movement to materialize for elder-care services? Is it reasonable to predict a more consequential response by employers or government to employees' elder-care obligations than to their child-care needs? More likely, the women who somehow manage two full-time jobs, combining child care with paid work, will simply be expected to add elder care as well, as indeed they already do. Then all the constraints on family care provision and resulting family perceptions of advantages to death control, as discussed in Chapter 5, will come into play.[80]

In *The Feminization of America*, Elinor Lenz and Barbara Myerhoff examine how women's values are changing both public and private life in America. They claim that the women's movement fosters "the emergence of a new social consciousness and a growing awareness of the need for a more balanced, more compassionate society."[81] Will it also facilitate increasing acceptance of death control? Since women are the primary caregivers to frail elders in both the formal and informal sectors, they often witness their suffering at first hand; they are also disproportionately burdened with caregiving obligations under the current system, and often victimized by the system as well. Finally, women are the primary *recipients* of long-term care. For all these reasons, women have a large stake in death control outcomes. Hence there would seem to be scope for social change in the direction of greater compliance with individual preferences for aid-in-dying if women's values hold sway.

Will growth in the number of women physicians—from 7.5 percent of medical school graduates in 1969 to over 33 percent by 1989—help discourage the excesses of technological medicine? Among medical students, women are initially more interested in patients and their emotional problems than men are. But these gender differences tend to disappear as medical education progresses. Attitudes toward patients converge in a "male" direction, as women's interest in the social and pyschological aspects of patient care declines. Thus expectations that more women in medicine would resolve problems of distance and impersonality remain unfulfilled—the documented trend thus far has been in the opposite direction.[82]

On the other hand, women physicians are more likely to practice in primary care specialties, with their emphasis on close personal contact and communication with patients; they also spend more time with individual patients and seem to value openness and honesty with them more than their male counterparts do. All these attributes can also facilitate decisions to let die or to help die, as well as more caring attitudes in general. However, neither the frequency of deliberate death nor qualitative differences in the care provided to frail elders by the gender of the provider have been investigated, so there are no empirical data on patient outcomes on which to base conclusions. According to the few published reports available, the American physicians who have provided aid-in-dying to patients are exclusively male. Women physicians are still underrepresented in positions of power within medicine, limiting their influence at the societal level. But women's values, insofar as they gain greater sway in American society, are quite consistent with choices for deliberate death as part of an improved emphasis on caring and personal autonomy.[83]

The Compression of Morbidity

Pessimistic evaluations of science's potential for solving human problems have often been proved wrong. So should we be too quick to dismiss the possibility that some combination of medical advances, technological gains, changes in individual behavior and life-style, and disease prevention efforts will extend the disability-free period of life, while the period of morbidity, extreme frailty, and terminal decline is "compressed" into a much shorter interval? This would reduce the need for both medical care and long-term chronic-care services and their associated personal, family, and societal costs. How close are we to an ideal scenario where everyone remains healthy and independent for many years and then dies quietly (and quickly and cheaply) in his sleep? Future changes in this direction will not help the many who are now suffering, of course, but what of generations to come? Are the problems of extreme frailty and prolonged dying just a temporary aberration in the long view of history? Will they eventually solve themselves, with the help of the scientists?

Most studies of the potential for morbidity compression are not optimistic; in fact, they suggest that the prevalence of serious functional disabilities in the older population will increase in the foreseeable future. Improvements in medicine and life style may indeed help postpone the onset of potentially *fatal* diseases, such as cancer or heart disease, and enhance survival prospects for their victims, as is already happening. But longer survival does not mean the condition is, or can be, cured. Often, it is just *managed* better than in the past, with drugs and surgery, for example. In contrast to these gains in the control of potentially fatal ailments, there is no clinical evidence to support the notion that the chronic, *nonfatal* diseases of aging may be prevented or postponed by medical advances. Examples of such disabling but nonfatal conditions are degenerative arthritis and the various senile dementias. Little is known about the causes of these conditions, and they are difficult or impossible to prevent. Furthermore, the *severity* of such disabling conditions increases as individuals age, and researchers now see little hope that medical advances can change this either. Finally, longer lives are also characterized by the simultaneous presence of *several* serious health problems, not just one.[84]

Life expectancy has risen dramatically in the United States in the twentieth century and is expected to continue increasing for perhaps the next fifty years. This means that the period of time from the onset of a disability until death may increase, not decrease, as proponents of "compression" hope. And as sick people live longer without being cured, disabilities will become more concentrated among the oldest old—where they are difficult to manage without considerable help from others. Increasing pressures on acute-care hospitals, long-term care institutions, and other health resources are likely too, as the absolute size of the disabled population increases.[85]

The improved survival of persons with debilitating diseases and functional impairments gives them (and their caregiving relatives) time to develop new, additional debilitating conditions, time for existing conditions to worsen, and time also to deplete the psychic and monetary resources essential for coping with their situation. Hence quality of life at the oldest ages may not improve because the intensity and duration of disability and dependency threaten to increase, not decline, with gains in average life expectancy. Greater reliance on public services and public funds seems inevitable. Because a compression of morbidity is too far in the future for anyone now alive to anticipate, we must return to where we started: growing perceptions of advantages to death control.[86]

Implications for Death Control

As we have seen, current long-term care options are sorely inadequate and meaningful reforms slow, difficult, and expensive. Although debates about long-term care have intensified in recent years, there is little consensus regarding how it should be organized, delivered, or financed as a coherent national policy and none seems to be forthcoming.[87] What can we expect if substantial improvements in formal care services, which I believe are unlikely to materialize soon, prove to be achievable after all? What if good-quality home care is accessible to all who need it? If more nursing homes are built, amply staffed, and effectively regulated? If hospice care is available to everyone who wants it, regardless of how prolonged or costly his needs are? If enough humane, loving caregivers are trained? If caring is rewarded with prestige and promotions at least as much as curing is? If stress and burnout are virtually eliminated?

In the final analysis, improved services and better institutions are only stopgap measures—postponing but not resolving critical decisions about the timing and circumstances of death. More and better caregivers and more and better institutions may mean *greater* resort to deliberate death, not less, as "caring" becomes more consistent with "letting go" and, if necessary, "helping go."

Some caregivers are already convinced by their own experience, and more will follow. A good example is Dr. Howard Caplan, who recommends legalizing "active" euthanasia because "ten years of practice in geriatrics have convinced me that a proper death is a humane death. That's either in your sleep or being *put* to sleep."[88] More caring caregivers and more humane institutions thus may well facilitate more timely deaths in accord with individual and family preferences.

The "mores and betters" have not yet become a reality, however, nor are we well on the way to becoming a nation where caring is on an equal footing with curing, let alone preeminent. Those who advocate a person-centered, caring medical system, unfortunately, provide few instructions for the appealing transformations they envision.[89] Since so much caring work, especially with the frail elderly, is poorly remunerated, barely acknowledged, and performed largely by the most disadvantaged workers, one must ask if the combined characteristics of care providers and care recipients explain the paucity of meaningful reforms: the majority on both sides are poor, weak, and powerless; most care recipients are further disadvantaged by gender identity (they are preponderantly female), advanced age, and frailty itself; providers are often both female and members of disadvantaged minority groups. Trapped in a health system, and a nation, run largely by healthy, wealthy, white men, the chances for significant change seem slight until and unless these marginal, disvalued groups somehow become socially valued or powerful enough to command the necessary resources. Since this seems improbable in the short run, it is likely that society will continue to perceive advantages in condoning explicitly or implicitly (by failing to discourage) attitudes and behavior that facilitate more timely dying as one way to ration scarce resources and control public spending. Thus, *success* in creating the "mores and betters" may increase the acceptability of a deliberate, quicker death as an act of caring and compassion. Likewise, our continued *failure* to produce them promises to result in the same end—increasing tolerance for deliberate, quicker death—but for different, less admirable reasons.

Hazards of Death Control

Problems of increasing frailty, prolonged dependence, and lingering death necessitate appropriate responses for coping with them. Clearly, individual attitudes and behavior must change, and social institutions with them. Growing perceptions of individual, family, and societal advantages point to a solution: increased resort to deliberate death and a move to more humane, gentler, and quicker means. Ideally, competent individuals will freely decide the timing and circumstances of their own death. Barring that, a proxy will act responsibly in accordance with the prior instructions and best interests of the patient. However, as the discussion of advance directives in Chapter 6 suggests, these ideals are very hard to achieve in the real world. Here I elaborate on other limitations of the death control "solution"—its shortcomings, dangers, and the new problems that come in its wake.

Whatever the option, in a diverse society divided along lines of gender, race, class, and culture, not everyone has an equal chance of obtaining it. Are some people more likely to have their preferences respected (or sought) than others? Are medical personnel prone to giving up more readily in some cases? Are other patients kept alive too long? Will treatment be withheld or withdrawn for the wrong reasons? Will the choices offered to patients vary, based on their ability to pay or social standing, for instance? Who may be protected with advance directives and who may be left out? No one knows the answers to such questions, because they have rarely been asked, despite the national ferment surrounding other death control issues. Even in the Netherlands, where euthanasia is more freely practiced, there is a paucity of empirical research, the government publishes no regular statistics, and doctors rarely record cases of euthanasia on the death certificate. This means that no one really knows the extent of the practice or the characteristics of the recipients.[1] Nor do we know how many requests are denied. The atmosphere of secrecy that now surrounds negotiated death thus not only assures privacy to all parties, but allows scope for abuse in the form of premature death or delayed death.

Gerontologists, social workers, and historians, among others, have long suspected that sex, race, class, and other factors beyond an individual's control affect diagnosis and medical treatment. For example, even when clear-cut, "objective" diagnostic criteria are available, cultural stereotypes based on sex and race influence psychiatric diagnoses and, presumably, treatment. If a patient with a legitimate physical complaint is dismissed with a prescription for sedatives because "it's all in her head," the real problem may not be diagnosed or diagnosed too late. Doctors often use strongly pejorative terms such as "turkey," "crock," or "brain stem preparation" for patients who, in their opinion, are of low social worth, suffer from chronic or self-inflicted illnesses, or have diminished mental capacity. Doctors clearly believe that such people would be better off dead, but the patients do not die; on the other hand, they do not get better either—hence the extreme frustration of caring for them. So doctors try to "get rid of" them in other ways, as detailed in recent descriptions of medical training and practice; for example, they may transfer them to another department or to a different hospital, where staff, in their turn, try to move them elsewhere or back to the first institution. Some experts believe that these behaviors represent healthy coping mechanisms that allow physicians to handle the frustrations of their work. Others contend that "medical slang displays a blunted capacity to care and a deeply dehumanizing orientation to patients which blames them for their illness, views them as potential learning material, and jeopardizes their care." But direct observation of interactions between doctors and patients is a relatively new area of research, little more than a decade old, so we do not know nearly as much as we should about these life-and-death encounters.[2]

Questions of race, class, and gender have been particularly neglected in accounts of doctor-patient interactions. But we do know that the doctor's power as an authority figure is greater when the patient is female, poor, or nonwhite than it is for the opposite categories, and we can infer from this some potential hazards of death control. In all societies, whether "primitive" or "modern," those with few or no resources are at greater risk of maltreatment. Just as "the elderly" are not a homogeneous group, neither are "the frail elderly." Thus we focus now on possibilities of premature death or delayed death that may derive from characteristics of the care recipient or his surrogate, in particular gender, class, and ethnicity. Note that these are not discrete categories, but overlap, creating potential for additional risk among those with a combination of disvalued characteristics. For example, women are the majority of frail elders and are more likely than men to be poor and spouseless in old age, and some minorities suffer disproportionately from poverty and ill health. We begin with gender issues, followed by discussions of class and ethnicity.[3]

Gender Issues

Biological factors and lifelong behavioral differences tend to produce different health problems for the two sexes in old age. From birth on, boys in our society are socialized to be strong and stoic; girls are expected to be physically weaker, more emotional, and more expressive about their feelings. These stereotyped expectations imply that one sex is "allowed" to complain about health problems and take on the "sick role" rather readily, whereas the other is "encouraged" not to. By adulthood, male socialization may lead some men to delay seeking medical assistance, so their health problems may be more advanced, and hence more life-threatening, by the time treatment begins. In contrast, women visit physicians more often; they receive more diagnostic services, more lab tests, more prescriptions, and more follow-up care. Women may request more services or physicians may offer more because they think this is what women want, what they will tolerate, or what they are willing to pay for.[4]

In the American health care system, reports of disrespect for women are frequent because health workers often reflect the disregard for women so prevalent in the larger culture. Many women receive most of their health care from gynecologists, most of whom are men. One critic, himself a gynecologist, reports that his colleagues, like male physicians generally, "bring their male prejudice against females and their need to be dominating and controlling to the doctor-patient relationship." Moreover, the attitudes about women that they absorb while growing up are often reinforced during medical training. The result, according to the same insider, is that "it is common and acceptable among practicing gynecologists to speak about their patients and their patient's bodies, sexual behavior, or medical problems indiscriminately, in terms that are demeaning and reflect a lack of simple kindness and respect." Images of women in advertisements in medical journals are highly distorted: women are often negatively portrayed as "depressed, dependent, emotional, submissive, excitable, passive, home-oriented, lacking in self-confidence, and as sex objects"; older women "are characterized as disturbed." There are also differences in the way men and women are diagnosed and treated. For instance, women suffering from end-stage renal disease are less likely to receive dialysis than men with the same condition; this is primarily due to the fact that women patients are older, on average, than men patients. Further, women on dialysis are 30 percent less likely to get a kidney transplant (considered superior to lifelong dialysis). There is also evidence that cardiovascular disease in women may not be diagnosed or treated early enough. Widespread cultural misperceptions, shared by medical professionals, that men's social roles are more important and their contributions to society greater than women's may well contribute to such discrepancies. Hence it would be premature to conclude that the American medical system is gender-neutral.[5]

Critics also suggest that many physicians believe that women are more demanding and more burdensome patients, and that they are harder to care for than men. But studies of physicians' attitudes toward male versus female patients are relatively rare and their results have been inconclusive, in part because attitudes are very difficult to measure. When questioned, for example, doctors may "censor" their responses and give answers that are "socially acceptable," but not entirely truthful. Our lack of knowledge on this crucial aspect of medicine itself constitutes a potential hazard for patients. Sex bias and physician stereotyping may disadvantage both sexes: assuming a woman's physical problem is an emotional or psychosomatic one is poor medicine, but so is treating a man's emotional problem as a physical ailment, an assumption which may cause the physician to deny him emotional support or psychiatric care. Like the rest of us, if physicians fall prey to social stereotypes, they fail to see each person as a unique individual. The need to rise above stereotypes is never more important than near the end of life, when death control decisions are made.[6]

Men have higher death rates than women at every age and the average man dies seven years sooner than the average woman. This gender gap in life expectancy is expected to continue into the foreseeable future. Hence women dramatically outnumber men among the elderly, and the female proportion continues to increase with each successive increment in age. More years of life are not always a blessing, however, since every added year allows an existing malady to worsen or an additional problem to develop. When several chronic diseases coexist, there are serious negative effects on the person's independence, happiness, and outlook on life. Women are much more likely to survive to the extreme ages where multiple chronic conditions have accumulated; men, in contrast, are more likely to die at younger ages, following illnesses of relatively short duration. Greater female longevity is particularly important with regard to the prevalence of dementing disorders, since dementia patients constitute the largest definable population of long-term care recipients.[7]

Table 9-1 documents sex differences in morbidity for community-based (noninstitutionalized) elders. The data indicate a greater extent of difficulties among aged women than among men. There is also substantial worsening with age for both sexes. Within each age category, and for virtually every type of activity listed, the percentage having difficulty in performing it is higher for women than for men. By age 85, for example, more than four in ten women have trouble walking and about three in ten report difficulty in getting outside, bathing or showering, or preparing meals. Among very old men, in contrast, about three in ten have trouble walking, whereas about two in ten experience difficulty in getting outside, bathing or showering, or preparing meals.

Frail old people unable to remain in the community must transfer to long-term care institutions and rely more heavily on the formal care system. Table 9-2 presents data on the functional status

TABLE 9-1

Percentage of Community-Based Elderly with Difficulty in
Selected Life Activities, By Age and Sex: United States, 1984

Difficulty in	65–74 Male	65–74 Female	75–84 Male	75–84 Female	85+ Male	85+ Female
Walking	12.9	15.1	18.3	25.7	32.2	43.3
Getting outside	4.5	6.5	7.5	15.3	21.8	35.4
Getting in/out of bed or chair	4.8	7.0	5.9	11.2	12.7	22.2
Bathing/showering	5.6	6.9	9.2	14.2	23.1	30.1
Eating	1.5	0.9	2.5	2.4	4.3	4.4
Dressing	4.4	4.2	7.3	7.7	14.1	17.7
Using toilet	2.4	2.7	3.6	6.5	10.0	15.9
Controlling urination	5.0	6.8	8.8	11.2	13.0	19.6
Preparing Meals	3.0	4.8	6.0	10.5	18.4	29.5
Shopping	4.6	7.8	9.6	18.4	26.8	41.6
Managing money	2.8	1.8	5.4	6.8	19.0	26.2
Heavy housework	11.2	24.3	15.9	36.4	33.3	54.2
Light housework	3.5	5.0	6.2	10.5	15.2	27.4
Number (000s)	7,075	9,213	3,128	5,121	585	1,312

SOURCE: National Health Interview Survey, 1984 Supplement on Aging, adapted from Tables 38-44 in R. J. Havlik, B. M. Liu, M. G. Kovar, et al., "Health Statistics on Older Persons, United States, 1986," *Vital and Health Statistics*, Series 3, No. 25 (Washington, DC: U.S. Government Printing Office, 1987).

TABLE 9-2

Nursing Home Residents Age 65 and Over by Sex, Age, and Functional Status: United States, 1985

Functional status	65–74		75–84		85+	
	Male	Female	Male	Female	Male	Female
Needs help in dressing	64.2	73.8	71.1	77.7	77.3	82.9
Needs help in using toilet room	42.5	47.8	45.9	48.5	50.8	57.3
Difficulty controlling bladder	6.4	7.0	11.0	11.0	13.6	11.7
Difficulty controlling bowels and bladder	24.1	29.6	31.3	34.5	33.9	36.4
Can walk with help	17.2	22.4	23.4	25.3	30.5	29.5
Chairfast	33.4	33.9	36.3	39.6	43.0	45.9
Bedfast	4.4	7.5	4.9	6.6	4.2	7.5
Needs help in eating	32.9	33.8	32.3	41.7	39.2	45.1
Vision partially impaired	8.7	10.8	16.8	13.2	17.0	19.7
Vision severely impaired or lost	4.2	6.5	6.5	6.0	10.6	11.9
Hearing partially impaired	7.6	7.3	19.4	13.0	27.7	24.8
Hearing severely impaired or lost	0.6	2.0	2.2	2.1	9.9	7.2
Number	80,220	131,880	140,630	368,370	111,230	483,470

SOURCE: 1985 National Nursing Home Survey, calculated from data in Tables 57 and 59 in R. J. Havlik, B. M. Liu, M. G. Kovar, et al., "Health Statistics on Older Persons, United States, 1986," *Vital and Health Statistics*, Series 3, No. 25 (Washington, DC: U.S. Government Printing Office, 1987).

of elders confined to nursing homes, the majority of whom are women. These data confirm that many institutionalized elders cannot manage the most fundamental life activities without assistance. Again, women tend to be worse off than men on many of the measures listed.

The statistics in these two tables indicate that women are the primary recipients of long-term care, both formal and informal. Data from the 1982 Long-Term Care Survey show that 1.6 million non-institutionalized disabled elders received unpaid assistance; six in ten were women. They may require the help of others for years, even decades, and so are vulnerable to all the negative repercussions (social, psychological, economic) of prolonged dependency, as both ageism and sexism operate in tandem. Their greater longevity and consequent accumulation of chronic, disabling conditions, amid rising concern with the costs of medical and long-term chronic care, suggest that women will be disproportionately affected by public cost-containment measures and implicit health care rationing. In a context of continuing negative stereotypes and persistent social devaluation of women within medicine and in society, the facts suggest that frail aged women are more vulnerable than their male counterparts to death-hastening decisions made by others. Hence death control issues are particularly salient for women.[8]

Because women generally marry older men, because men die sooner, and because women are less likely to remarry following widowhood or divorce, spouses (the first line of defense when care is needed) are less available to them. Hence they are more likely to have to rely on children or nonkin for necessary care. Such care is generally more perfunctory and also more easily relinquished when it becomes burdensome. And it is more likely to *become* seriously burdensome in the first place because women live longer and accumulate more chronic health problems; since these tend to become increasingly severe over time, they necessitate more complicated and prolonged care and hence greater demands on providers. Nonspousal caregivers, including adult children, are better able to withdraw from the patient, physically or psychologically, as her condition deteriorates, she becomes more demanding, or role conflicts or sense of burden intensify—all circumstances that make institutionalization more likely and help to explain why women predominate among residents of long-term care facilities.[9]

"By all attributes of status, the very frail old woman is among the most powerless of persons, vulnerable to all the indignities of age, poor health, the lower social status accorded females, and uselessness." Those in poor health, especially the cognitively impaired, are much more likely to be abused, including abuse by family members. Most studies suggest that women are more likely than men to be victimized by serious elder abuse, both at home and in institutions. Neglect is also concentrated among the oldest and most impaired elderly. Since women live longer and thus tend to be more impaired, especially by dementias, they are particularly vulnerable. Yet the major geriatrics textbooks devote little attention to the medical implications of women's longer lives.[10]

Some particular problems in the American health care system affect the two sexes differently, as shown below.

The Acute-Care Bias

The acute-care orientation of health programs and institutions disadvantages older women disproportionately compared to men. The serious mismatch between the types of services needed by frail elders and the services generally available has already been noted. But Medicare's exclusion of chronic care services burdens women far more than it does men, and its bias toward inpatient hospital services means that proportionately fewer of the health care needs of aged women are covered. In consequence, women are exposed to greater financial liability because they must pay for needed services themselves. Government unwillingness to address or redress these imbalances and societal tolerance of the inequities help reinforce women's second-class citizenship. Recent proposals in Congress to reform America's health care system are likely to overhaul the troubled acute-care system first, according to congressional observers, postponing long-term care reforms to some indefinite future date.[11]

Physical health problems are consistently associated with a higher risk of suicide—the primary form of premature death—at the older ages. Men have long had higher rates of suicide than women; the gender difference is greatest in old age. But the gender gap in suicide rates may be smaller than it appears, for two reasons. First, official figures are likely to be extreme understatements because, unless the evidence for suicide is overwhelming, doubtful cases are attributed to some other cause of death. Second, women outnumber men in suicide attempts that are unsuccessful, perhaps because women are more averse to such proven lethal instruments as guns. In nursing homes, men are more likely to engage in *direct* suicide attempts (slashing their wrists, for example) whereas women typically choose *indirect* forms of death-risking behavior, such as refusing to eat or to take prescribed medication. In short, the two sexes may be equally desirous to end their lives, but women seem to prefer gentler, more passive means, which are also less effective. Since sleeping pills take time to work, for example, someone may find the suicide attempter, rush her to the nearest emergency room, and so "save" her from death. Interestingly, the eight people who have committed suicide with Dr. Kevorkian's help (with or without his famous "suicide machine") have all been women. Since physician-assisted dying is both gentle and highly effective, it is reasonable to expect that more women will successfully end their lives if this choice becomes more readily available. This will reduce or eliminate any gender gap that now exists.[12]

In other contexts, existing medical technology that could prolong life or improve its quality (and perhaps prevent suicide) may not be made available to some elders because of "medical discrimination" that views such care as futile; older men with prostate cancer, for example, are less likely to receive the best available treatment than their younger counterparts. Other options may not be presented because the patient has limited ability to pay for them.[13]

Chronic Care in Home and Community

Elders of both sexes strongly prefer remaining in their own homes to any form of institutionalization, but health programs that depend heavily on families to provide care are more disadvantageous to women. Home care requires capable and willing assistants, and women are less likely than men to have a spouse or other supportive family member available to help them remain in the community, especially at the oldest ages. The feasibility of home care also varies with the patient's condition and the specific types of help required; again, women are relatively disadvantaged because their greater longevity allows the accumulation of more chronic conditions, which, in turn, complicate care provision. Owing to their higher incidence of poverty in old age, women also have less ability to pay a nonrelative for necessary services not covered by insurance (and most supportive services are not covered). As frail women live on to very advanced ages, their informal care providers, usually other women, are also aging and may be accumulating chronic conditions themselves that can impede continued caregiving. For all these reasons, women's preferences for remaining at home are less likely to be met than those of men, and they are much more likely to be institutionalized. Of course, community-provided home care and home health care are not without serious difficulties either, as discussed earlier. The quality of the care provided and the extent of mistreatment sustained by home care clients are hard to document. But, other things being equal, women are more vulnerable to abuse and neglect.

Long-Term Care Institutions

Approximately three out of four nursing home residents aged 65 or older are female, and the proportion female rises substantially with age. Women are six in ten of all residents aged 65 to 74 but seven in ten of those 75 to 84 and eight in ten of those 85 or older. At ages 85 and over, one in four American women, compared to one in seven men, lives in a nursing home. Some never married, and most of the rest are widows. One in three residents has no living children, and the children of the oldest patients may well be elderly themselves. So, as for the problems of old age in general, the problems of long-term care institutions are primarily women's problems.[14]

Awareness of one's low-priority status, exacerbated by age and frailty, has physical, social, and emotional consequences for quality of life and will to live. Women who spent their lives as housewives, mothers, or marginal workers may continue to be devalued in the institutional setting, whereas former "productive" workers (primarily men) may be seen as more deserving of sympathy and support on the basis of past contributions. Recall also that the oldest and most helpless patients, especially if mentally impaired, are those most likely to be victimized in institutions. Since elderly female nursing home residents suffer proportionately more memory impairment, disorientation, senile dementia, and chronic organic brain syndrome than men, they are disproportionately at risk. We know little about the circumstances surrounding the use of life-sustaining treatments in nursing homes, but a number of small studies suggest that nursing home residents are less likely to receive treatment than patients in acute-care hospitals; older residents, those who are cognitively impaired, and those without family, along with those having multiple diseases—all more likely to be women—are at greater risk of nontreatment and possibly premature death.[15]

Hospice

In-home hospice care, increasingly emphasized in public policy because it is less expensive than institutional hospice, requires a supportive, cooperative family which, for reasons noted above, women are more likely to lack. With its emphasis on palliative as opposed to curative therapy, moreover, hospice care, regardless of locus, may encourage patients to accept death too readily or to reject life-sustaining therapies too soon if it seems that professionals have "given up" on them.[16] If differential socialization produces women patients who are more passive, more susceptible to authority, or more anxious to please, particularly with respect to male physicians, they are especially vulnerable to the risk of premature death in the hospice setting. The same risks, of course, apply to incapacitated relatives of either sex for whom women ostensibly make end-of-life treatment choices.

Rationing

Within the elderly population, frail elders require a disproportionate number of health dollars and caregiving hours. There are important gender differences in ability to pay for care, whether home-based or institutional services are sought. Older women have less in the way of personal financial resources and are less likely to have private health insurance than their male counterparts.[17] They are not only more likely than men to be widowed but also more likely to have spent down the couple's joint assets on expenses associated with the husband's final illness. If they limited paid work to provide care to relatives (including children) in the past, they also inadvertently jeopardized their long-term economic security.

Spending down to qualify for Medicaid also affects the two sexes differently. Since Medicaid policies require that spouses be economically responsible for one another, the surviving spouse (typically the wife) is very likely to find herself on the Medicaid rolls, particularly if her institutionalization becomes necessary. The longer the duration of stay in a nursing home, the greater the risk of impoverishment and reliance on public funds. In turn, the lack of personal resources has a negative impact on the quality of care received. As one 74-year-old woman put it: "All the financial security I had when I came in here ... vanished down the drain.... When the last penny was gone, I became a Medicaid patient." She describes the humiliation, inferior medical and dental care, and decline in living conditions that her reduced circumstances entailed.[18]

Since women predominate among frail elders, it is primarily women for whom funding would be curtailed or access denied in cost-containment or rationing schemes. Rationing on the basis of age, which is seriously considered by some policy makers, will inevitably disadvantage old women as a group more than men, since the former are more likely to survive to the extreme ages and rely more heavily on publicly financed health care. The combination of societywide economic woes and continuing social devaluation of aged women may thus lead to unnecessary suffering, untreated (but treatable) conditions, and premature death, as health care cost concerns become more pressing. Restriction or denial of medical care may also encourage suicide among the elderly of both sexes if they are left to choose between deprivation and death.[19]

Questions of Competence

Experts agree that appointment of a guardian is biased against elders who are simply eccentric or noncompliant rather than mentally incapacitated. Again women may be more disadvantaged than men. Cultural images of women as helpless, childlike, irresponsible in money matters, and easy prey for swindlers and con artists may help make declarations of incompetence and petitions for guardianship more likely for them than for their male counterparts, thus opening the door for further decision making by surrogates. It would be serendipitous indeed if proxy decision makers always knew the "best interests" of the patient with respect to life-sustaining treatments and, knowing them, acted accordingly. But, in fact, the congruence of proxy decisions with the real wishes of the patient has been called into question, as shown in Chapter 6. Without specific action to prevent abuse, then, growing numbers of elders are at grave risk of having their most intimate decisions—literally, life or death—made by others. It is worth reiterating here that frail aged men are more likely to have such decisions made by their spouse, who is presumably the person best acquainted with their preferences, whereas more distant kin or outsiders will often decide for women.[20]

Expert Advice

Health policy, planning, laws, administration, and research are all dominated by men or male-centered thinking, as is the delivery of many medical services. In sharp contrast, hands-on personal care—bathing, feeding, and toileting, for example—is typically the province of women workers. Despite recent shifts in the American occupational structure, privileged white men still constitute the majority of lawyers, doctors, legislators, and other experts whose actions influence people's lives. Their views of women's best interests, however well intentioned, may correspond poorly or not at all to women's own views. Gender disparities in clinical decision making, for example, have been reported in the medical literature, as noted earlier; these work to women's disadvantage. Moreover, even the mass-based aging organizations (predominantly male-led) "have typically not separated out the unique needs or interests of older women." For example, although programs like Medicaid, Supplemental Security Income (SSI), and food stamps are especially salient to older women, they receive little attention from the old-age lobby. And the Medicare Catastrophic Coverage Act, which would have benefitted low-income elders (a population that is disproportionately female) was quickly repealed due to the vociferous objections of well-off elders, who would have had to pay more under the plan.[21]

In recent popular and scholarly literature, experts from a variety of disciplines have stressed the obligations of elders to the rest of society, including, in some cases, their duty to die.[22] Women have long been socialized to heed the advice of "experts," especially male physicians, to put others' needs above their own, and to take the more passive role in social interactions. Historically, they have been responsible for the physical health and emotional well-being of family members. Since many new life-sustaining technologies and long-term care generally are expensive, their use has consequences for the larger society, raising issues of distributive justice and generational equity, for instance, that are widely disseminated in the popular media. Women may be more responsive to such concerns than men: given the emphasis on selflessness in female socialization, they may continue to be altruistic in the final stage of life. They may also be more vulnerable to suggestions for "letting go," including nonverbal cues. It is easy to envision a variety of situations in which death occurs too soon owing to a combination of past socialization, poor health, and weak resistance.

On the other hand, the limited evidence available to date indicates that women are less approving of euthanasia and suicide than men are. This may be because men are socialized to take action in undesirable situations, whereas women are socialized to tolerate them. Differential socialization may also account for the fact that in "mercy killing" cases that reach the judicial system, men predominate in the active "killing" role, whereas women tend to occupy the passive role of recipient. This seems to hold also for cases of "mercy killing" and assisted suicide that never enter the courts. For example, *Jean's Way* is Derek Humphry's account of how he aided the suicide of his first wife. The book is a good illustration of the paternalism characteristic of many husband-wife relationships. Jean's husband knows, for example, that running a shop "would provide the right kind of vocation for [her] now that our sons were about to start their own adult lives"—a "healthy preoccupation" that would keep her from becoming "agitated" about her cancer. When she objects to his placement of a large mirror where she can see her mastectomy scar too vividly, he tells the reader: "I decided it would be bad for her psychologically if I accepted her argument . . . by now, she ought to have accepted the scar. . . . It only needed this bit of prodding and firmness for her to acquiesce." Jean never mentioned the matter again, he adds. Finally, when Jean asks, "Is this the day?" (when she should swallow the fatal dose that would end her life), he responds that it is. He then adds, "I asked myself if I should cross-examine her about the correctness of her part of the decision. However, I resisted this because it was so apparent that she was depending on me for judgement." I know of no parallel instance in which a husband was equally reliant on his wife to tell him when to die.[23]

Because they have been socialized to be submissive, especially to their husbands, some women may hesitate to make any choice at all, let alone the one that best fits the situation. Alternatively, women who are primary caregivers for others, especially incompetent patients, may hesitate to act on their charge's behalf. There is evidence, for example, that the coping mechanisms of female caregivers are generally more passive than those of males.[24] Thus suffering can be prolonged as death is delayed for a frail relative because of indecisiveness on the part of the caregiver; alternatively, death may be hastened by undue pressures from third parties, such as those arising from efforts to control costs. Both as patients and as care providers, then, women may defer overmuch to male decision makers—doctors, lawyers, ethicists, or relatives. Men, in contrast, may tend to act precipitately, without due regard for their unequal power relationships with women or the real wishes of the patient.

Especially where the right to choose death is concerned, the health care system intersects with the legal system, also male-dominated. Women's preferences with regard to life-sustaining treatment are either not considered by the courts, subjected to a higher burden of proof (relative to men), or rejected outright. The courts view earlier statements of very ill, now incompetent male patients as rational, but see women's remarks as "unreflective, emotional, or immature." A case in point is an elderly retired hospital administrator who became profoundly disabled following a series of strokes. Her vast hospital experience and many prior remarks regarding her wishes that life support not be used were dismissed by a New York court in a 1988 decision characterized by a condescending view of women's "emotionalism." Treatment continued over the objections of her daughters as well, both of them nurses who had cared for their mother throughout her illness, as the court deferred to the physician's judgment. Such gender patterned reasoning by paternalistic judges puts women at risk of having important decisions about their care expropriated by professional or civic decision makers.[25]

Experts also play a role on the other side of the caregiving equation, cautioning adult children not to try to do too much for their aged parents. As we have seen, aged women are less likely to have a spouse available to provide needed care, leaving them more reliant on their children. So to the extent such advice is heeded by families who feel constrained in their efforts to provide care, aged women in need of help will be less able to count on assistance from relatives. Yet community and institutional alternatives are risky and inadequate, and the average woman must pay for them out of a smaller income than her male counterpart. The attractions of "death with dignity" may increase accordingly.

The Women's Movement

Historically, the desire for birth control came predominantly from women, who stood to gain more than men because it was their bodies and minds that had to endure the ill effects of uncontrolled childbearing. More recently, women have expressed discontent and anger over their exclusion from health-care decision making, an exclusion that reflects their subordinate position in American society generally. They criticize the male-dominated health care system for its technological emphasis, depersonalization of the individual, and the unnecessary, uninformed, or intrusive treatments it has encouraged.[26] Thus far, women's criticisms and health reform efforts have focused on reproductive issues (contraception, abortion, and childbirth in particular). But clearly their concern may easily expand to encompass elder care, aging, death, and dying, and to women's special interests in these issues both as patients and as care providers. Because women constitute a growing fraction of the older population and have disproportionate needs, and frail elders of both sexes are highly vulnerable, they are prime candidates for a more humanistic, caring approach to their needs.

Feminist critiques of the health care system have focused on several interrelated problems that can logically be extended to decisions about forgoing life-sustaining treatment and about deliberate death. First, to the extent that physicians are influenced by negative stereotypes of old people, questions may arise regarding control, authority, and power in their relationships with patients. "Fatherly physicians and paternal surgeons cannot be trusted," critics maintain, and conflicts occur over issues of informed consent, self-determination, and access to alternatives.[27] If women patients, for example, are not given full information about their condition and treatment options because of negative stereotyping, are labeled "problem patients" when they persist in asking questions, or their ability to choose for themselves is distrusted, control over their fate may be usurped by medical professionals.

Women in America are still widely perceived as inferior to men. Social attitudes influence how many women (including, presumably, women physicians) see themselves and how they cope with illness and disability, their own or that of others. If they feel inadequate or incompetent, passive or dependent, their decision-making ability in all areas of life is compromised. A medical system that also views them as frail, weak, and inferior may not afford them sufficient opportunities to exercise freedom of choice. For the same reasons, the care they receive may be inadequate or indifferent, carrying the risk of premature death or unnecessary suffering if death is delayed. Subject to the whims of the same system, overly passive women caregivers may put the welfare of their charges, male or female, in jeopardy.

The efforts of women health activists stress self-determination in matters of health care, a demand that includes both the right and the responsibility to be involved in crucial decision making and entails full knowledge of the risks and benefits of medical procedures.[28] Self-determination, full knowledge, and involvement in decision making are also at the heart of debates about the right to choose death. If the battle for reproductive freedom is any guide, the active role of deciding for themselves would seem one that most would prefer.

Class Differences

Class differences are also likely to operate in the death control arena. Social class figured strongly in determining access to birth control (as it still does to some extent). Most doctors in the nineteenth and early twentieth centuries publicly opposed contraception. But well-to-do women, who knew their doctors better because they saw them more often, were more successful in getting the information they wanted. Poor women, on the rare occasions when they saw a doctor, were unsuccessful in the same endeavor. In other words, the private doctors who could make "exceptions" for their upper-class clientele found themselves unable to do the same for the mass of women. As late as 1937, when a poll showed that 79 percent of American women believed in birth control, those who lacked regular access to a private physician also lacked access to contraceptive information. So involuntary childbearing, which burdened all women, burdened poor women most.[29]

The three elements that constitute class, or socioeconomic status, are income, education, and occupation. With respect to occupation, of course, only the former occupation is relevant for frail elders, with whatever current income it continues to produce in the form of savings accounts, interest on investments, or pension benefits, for example. Social class of one's family of origin affects early socialization, educational attainment, occupation, lifestyle, diet and health habits, and access to preventive and diagnostic care, and so affects well-being in the last stage of life as well as the life course generally. Similar statements may be made about the influences of gender and ethnicity, which operate in tandem with social class to affect well-being in old age. Income from private pensions and Social Security, for example, is a product of lifetime work patterns, which typically differ greatly for men versus women and for minorities versus the majority. And minority status and the discrimination that often accompanies it undoubtedly contribute to lower socioeconomic standing.[30]

One view, the "age as leveler" perspective, "argues that the aging process is so pervasive and powerful that it mediates any racial, ethnic, or social class differences that might exist among older people." Another view, "double jeopardy," suggests instead that lifetime disadvantages are not only carried over into old age, but compounded by the aging process, with some people continuing to be disadvantaged in their frailty as they were throughout life. For those concerned about possibly discriminatory application of new death control options, neither bodes well for frail elders. Whereas the "age as leveler" perspective implies that they are equally at risk of undesirable outcomes, "double jeopardy" implies a continuation of a lifetime of injustices for those already hurt by a discriminatory system.[31]

"Social value" criteria, which consider the impact on society of saving or not saving a particular life, may be differentially applied to the poor. Although many objections have been made to their use, factors such as income, occupation, community service, and education—all unequally distributed in our society—have had a significant impact on patient selection decisions for many years. When choices must be made, lifesaving medical resources typically go to those who, in the judgment of the deciders, are most likely to benefit society in the future. Inevitably, of course, such criteria disadvantage the oldest and frailest, who must qualify on the basis of past contributions, not future ones. But perceptions of social value are affected by other biases of the deciders too. There is some evidence that white men are favored over blacks and women when choices are made. For example, white Medicare patients are 3.5 times more likely to have heart bypass surgery than black patients covered by the same program. Racial differences in the incidence of heart disease do not explain the variations, but racial prejudice among physicians and lack of medigap insurance (to pay for services not covered under Medicare) are possible explanations. Those hurt by such decisions may be unaware of the fact or, being aware, may be unable to act on their knowledge. On the other hand, the fact that some patients are relatively wealthy and have private insurance coverage in addition to Medicare may put them at risk of overtreatment by greedy practitioners seeking to increase their income.[32]

American aging policy has consistently favored "haves" over "have nots" in the distribution of benefits. Tax expenditures for the elderly, such as the exclusion of Social Security income from taxation for retirees, their dependents, and survivors, are heavily weighted in favor of a small, well-off elite. "Deservingness" is the concept underlying this uneven distribution of benefits. For example, those whose lives were characterized by steady employment and high earnings are deemed more "deserving" in old age than people whose employment history was erratic and whose earnings were low. Public policies such as Medicaid and Supplemental Security Income serve the less "deserving." Because these programs involve a great deal of state discretion in setting eligibility criteria and benefit levels, they are more vulnerable to cutbacks than are federal programs, depending on the state's fiscal strength and its willingness to fund them. When budgets are cut, it is the poor who suffer most.[33]

As we have seen, the frail elderly have often been treated as low priority, their admittedly great needs balanced against society's limited resources, their already long lives, and the legitimate claims of other groups. But differences *within* the frail category are substantial: all are physically or mentally weak, but some unfortunates are more vulnerable than others. To illustrate, about eight million older Americans have incomes near or below poverty, and income inequality seems to be greater among the aged than among those under 65, yet a new popular stereotype of American elders as "greedy geezers," bent exclusively on pursuing their own selfish interests, helps render these disparities invisible. But the fact remains that monetary resources are unevenly distributed among frail elders, affecting their ability to obtain needed services. The categories of elders most likely to be poor are also the fastest growing—women, disadvantaged minorities, and the oldest old.[34]

Moreover, in practice, the equal benefits defined under Medicare are not equal. Higher-income elders, and their advisors and caregivers, are more sophisticated in manipulating the system to obtain good care. They can better afford deductibles, copayments, and medigap policies and thus are more attractive clients to doctors, hospitals, and nursing homes. Within institutions, they receive better care and enjoy pleasanter surroundings and more autonomy than their counterparts on Medicaid. They can better afford the home care services that allow them to remain in their own home, since many such services must be paid for privately or forgone. They can command more respect from professional providers and they, or their relatives, can complain more effectively about mistreatment or overtreatment. Finally, their caregiving relatives have greater access to respite and other support services not reimbursed by third-party payers that, in turn, help the better-off to implement their personal choices about the locus of treatment.[35]

Trends toward corporate medicine and for-profit health care institutions threaten to exacerbate existing class disparities in access to high-quality care. Profit-making hospital chains, for instance, do not want to locate in depressed neighborhoods and strongly prefer privately insured patients to those on Medicaid.[36] Further, to the extent that health care for the poor is crisis-oriented and they lack a regular doctor, they are more dependent on the care of strangers—those less likely, and often too busy, to appreciate their personal history, needs, or preferences. The hospitals and emergency rooms where the poor are served tend to be crowded, their staff more harassed, and their budgets more constrained. They may be chronically understaffed and suffer from rapid turnover. To the extent that such facilities are staffed by less well-trained or less experienced personnel, clients are further disadvantaged.

Health and socioeconomic status are highly interdependent. In 1989, for instance, 15.6 percent of elders with family income under $10,000 rated their health as poor, compared to only 5.1 percent of those whose family income was $35,000 or more. Those in the lower socioeconomic strata are typically sicker, have more coexisting health problems, and may be sicker longer; thus they are often more expensive to treat than their higher-status counterparts. People needing long-term care are also disproportionately likely to be poor. By definition, of course, the poor have few resources to exchange for needed services. In fact, two-thirds of poor elders are not even protected by Medicaid, a program specifically designed to cover the poor and medically indigent; only 34 percent of poor elders have supplemental (medigap) insurance. According to a recent report by the Congressional Budget Office, some physicians refuse to treat Medicaid patients, and some hospitals may discourage doctors from admitting them owing to the relatively low reimbursement rates for their care. So access to care may be limited even for the poor elders who do qualify for the program.[37]

There are also elders who are not poor enough: their incomes are too high to qualify them for Medicaid assistance, yet they cannot afford institutionalization or other long-term care services as private-pay clients. Only one in ten of the near-poor (those barely above the official poverty line), has Medicaid coverage. This means that many elders, regardless of the severity of their health problems, are excluded from publicly paid services. In Florida, for example, some wives have had to move very ill husbands out of a nursing home because they could not afford the costs of care; this despite their very limited ability to care adequately for the spouse at home.[38]

Patients and their caregiving relatives depend on the judgments of professionals for information on treatment options, interest, compassion, and concern. Patients are entitled to expect advice, not merely neutral information on risks and benefits, from medical personnel. But the advice itself and the way it is presented differ substantially from doctor to doctor and patient to patient, depending on their personality styles and each party's assessment of the situation, and of each other. Separating legitimate influence from that which is coercive, biased, deceitful, or otherwise not in the patient's best interests is exceedingly difficult.[39] Differences in educational attainment, an important element of social class, affect physician-patient relationships and operate in meetings with other health care personnel as well. One's place in the social order affects the lifetime accumulation of knowledge, the ability to successfully question or challenge expert opinions, to demand or reject treatment, and to make choices for oneself instead of humbly deferring to those made by others.

Medical exchanges are automatically weighted in favor of the expert, especially the physician, but the power imbalance is worse for some patients than others. The poor and less educated are at more of a disadvantage than the wealthy and highly educated. Consent forms for surgery, for example, typically require college-level reading skills; persons whose reading ability is inadequate for the task must depend on others for sufficient information about the relative risks and benefits of the procedure. Not surprisingly, younger and better-educated respondents are those most likely to challenge their physician. The willingness of patient or proxy to say "no," to risk displeasing the doctor, or to question his authority are thus conditioned by the social gap between them. On the practitioner's part, decisions to hospitalize, perform surgery, or institute expensive technologies may be subtly influenced by inappropriate characteristics of patients, such as sex, race, ability to pay, or even how they speak or dress. Even the lowliest aide in the worst nursing home exercises some discretionary power over very vulnerable clients, for example in deciding whether to call for help in the middle of the night for a patient she dislikes. Because meaningful consent to, or refusal of, life-sustaining medical interventions requires adequate information conveyed by practitioners in the best interests of the patient, it is crucial to consider the disproportionate risks that disadvantaged individuals, or their surrogate decision makers, face in negotiating the health care system. In particular, inadequate communication due to educational disparities between providers and patients may have tragic results.[40]

Higher education is associated with more favorable attitudes toward death control, implying that better-educated individuals are more likely to draw up advance directives than the less-educated because they are more aware of the risks and hence more motivated to avoid unwanted outcomes. For example, when elderly hospital patients were asked about their preferences regarding life-sustaining treatment, those with a "never treat" pattern averaged 14.8 years of formal education, compared to a mean of 12.5 years for those with an "always treat" pattern. Perhaps an even more telling finding in the same study is that those who had not formed *any* opinion (12 percent of the sample) were the least educated, averaging only 10.8 years. Thus lower levels of education seem to be associated with less awareness of the limitations of medical practice. It follows that to the extent that advance directives achieve their intended purpose, the better-educated have improved odds of having their preferences respected. They can more effectively exercise their right to choose to die in their own way, at their own time. In sharp contrast, practitioners may assume, with some justification, that those who did *not* sign an advance directive want all available medical means employed to prolong their life; their failure to document their wishes thus places them in grave danger of overtreatment should they become incapacitated, assuming, of course, that other characteristics, such as ability to pay, do not operate to hasten death when outsiders make the decisions.[41]

Long-term care is expensive, limited in quality and quantity, and meagerly funded with public monies; only the financially well-off can afford the best of what is available, and that may still be inadequate. For those who were always poor, and those who become poor in old age, the new Patient Self-Determination Act, which became effective in December 1991, may not constitute an enhancement of self-determination but instead convey a different message: many elders may wonder whether the new documents they are being encouraged to sign will limit their medical treatment in order to cut costs, under the guise of enhancing their autonomy.[42]

TABLE 9-3

Projected Growth of the Older Population, by Race: 1990–2050 (Numbers in Thousands)

Year	Total	65+ White	Black	Other races
1990	31,559	28,344	2,612	603
	(100.0)	(89.8)	(8.3)	(1.9)
2000	34,882	30,776	3,131	975
	(100.0)	(88.2)	(9.0)	(2.8)
2010	39,362	33,984	3,860	1,518
	(100.0)	(86.3)	(9.8)	(3.9)
2020	52,067	44,084	5,587	2,396
	(100.0)	(84.7)	(10.7)	(4.6)
2030	65,604	54,460	7,784	3,360
	(100.0)	(83.0)	(11.9)	(5.1)
2040	68,109	55,159	8,778	4,172
	(100.0)	(81.0)	(12.9)	(6.1)
2050	68,532	53,925	9,571	5,036
	(100.0)	(78.7)	(14.0)	(7.3)
		85+		
1990	3,254	2,962	251	41
	(100.0)	(91.0)	(7.7)	(1.3)
2000	4,622	4,186	354	82
	(100.0)	(90.6)	(7.7)	(1.7)
2010	6,115	5,476	478	161
	(100.0)	(89.6)	(7.8)	(2.6)
2020	6,651	5,787	600	264
	(100.0)	(87.0)	(9.0)	(4.0)
2030	8,129	6,923	788	418
	(100.0)	(85.2)	(9.7)	(5.1)
2040	12,251	10,274	1,287	690
	(100.0)	(83.9)	(10.5)	(5.6)
2050	15,287	12,534	1,817	936
	(100.0)	(82.0)	(11.9)	(6.1)

SOURCE: U. S. Bureau of the Census, Current Population Reports, Series P-25, No. 1018, *Projections of the Population of the United States by Age, Sex, and Race: 1988–2080* (Series 14 - Middle Series) (Washington, DC: U. S. Government Printing Office, 1989), by Gregory Spencer.

Those disadvantaged, neglected, or abused by the system in the past have reason for concern about continuing inequities.

Ethnic Dimensions

The United States is a multicultural society, and minorities will comprise a growing proportion of the total aged population in decades to come (Table 9-3). Note that if Hispanics were included among the minority groups shown in the table, the proportion of minorities would be greater yet: instead of the 17 percent included as blacks and other races for the year 2030, for example, inclusion of Hispanics would raise the total minority proportion to 24 percent.[43]

The concept of ethnicity incorporates both race and national origin. Shared origins, histories, and values play some role in the aging process, the prevalence of chronic illnesses and functional disabilities, how sicknesses are defined and how they are managed, and the way caregiving is perceived and carried out. Ethnic background also affects the public services available to minority elders and their caregiving relatives. Service provision, in turn, may be influenced by ethnic stereotyping, ignorance or misunderstanding of a group's unique needs, and unwarranted assumptions about the strength of family ties. Ethnic differences also influence what services are requested or sought out, and the barriers—such as class background and command of the English language—which inhibit their use. Potential clients are less likely to use a particular service if the providers or other users are conspicuously different from themselves; their hesitation may be due to past experiences of overt discrimination or simply discomfort and suspicion of unknown cultures. Older blacks, for example, lived much of their lives prior to the civil rights movement, in a system that barred their access to a variety of public facilities and relegated them to separate, inferior services.[44] Finally, it is important to keep in mind that there are enormous differences *within* ethnic groups as well as between them. All these interacting factors, in turn, affect how death and the dying process are handled and influence the end-of-life treatment choices made by individuals, families, and caregivers in the formal sector.

In terms of income, educational attainment, housing quality, and health status, the minority aged are disadvantaged compared to other older Americans. The eight million elders whose incomes are near or below the official poverty threshold include a disproportionate number of blacks, for example. The Hispanic population is extremely diverse, with important subgroup variations that affect health, education, and financial status. Higher proportions of black and Hispanic elders are not covered by Medicare or any other health insurance; they also tend to have fewer resources, such as private pensions or substantial assets.[45]

Blacks are more likely than whites to suffer from major health problems, such as circulatory diseases and cancer. Their conditions are often more serious too, in part because of delays in diagnosis and treatment. With respect to cancer, for example, blacks, especially if they are poor, are less likely to receive health services such as pap smears or prostate examinations, which aid in early diagnosis; they are also less knowledgeable of cancer's early warning signs and more pessimistic about treatment outcomes. Overall, noninstitutionalized older blacks of both sexes are proportionally more disabled than community-dwelling whites. Their rate of hospitalization is higher and length of stay longer, on average. Other minorities are often health-disadvantaged too. Like many older blacks, older Hispanics and Native Americans tend to have relatively low educational attainment and are disproportionately poor, characteristics that limit their access to health care and prospects for self-determination with respect to life-sustaining treatment.[46]

Because minority elders are often sicker than whites and because they are less able to afford paid alternatives, they are more dependent on informal caregivers, primarily relatives. Since the family is often poor too, such dependence may be risky for vulnerable elders. Physicians working for the Indian Health Service, for instance, report cyclical patterns of hospitalization and returns to inadequate home care situations for older Indians, as their chronic health problems are repeatedly exacerbated in the home setting-by poor diet, for example. Their caregiving relatives are disproportionately burdened, too. Families sometimes hospitalize frail relatives in order to give themselves some respite from caregiving, delivering the elder to the hospital on Friday afternoon with a list of vague complaints and returning on Monday to resume their tasks. Support groups, such as those for Alzheimer's disease, rarely extend services to minority caregivers. More generally, advocacy groups have tended to focus on the needs of the majority despite the different, potentially greater needs of the minority.[47]

Blacks and Hispanics are less often institutionalized, owing more to their poverty and institutional discrimination than to different care preferences. The same is true for American Indians, who experience the additional constraint that existing facilities tend to be at a considerable distance from their homes; this inhibits frequent visiting by friends and family and any "watchdog" effects such visits may have on the quality of institutional care. Lower rates of institutionalization also suggest that caregiving obligations weigh more heavily on minority family caregivers relative to their counterparts in the majority.[48]

Because nursing homes prefer private-pay patients whenever possible, owing to Medicaid's low reimbursement rates, Medicaid patients must wait longer for institutional placement and the homes they end up in are of lower quality. Since blacks, for example, are far more likely to rely on Medicaid from the beginning, they are more likely to experience these institutional prejudices. Because nursing homes also select against "heavy care" cases, the institutionalization option is again less available to older blacks since, on average, they are sicker than whites. Finally, nonwhite elders are more likely to be diagnosed as mentally ill rather than simply old and frail. In 1976, for example, 26 percent of institutionalized aged nonwhites were classified as wards of the institution, the state, or a court, implying they were incompetent; the figure for whites was only 12 percent. This suggests that nonwhites are more vulnerable to the risks of proxy decision making regarding end-of-life treatments.[49]

Access to high-quality care for minorities is also hindered by shortages of personnel and finances. Facilities in inner-city neighborhoods, small towns, or remote rural areas, where many minority elders live, face greater difficulties in hiring and retaining staff. For example, a survey of nursing homes on American Indian reservations revealed serious problems: noncompetitive salaries and benefits and an absence of supportive services were not attractive to professionals, whereas nonprofessional staff members suffered from alcohol-related problems and frequent absenteeism.[50]

Other problems disproportionately affect minority caregivers, especially women, in the informal sector: simultaneous care responsibilities to two generations (children and frail elders); low income; discrimination in the labor force that limits earnings and thus affects ability to pay for supportive services; discrimination in the services available to poor people or in poor neighborhoods; cultural and language barriers that hamper communication with better-educated service providers. Disadvantaged minority women workers are heavily overrepresented in the lowest-level jobs in the formal care sector, such as nurses' aides and home care attendants. On the one hand, this leaves them disproportionately vulnerable to the "contagion stress" that results from exposure to high-stress situations both at work and at home. On the other hand, their frail charges, whether they are relatives or clients in the formal care sector, may be more at risk too. The harsh facts of life for many minority group members help create the high-risk elders, high-risk caregivers, and high-risk family systems that contribute to elder neglect and abuse, as well as harmful outcomes for the caregivers themselves. And these, in turn, are likely to influence the choices made by, with, and for frail elders in the final stage of life.[51]

Yet, ironically, an idealized image of ethnic subcultures among policy makers and service providers has exaggerated the potential for informal support in minority families. For example, it is often assumed that aged Mexican-Americans are well cared for in their extended families, a misleading notion that may serve as an excuse not to offer social services to this group. In the real world, elders who live in an ethnic enclave, surrounded by relatives, are not guaranteed a blissful old age. In fact, the evidence suggests that ethnic families have limited capacity for dealing with the difficult problems of frail elders. Hence if the "mores and betters" discussed in the previous two chapters are to deter greater resort to deliberate death, they must also take account of the unequal risks confronted by a rapidly growing population of ethnic elders, unconscionable caregiving demands on their already disadvantaged relatives, and more limited access to even the poor long-term care options available to the majority.[52]

Summary

Gender, class, and ethnic identity affect one's definition of a problem, knowledge of the availability of solutions, their acceptability, and perceived advantages to new behavior. They bear on the judgments people make for themselves and for one another, and on those they are permitted to make. Decisions about treatment based on patients' nonmedical characteristics may reflect professionals' conscious or unconscious estimations of "social worth" and hence the choices considered for or offered to the patient. Such influences are hard to measure, and empirical data on variations in long-term care and end-of-life treatment by sex, class, and ethnicity are lacking. Nonetheless, these characteristics of frail elders and their caregiving relatives are likely to affect death control outcomes directly or indirectly. Within each religious group, for example, blacks are much less likely to approve of euthanasia than whites, perhaps because relatively powerless groups feel more threatened by possible abuses. Inferior treatment by formal service providers may seem to justify their concern and increase distrust between minority patients and their health care providers. But powerless patients may find it difficult to avoid victimization. In seeking to deter undertreatment, for instance, they may inadvertently risk overtreatment, and delayed death, by insisting on procedures that are unwarranted or futile.[53]

Clearly, the gaps in our knowledge of differential treatment outcomes based on patients' nonmedical characteristics represent a hazard with respect to the practice of death control. But given what we already know of overt and covert discrimination in the health care system, we should expect that persons unable to exercise their rights with respect to health care decision making will include disproportionate numbers of minorities, women, and the poor. Many physicians are also reluctant to relinquish their discretionary authority. But they are more likely to retain it with some categories of patients than with others, so we may fully expect end-of-life treatment discrepancies along class, sex, and ethnic lines. Differential application of "no codes" and "slow codes" and undue manipulation of individual and family decision making, based on criteria that should be irrelevant, such as ability to pay, are not unlikely, and will hasten death for some patients. As for delayed death, some patients are subjected to unproductive or painful treatments simply because they can afford to pay. In the words of one doctor, "If DNR meant, 'Do Not Reimburse' instead of 'Do Not Resuscitate,' far fewer of the terminally and hopelessly ill would receive pointless treatment." Other patients are overtreated in order to shield doctors and hospitals from prosecution, in response to the demands of family members, or even in the interest of training new doctors or completing a research protocol. According to one expert on health law, for example, doctors learn in the course of their medical training that their clinical superiors expect them to take advantage of every opportunity to practice surgical techniques, despite the lack of patient consent or the likelihood of benefit. It behooves us to ask which patients might be likely to endure these experiences—the rich, the highly educated, the planners? Or those who are poor, ignorant, and powerless? Those whose proxy decision makers are well informed and articulate, or those who are timid, fearful, or overly trusting? The secrecy that now surrounds death control proceedings may already conceal a variety of abuses.[54]

The future will see an increasing concentration of infirmities in advanced old age, especially among women.[55] As Table 9-3 shows, the proportion of disadvantaged minorities in the older population and among the oldest old will also grow substantially. Income disparities within the frail elderly category are significant, and an early end to cost-containment efforts in public policy for long-term care is unlikely. Thus the problems of gender, class, and ethnicity discussed here will not go away and are likely to worsen. Without specific efforts by policy makers and health care providers to eliminate discriminatory treatment, advance directives, insofar as they protect at all, will protect only those segments of the population that are already advantaged. The absence of efforts to change the unsatisfactory *status quo*, however, will in no way reduce the need to make hard choices about the timing and circumstances of death.

Last Rights and Responsibilities

Weighing the Risks and Benefits of Death Control

When 26-year-old Pat Moore put on wrinkled latex "skin," donned a gray wig, and walked with a cane to become 80-year-old "Grandma Moore" for a graduate studies project, she received a frightening foretaste of the "golden years." Over the three years the experiment lasted, she was alternately ignored, shoved, jostled, robbed, and otherwise assaulted; one day she was pushed down a flight of stairs and on another she was brutally beaten by a gang of young boys. Treatment was generally much better when she dressed as a well-off woman than as a poor one, but her accounts would persuade no one of Americans' benevolence towards frail old people.[1]

Unlike this feigned Grandma, who could shed her skin and become young again (at least temporarily), there are all too many real elders suffering ill treatment they do not deserve. In fact, the world has never seen a society in which so many frail elders needed so much for so long. Collectively, they are the oldest, the sickest, and often the poorest. That Americans kill them, directly or indirectly, is beyond dispute. That some at least are ready for death, perhaps longing for it, is also certain. That some deaths are unduly hastened is equally undeniable. The problems of frail elders are everyone's problems; they will be our personal problems if we live long enough. But while social workers invent pleasant activities for demented elders and health workers infantilize and toddlerize others, few think to ask if this kind of life—where the frail have lost much of their human dignity, where they may no longer be able to reject such "help" or ask for the kinds of help they really need, and are too often mistreated—is one that anyone would ever want.

Throughout history, important distinctions have been made between the intact and the decrepit, between biological life and biographical life, between reciprocity and prolonged one-way dependence, with treatment of old people varying accordingly. Examples from societies at every stage of development confirm that death hastening is not directed toward "the old" as a class, but to a specific subgroup—those so frail that they are no longer able to contribute to the well-being of others in exchange for support received. If they are poor and familyless, their death is even more likely to be rushed. Intact elders typically experience quite different treatment. To believe that late-twentieth-century Americans invented this dichotomization of treatments, or that we are unique in this regard, is to delude ourselves. People everywhere have disvalued frailty and set tolerable limits on unreciprocated support. Clearly, we Americans need to recognize that "the old" are not all alike: while some must be helped to live their lives to the fullest, others must be helped to die. It is reassuring that change in the direction of greater openness about the realities of frailty and death has been occurring in recent years, thanks to the sorrowful examples of patients like Karen Ann Quinlan and Nancy Cruzan and to pioneers in the death control movement who have forced the problems to the forefront of national consciousness.[2]

The Demographic Imperative

Social institutions have been very slow to respond to dramatic changes in human longevity, especially the long-term morbidity, suffering, and dependency that it may entail. But the population at risk of prolonged dying is growing steadily, despite lack of institutional preparedness, and morbidity prevalence is increasing as death rates continue to decline. Even optimistic forecasts suggest that illnesses during the last stage of life will continue to resist treatment and defy cure.[3] Meanwhile, the greater control over life and death that medical technology now allows forces us to confront difficult questions about the meaning of life and the nature and extent of caregiving obligations, including whether and how death should be facilitated. The continuing proliferation of new life-extending technologies and escalating demands on the long-term care system ensure that hard choices will be more necessary in the future than they are today. Meanwhile, the gender gap in life expectancy ensures that greater proportions of women than men will survive to the older ages where multiple chronic conditions, dementias in particular, complicate care requirements and increase the duration of need. And disadvantaged minorities, with their greater vulnerability to both ill health and poverty, will constitute a growing proportion of the total elderly population in decades to come. Unprecedented burdens of morbidity for individuals and unprecedented needs for care from family members and paid providers are the predictable result. New demographic realities are helping to fuel demands for social change to cope with them.

The Social Imperative

The desire to escape, minimize, or end useless suffering—our own or that of others—is an inherent human characteristic, found in all times and places. Chapter 2 established that extreme frailty and prolonged dependency have always been disvalued. Mere biological survival is not the point, and never was, in the long view of human history. Yet faith in scientific medicine, where the possibilities for miracles came to seem limitless in the twentieth century, led us to temporarily overrate medicine's potential. By emphasizing the extension of biological life, we gave short shrift to life's social dimension—the biographical component that distinguishes human beings from other life forms. The death control movement is attempting to restore the balance. In this reordering, the appropriate time for death is when permanent loss of the capacity for meaningful interaction with others has occurred or seems imminent.

When the capacity for social interaction has been irreparably eroded, nonsupportive treatment, including such "active" forms of death hastening as strangling frail elders or burying them alive, has been far more common around the world than most people realize. Because extreme frailty and prolonged dependency continue to be highly disvalued in modern industrial societies like the United

States, many forms of nonsupportive treatment and death hastening exist in our midst as well. The new powers of medicine prolong biological life, adding a formidable new problem in the form
of death delayed beyond the point where a meaningful life is possible. Prolonged dying has increased care burdens for individuals,
their families, health care workers, and society, while other aspects
of modernization, such as the separation of home and work and
the movement of women into the paid workforce, have put new
constraints on care provision.

It is unlikely that death hastening reflects a desire to deliberately
hurt or kill a helpless victim. Instead it reflects the priority of the
biographical over the biological component of life. Given that
time, energy, and other resources are always limited, the wish not
to continue lives of poor quality, when there is no promise of
meaningful return to the human community, is eminently rational.
Prioritizing is essential for society to survive, especially when the
nonfrail may be seriously harmed by their efforts to provide for
the frail, perhaps becoming prematurely frail themselves as a direct
result of their efforts.

The existence of the three preconditions—acceptability of the
idea of control, the perception of advantages accruing to new attitudes and behavior, and the availability of appropriate means for
accomplishing new goals (or, more accurately, new variations on
old goals) points to increased resort to death control.
Extraordinary changes in acceptability have occurred over a relatively short time. The wide acceptance of "passive" euthanasia by
the 1970s, for example, would have been thought impossible
twenty years earlier.[4] Advantages for the individual, the family,
health care workers, and the larger society are undeniable. The potential for gentler means of deliberate death also exists, and a majority of Americans favor their use. According to a Roper Poll
conducted in 1991, 54 percent of Americans said that physicians
should be allowed by law to administer lethal drugs to help a patient die (see Table 4-1); one in three (36 percent) opposed the
idea, and the rest were undecided. These percentages suggest that a
further tilt toward acceptance is likely: the fact that a majority already approves will make it easier for others to follow in the same
direction. Just as the pill is preferred to vaginal plugs made with
crocodile dung, and condoms to abstinence, for preventing con-

ception, so will many dying elders and their significant others prefer a lethal injection from a trusted physician to slow self-starvation in the back room of a nursing home, a violent end with gun or knife, or the lost world of senile dementia, where care providers await a medical crisis that will "allow" death to come when treatment is withheld.

But as matters now stand in this country, too few get the gentle death they long for. Current laws, ambiguous and contradictory, provide little guidance. Advance directives offer some protection, but relatively few Americans have resorted to them thus far. Even when there is a directive, however, the health team may be unaware of its existence, there may not be time to inquire about or interpret it in an emergency, or the document may not cover the specific situation. Health workers and hospitals want to protect themselves from liability, and they still see aggressive treatment as the best route for doing so. And health workers may indeed know best in the situation at hand—if they follow their own instincts they may be able to preserve a life of acceptable quality for the patient despite the "let me die" instructions contained in an advance directive.

In an emergency, when clear thinking is most required, it is also most difficult to do. Hence despite the best intentions of the most loving proxy decision makers, outcomes may not coincide with patient preferences. Those who are less lucky—the familyless, the poor, or the uneducated—will die when and how strangers decide they will, perhaps unaware that there were ever choices to be made. Thus, although in recent years we have witnessed a powerful endorsement of patient autmony, practice continues to fall far short of the ideal.[5] A bias to treat still exists and doctors often remain the primary decision makers, especially for familyless elders. The paucity of alternative care arrangements speeds death unduly in some cases, while other deaths are more often violent (shooting, stabbing) than gentle.

Even the *Cruzan* case, the first right-to-die case decided by the Supreme Court, "provides uncertain protection for the rights of autonomous patients and virtually removes any constitutional protection once a person is declared incompetent." And despite the fact that suicide has been decriminalized in the United States, it is still against the law in many states to help someone do what they have the legal right to do. In some extreme cases, medication is withheld from patients in severe pain due to providers' fears that they might save up enough pills to commit suicide. Do we really want desperate people to move from state to state in the hope of having their final wishes respected? For example, in order to die before she lost her dignity and her personhood to Alzheimer's, Janet Adkins had to travel to a different state and die in the back of an old van in a county park. She urged her husband to stay away lest he be implicated for violating the law, so she had to die alone, far from home and separated from those she loved. "Society forced Janet into that van," said her husband and, we might add, kept him out of it, depriving them both of comfort and peace. This is what our legal and medical systems have produced. But is it what we really want?[6]

We need a consensus on how our right to choose death may best be implemented, and rules, formal and informal, must be changed to better fit new realities of frailty and prolonged dying. Since many reasonable people see no meaningful distinction between the two, we must reconsider the wisdom of regarding "passive" assistance as acceptable in law and medical practice while "active" assistance is generally discouraged. If brutal killing in a "just war" is allowed, and capital punishment is tolerated by many Americans, why should we hesitate to help very sick old people to die? A peculiar situation indeed, when deaths with no element of voluntariness or mercy, and obviously not in accord with either the preferences or best interests of the decedent, are acceptable while assisted dying for those who have good cause for wishing to die, and who can no longer help themselves, is prohibited. In another analogy, why do we praise our actions when a beloved pet, sick or injured, is "put to sleep," and attach an entirely different meaning to identical actions, identically motivated, when the recipient is our parent, our spouse, or our patient? It is obvious that our right to choose death is worthless if assistants are prevented from cooperating. This is equivalent to granting citizens the right to have a broken arm set, but making it illegal for health personnel to set it, or claiming that people have reproductive rights while enjoining doctors from prescribing contraceptives and arresting pharmacists for selling condoms.

Recently, opponents of "active" euthanasia have argued that

"caring" should supersede "curing" in the American health care system and that this will abrogate any need to deliberately choose a quicker death. The historical record and recent experience suggest otherwise, as I have argued throughout this book. When intensive care is needed, as it always is by some, it is highly valued, and rewarding to the providers, only if it is relatively short in duration and the recipient is expected to return to meaningful social roles. There is no indication that this prioritizing has changed over time.

Consider also the conditions necessary for informal elder care to be highly rewarding today, as outlined by an expert on elder-care issues: (1) the experience must be freely chosen; (2) caregivers must get support from their family, the medical profession, and others as needed, so that they are neither overburdened nor impoverished; (3) excellent institutional care must be available if needed; and (4) the caregiver must not be made to feel guilty for choosing institutional care. With this combination of circumstances, "caregiving can be a meaningful close to a loving relationship. It can be a rich, deep connection to the cycles of life and an experience that many people would not want to miss."[7]

But extensive social supports like these, which might make caregiving to frail elders a valued role, do not exist in America today, nor do they exist anywhere else in the world, nor could they have been found in some idealized past. Moreover, it is very doubtful that they can now be created, because characteristics of frail elders and the nature and duration of their needs strongly militate against protracted devotion from providers—stress, burnout, and "compassion fatigue" are inevitable when care demands seem endless and the potential for reward slim. When the recipient cannot get better, providers must eventually ask why they are trying so hard. The patient too, if still competent, must ask the same question. New caring goals are a predictable result of such questioning.

The "mores and betters" that might produce a caring society adequate to deal with the new realities of advanced age and extreme frailty are unlikely to appear soon. Moreover, the current fragmented system creates many victims. First and foremost, it endangers frail elders, especially disadvantaged minorities, women, and the poor, owing to its manifold shortcomings in both the caring and the curing realm. Caregiving relatives may also be victimized.

Social norms leave them little choice but to provide care, yet the long-term care system offers few supportive services or alternative forms of care when family capacities are exhausted. Impaired health, impoverishment, misery, and even premature death may result. Providers in the formal system, from the highest-paid professionals to the lowliest attendants in nursing homes, face problems of stress and burnout in consequence of their efforts on behalf of patients who cannot get better regardless of the effort expended; they are witnesses to the suffering involved and may contribute to it out of fear, malice, or ignorance. They too are victims of the system.

Moreover, in the final analysis, more and better long-term care services will merely postpone decisions about death; they cannot ultimately avoid them. In the unlikely event that it does materialize, however, more and better caring is entirely consistent with earlier, deliberate, "active" forms of death control. A hospice-type emphasis on compassion, preservation of the patient's dignity, and attention to the caregivers' needs, for example, can be wholly compatible with "active" aid-in-dying. Renewed emphasis in recent years on the social dimensions of life suggests that this will continue to be a focal point for further changes to come. Precedents and parallels throughout history suggest that there will be no lessening of individuals' desires to avoid suffering and control their dying, as they have long attempted to control their living. It is increasingly apparent to many that maximizing biological longevity in the absence of biographical considerations is not good enough.

The Economic Imperative

As we have seen, caregiving to frail elders has tremendous economic costs, even disregarding the opportunity costs to family members, primarily women, who must limit or forgo paid work in order to provide care. With a growing population in need of care, economic costs promise to grow in years to come, but will grow less if service levels are kept constant than if they are increased. Yet many frail elders and their informal caregivers are currently underserved, and severe limitations in formal services are more the rule than the exception. Other, hidden costs of long-term care have received little attention. For example, our society now plainly needs caregivers to care for the caregivers, both in the formal and informal sectors, a phenomenon I referred to as "caregiving involution." Presumably, many caregivers would be engaged in other productive pursuits if caregiving requirements were less, pursuits conceivably more to their liking or where their talents could be more efficiently utilized. Caregiving and caregiving involution, in other words, have opportunity costs in that they draw workers away from other important roles. The effects on individual morale and national welfare, which may be substantial, are not yet the focus of scholarly interest or governmental concern. Few have addressed the fundamental issue of how much of society's resources should go to health care versus many other socially valued goods and services.[8]

"Bed and body" workers, usually women and minorities at the bottom of the job hierarchy, are those likely to be most in demand as care needs escalate in coming years. But such jobs are historically those least able to attract and keep workers, and the same may be true of other fields where most of the work involves extremely frail or dying patients. Thus they may continue to attract only the most desperate job seekers. What will make such jobs more appealing to workers? How will workers who are compassionate and truly caring be retained? Assuming pay and benefits are substantially improved, there is no necessary connection with a reduction in worker stress and burnout, or an improved caring environment, since the clients' problems are largely intractable. And how do we improve the professional jobs at the top of the hierarchy, where workers are already advantaged in terms of pay and prestige but may nonetheless suffer from stress and burnout?

Patients and their relatives may have other priorities than paying the bills for long-term care services and life-prolonging treatments that accomplish little in terms of quality of life for the recipients. Since the oldest and frailest are highly dependent on public funds, societal concerns are also justified. Taxpayers, for example, are entitled to ask what better uses there might be for their hard-earned tax dollars than expending them on futile or unwanted treatments for those who have lived long and are obviously suffering. We need to distinguish between public willingness to provide expensive programs for "the old" and willingness to finance open-ended "care" imposed on those longing to die.

Since the tolerance of taxpayers has a limit, the only other way to get more public funds allocated to the long-term care needs of frail elders is to divert them from somewhere else in the budget. This is far from impossible. After all, in 1986, a year when the United States was not at war, the Pentagon spent close to a billion dollars a day ($41 million an hour) on national defense. In the same year, the American military budget exceeded the gross national product of all but eight countries in the world.[9] If we are willing to divert some funds from the military, a move that many Americans favor, does that mean we want to divert them to frail elders? Or should they go to other pressing needs—schools, public transportation, wildlife conservation, or toxic waste cleanup, to name a few? Significantly, neither long-term care deficiencies nor the size of the defense budget are well-kept national secrets: both are prominent topics in the mass media. Yet there is no groundswell of public opinion demanding that one be reduced for the sake of the other, so presumably Americans have other uses in mind for any "peace dividend" that may materialize.

Do we need caring? Of course. Neither we as individuals nor our society can survive without it. Do we need better carers and better caregiving institutions? Assuredly. Should we spend more money in efforts to produce better care? Yes, certainly, if it enhances biographical life and deters premature death. But the nature of care and its goals should reflect our values and the needs of the people involved. The endurance expected of the old and the ill, for example, as well as the sacrifices expected of caregivers should have far more reasonable limits than they now do, in line with the wishes and capabilities of each party. We must bear in mind too that cost containment is a dangerous criterion to apply to caregiving. It is of paramount importance to maintain a sharp distinction between *support* for individual and family choices to facilitate death and unwarranted *promotion* of the death option (in the interest of cost containment rather than the best interests of patients and families, for example).

Of Rights and Responsibilities

Societies cannot entirely prevent death for citizens who are young, healthy, well educated, or exceptionally talented, let alone the aged, the ill, and the very frail. People who should know better drink and drive, neglect to fasten their seatbelts, ignore "safe sex" precautions, and step off the curb without looking in both directions first. Laws are enacted to try to protect them from the consequences of their behavior, but society does not try very hard to constrain our choices to harm ourselves. Indeed, sometimes our choices harm others—for example, when we drive under the influence of alcohol or when a pregnant woman takes illicit drugs. No society does all it could do to prevent this behavior either, because such ventures are costly and interfere too much with personal freedom. And they might not work. Thus, despite the manifest advantages of postponing death, other important values intervene to limit societal efforts.

Assuming we are sufficiently competent to make choices at all, our choices are limited to those we see available, if not necessarily to those within the letter of the law. We may not see (or seeing, decline to use) some options routinely used by our fellow citizens. Here we return once more to the comparison of death control with birth control. Many people today are oblivious to the extreme social coercion that limits their reproductive options: they make seemingly "voluntary" choices in a pronatalist environment that strongly discourages them from choosing nonmarriage, childlessness, or a one-child family.[10] Couples with excellent parenting skills are discouraged from having large families by fear of the disapproval, even scorn, of friends and neighbors. We abide by these unwritten rules because we are brought up to believe they are right, because we crave the approval of significant others and shrink from their censure, and because it is always easier to go along with the group than to be different—if everyone else does it, we need not trouble ourselves with thinking through the pros and cons in our own unique circumstances.

This is not to say that "going along with the crowd" is necessarily bad or that being different is necessarily desirable. But it is to say that we need to be aware of the social rules that limit free choice and be willing to reject them or change them if the situation warrants. Despite all the means of contraception currently available and the drastic impact of unwanted children on the children themselves, their parents, and the community, many unwanted births still occur in the United States. A few couples have never heard of contraception, some fail to use it for other reasons, and some use it ineffectively. Some "think" they want children when they have failed to think at all. Ignorance, passivity, and fear of criticism hurt some groups more than others—the less educated and the poor, for example. They pay the price in terms of dissatisfaction and personal misery.

For death control, we must first be mindful that there *are* choices. Then we must be clear about what the choices are. Healthy autonomy for frail elders is not on the list; even unhealthy but manageable autonomy is often not on the list either, nor is the possibility of a return to independent functioning. Some choices do remain, however: how and when to die, what to ask of caregivers, what image of oneself to leave behind, for example. One's death may be envied by survivors for its serenity and "goodness" or call forth a sigh of relief from exhausted caregivers, or fall anywhere between the two. One may die slowly, uncomfortably, or passively, as most now do. Or death can be relatively quick and painless if the person is capable of the necessary preparations or has assistants willing to risk prosecution. Competent individuals have choices at the end of life: we can take a big risk by doing nothing and trusting the system or our relatives to make the choices we would have made. Or we can discuss our preferences with our relatives and doctors well in advance of a crisis and appoint someone we trust to act for us if we become incapacitated. Or we can opt for still more active control and commit suicide while we are still capable, sacrificing some unknown amount of remaining lifetime in the process. If one waits too long, the last option will fade away. Each option thus has risks, even for those who remain competent. For the incompetent with no prior instructions, the risks of not dying as they might prefer are obviously greater.

In our roles as family members, whether as patients, care providers, or concerned onlookers, we also need to be clear about what the choices are. Curing is impossible. Prolonged caring is sometimes necessary but must be balanced by the needs of providers and those of other family members. Caregivers in the formal system also need to think critically about when heroic efforts may not be in the patient's best interests, when caring should take precedence over curing, and when "active" aid-in-dying may be fully justified as part of caring. The Hippocratic tradition is far from the only one for resolving ethical problems in medicine, and the oath itself is vague about the propriety of "active" aid-in-dying provided by doctors. For instance, does the injunction "to help the sick" sometimes include helping them achieve a quicker and more peaceful death? Does the promise to "do no harm" sometimes preclude the use of life-extending technologies that offer little real benefit to the patient? It is time to rethink the Hippocratic oath, either clarifying its vagueness or replacing it with more appropriate language, as some medical schools are already doing. However, as one ethicist put it, "it is entirely wrong to expect the members of one profession as a regular matter of course to jeopardize their whole careers by breaking the criminal law in order to save the rest of us the labour . . . of changing that law." The rest of us—patients and future patients, family members, and caregivers—must think for ourselves and set the necessary changes in motion.[11]

The birth control movement was an assertion of an individual's right to self-determination in reproductive matters, along with efforts to ensure that the means to exercise their choices were freely available to all. Today, the means to control the timing and circumstances of death are also at hand, though the legal system has yet to fully clarify the parameters of our right to choose death. Just as it is advantageous for couples to decide the number and spacing of their children, so it is advantageous to direct one's fate at many other points over the life course, including its ultimate end. Just as there are risks attached to the failure to learn about and exercise one's reproductive rights (unwanted children, for example), so there are penalties for ignorance, passivity, and neglect when it comes to death control options. Regardless of our aversion to risk, choices about the timing and circumstances of death can only be postponed, often at the cost of considerable suffering, but cannot be avoided in the end. Failing to choose is a choice of sorts, too—the riskiest of them all. Clearly, by not acting, we will be acted upon.

Continuing the analogy of death control with birth control, note that whatever the advantages of new reproductive behavior, however great the perceived need for it, there is always the potential for risk and abuse. Many contraceptive methods have undesirable side effects, for example. Moreover, if couples postpone childbearing too long with the new methods, they risk infertility or a greater threat of complications for mother and child. Others who limit family size find that tragic accidents or illnesses result in child deaths, and that it is too late in the life-cycle to have more children. On the abuse side, the mass media are replete with stories of forced vasectomies in India, injuries and deaths attributable to defective intrauterine devices, and the like.

Ideally, potential users of birth control should be aware of the risks and make their choices freely in light of full information and in the absence of coercion. In practice, of course, some risks will remain and occasional abuses will occur. Risks, including the risk of premature death, cannot be entirely eliminated when it comes to death control either, and the secrecy that now typically surrounds negotiated death actually invites abuse. Suggestions of an obligation to die or deliberate nontreatment for nonaltruistic reasons (due to efforts to contain costs, for example) may prove hard for some to resist. But the present system is full of abuses too, and the advantages of deliberate death are too appealing to simply go away if we ignore them.

But risks can be minimized. Good legislation can guard against abuses and punish those who violate the rules, and sensible safety precautions should include efforts to reduce secrecy and encourage public debate on the issues. If patients, doctors, and families are making life-and-death decisions every day, as we know they must, a wise society will insist that they act within the law and do so as openly as possible, rather than behind closed doors, employing unknown criteria. Those who are skeptical about opening up such sensitive proceedings should consider our experiences with birth control: few in the nineteenth century would have believed that the detailed statistics on methods used, reasons for choosing one method over another, and other forms of intimate personal behavior that scientists now routinely collect were even remotely possible. Increasingly tolerant attitudes and laws in years to come should likewise help produce better statistics and in turn allow better estimates of the extent of death control and its impact.

Unfortunately, however, in the United States today we are still practicing "back-alley" euthanasia, with all the dangers that go with it. Yet tremendous pressures for change are plainly present in American society, as death control issues are disseminated through the mass media. Already, decisions for deliberate death are leaving a well marked paper trail, as "Do Not Resuscitate" forms are used more openly and more frequently. New thinking and new behavior are already affecting policy decisions, and vice versa. Competent elders *can* reject medical treatment that merely prolongs suffering, and the law now supports their right to do so. Dedicated caregivers *can* make good decisions to help the incapacitated escape the bonds of biological life when they become too onerous. Doctors, health care workers generally, judges and juries, and ordinary citizens *can* distinguish between biological life and biographical life, between compassionate aid-in-dying and willful murder. Collectively, the well-publicized tragedies of others and the lively debates they inspire compel us to think critically about our values and priorities; ultimately, further social change will emerge from this clash of ideas and ideals.[12]

Consider again what has already happened, as illustrated by the following story: when an elderly woman was admitted to the hospital emergency room, the nurse, seeing a physician approach with medical equipment, drew him aside to tell him the woman did not wish to be resuscitated. How did the nurse know that, the doctor demanded. She responded, "I asked her if she wants us to pound on her chest when her heart stops, and she said no." "Good grief! You can't ask her that!" said the doctor. "This is an emergency room!"[13] The nurse who recounted this episode did not finish the story, so we cannot be sure whose wishes prevailed in this particular case. But the questions were raised, and that is definitely progress. We *can* ask that!

Notes

Preface

1. Andrew Malcolm, "Death, Ethics, and Choice," in *Aging & Health: Linking Research and Public Policy*, ed. Steven Lewis (Chelsea, MI: Lewis Publishers, 1989), p. 173; David J. Rothman, *Strangers at the Bedside: A History of How Law and Bioethics Transformed Medical Decision Making* (New York: Basic Books, 1991), p. 260; Derek Humphry, ed., *Compassionate Crimes, Broken Taboos* (Los Angeles: The Hemlock Society, 1986), pp. 5, 22; the advertisement for living wills appeared in the *New York Times Magazine*, September 30, 1990, p. 99; Gloria Borger, "The Shadows Lurking Behind Dr. Death," *U.S. News and World Report*, December 17, 1990, p. 31; Elisabeth Rosenthal, "In Matters of Life and Death, the Dying Take Control," *New York Times*, August 18, 1991; the "suicide manual" is Derek Humphry's *Final Exit*.
2. For the first application of these preconditions (to birth control), see Ansley J. Coale, "The Demographic Transition," in *The Population Debate: Dimensions and Perspectives* (New York: United Nations, 1975), p. 353; for their first application to death control, see Barbara J. Logue, "Death Control and the Elderly," *International Journal of Contemporary Sociology* 28 (1991): 27–56.

Chapter 1

1. For attempts to distinguish "acts" from "omissions," see President's Commission for the Study of Ethical Problems in Medicine and Biomedical and Behavioral Research, *Deciding to Forego Life-Sustaining Treatment* (Washington, DC: U.S. Government Printing Office, 1983), pp. 61–67.
2. This discussion draws on the work of James Rachels, in *The End of Life: Euthanasia and Morality* (Oxford: Oxford University Press, 1986), esp. pp. 5, 26–27, 32–33.
3. Quote is from Linda Gordon, in *Woman's Body, Woman's Right: A Social History of Birth Control in America* (New York: Grossman, 1976), p. 27.
4. U.S. Congress, Office of Technology Assessment, *Life-Sustaining Technologies and the Elderly* (Washington, DC: U.S. Government Printing Office, 1987), p. 197.
5. On the right to choose death, see Steven H. Miles and Allison August,

"Courts, Gender and 'The Right to Die,'" *Law, Medicine & Health Care* 18 (1990): 85; and President's Commission, *Deciding to Forego*, p. 63; statistics on quitting dialysis and negotiated death are in Andrew H. Malcolm, "What Medical Science Can't Seem to Learn: When to Call It Quits," *New York Times*, December 23, 1990. Suicide, assisted suicide, and the reactions of courts and juries are discussed by Derek Humphry and Ann Wickett in *The Right to Die: Understanding Euthanasia* (New York: Harper & Row, 1986), esp. pp. 131–140, 225.

6. On the history of euthanasia, see Margaret P. Battin, "Age Rationing and the Just Distribution of Health Care: Is There a Duty to Die?" in *Should Medical Care Be Rationed by Age?* ed. Timothy Smeeding (Totowa, NJ: Rowman & Littlefield, 1987), pp. 69–94; and Humphry and Wickett, *Right to Die*, passim; for parallels with birth control, see Gordon, *Woman's Body*, passim.

7. Kevin Kinsella, "Aging in the Third World," U.S. Bureau of the Census, *International Population Reports*, Series P–95, No. 79 (Washington, DC: U.S. Government Printing Office, 1988), pp. 14, 33, and passim.

8. U.S. Senate Special Committee on Aging, American Association of Retired Persons, Federal Council on the Aging, and U.S. Administration on Aging, *Aging America: Trends and Projections* (1987–1988 ed.) (Washington, DC: U.S. Government Printing Office, n.d.), p. 1; Dorothy P. Rice and Mitchell P. LaPlante, "Chronic Illness, Disability, and Increasing Longevity," in *The Economics and Ethics of Long–Term Care and Disability*, ed. Sean Sullivan and Marion Ein Lewin (Washington, DC: American Enterprise Institute for Public Policy Research, 1988), pp. 23–24.

9. U.S. Senate Special Committee on Aging, American Association of Retired Persons, Federal Council on the Aging, and U.S. Administration on Aging, *Aging America: Trends and Projections* (1991 ed.) (Washington, DC: U.S. Government Printing Office, n.d.), p. xxiv.

10. Barbara Boyle Torrey, "Sharing Increasing Costs on Declining Income: The Visible Dilemma of the Invisible Aged," *Milbank Memorial Fund Quarterly/Health and Society* 63 (1985): 392–393; Gordon F. Streib, "The Frail Elderly: Research Dilemmas and Research Opportunities," *The Gerontologist* 23 (1983): 40–41; for the importance of subgroup differences among the old, see Ira Rosenwaike and Barbara Logue, *The Extreme Aged in America: A Portrait of an Expanding Population* (Westport, CT: Greenwood Press, 1985), pp. 210–211; Jill Quadagno, Cebra Sims, D. Ann Squier, and Georgia Walker, in "Long–Term Care Community Services and Family Caregiving," in *Aging, Health, and Family: Long–Term Care*, ed. Timothy H. Brubaker (Newbury Park, CA: Sage Publications, 1987), pp. 119–120.

11. On "management" versus "curing," see Rice and LaPlante, "Chronic Illness"; James C. Riley, "The Risk of Being Sick: Morbidity Trends in Four Countries," *Population and Development Review* 16 (1990): 403–432; and Lois M. Verbrugge, "The Dynamics of Population Aging and Health,"

in *Aging & Health: Linking Research and Public Policy*, ed. Steven Lewis (Chelsea, MI: Lewis Publishers, 1989), pp. 23–40, esp. pp. 30–31; Verbrugge uses National Health Interview Survey data in "Longer Life but Worsening Health? Trends in Health and Mortality of Middle–aged and Older Persons," *Milbank Memorial Fund Quarterly/Health and Society* 62 (1984): 475–519.

12. U.S. Senate Special Committee on Aging et al., *Aging America* (1991 ed.), pp. 112, 115–116.

13. Berkeley Rice, "Death by Design: A Case in Point," in *Compassionate Crimes, Broken Taboos*, ed. Derek Humphry (Los Angeles: The Hemlock Society, 1986), p. 9.

14. The Florida man is quoted by Margaret Pabst Battin, in "Euthanasia Is Ethical," in *Euthanasia: Opposing Viewpoints*, ed. Neal Bernards (San Diego: Greenhaven Press), p. 20; on the double suicide, see Humphry, ed., *Compassionate Crimes*, p. 5.

15. Carolyn Wiener, Shizuko Fagerhaugh, Anselm Strauss, and Barbara Suczek, "What Price Chronic Illness?" in *Where Medicine Fails* (4th ed.), ed. Anselm L. Strauss (New Brunswick, NJ: Transaction Books, 1984), pp. 14–15; Congressional Budget Office, *Policy Choices for Long–Term Care* (Washington, DC: U.S. Government Printing Office, 1991), p. 5.

16. Marjorie H. Cantor, "Family and Community: Changing Roles in an Aging Society," *The Gerontologist* 31 (1991): 339; Dorothy P. Rice and Jacob J. Feldman, "Living Longer in the United States: Demographic Changes and Health Needs of the Elderly," *Milbank Memorial Fund Quarterly/Health and Society* 61 (1983): 372, 380.

17. Rice and Feldman, "Living Longer," esp. p. 363; Riley, "Risk of Being Sick," p. 407.

18. James F. Fries and Lawrence M. Crapo, *Vitality and Aging: Implications of the Rectangular Curve* (San Francisco: W. H. Freeman, 1981), p. 93.

19. U.S. Senate Special Committee on Aging, *Aging America* (1991 ed.), pp. 131, 133.

Chapter 2

1. Janice Reid, "'Going Up' or 'Going Down': The Status of Old People in an Australian Aboriginal Society," *Ageing and Society* 5 (1985): 76.

2. Jay Sokolovsky, "Introduction," in *The Cultural Context of Aging: Worldwide Perspectives*, ed. idem (New York: Bergin & Garvey, 1990), p. 10; Corinne N. Nydegger, "Family Ties of the Aged in Cross–Cultural Perspective," *The Gerontologist* 23 (1983): 26; Reid, "'Going Up,'" p. 84.

3. Accounts of the aged in premodern Europe and America may be found in W. Andrew Achenbaum and Peter N. Stearns, "Old Age and Modernization," *The Gerontologist* 18 (1978): esp. 309; W. Andrew Achenbaum, *Old Age in the New Land: The American Experience Since*

1790 (Baltimore: Johns Hopkins University Press, 1978); Peter N. Stearns, *Old Age in European Society: The Case of France* (New York: Holmes & Meier, 1976); idem, ed., *Old Age in Preindustrial Society* (New York: Holmes & Meier, 1982); idem, "Old Age Family Conflict: The Perspective of the Past," in *Elder Abuse: Conflict in the Family*, ed. Karl A. Pillemer and Rosalie S. Wolf (Dover, MA: Auburn House, 1986), pp. 3–24; David Van Tassel and Peter N. Stearns, *Old Age in a Bureaucratic Society: The Elderly, the Experts, and the State in American History* (Westport, CT: Greenwood Press, 1986); David H. Fischer, *Growing Old in America* (New York: Oxford University Press, 1977); Carole Haber, *Beyond Sixty–Five: The Dilemma of Old Age in America's Past* (Cambridge: Cambridge University Press, 1983); Jill S. Quadagno, *Aging in Early Industrial Society: Work, Family, and Social Policy in Nineteenth–Century England* (New York: Academic Press, 1982); idem, "The Transformation of Old Age Security," in *Old Age in a Bureaucratic Society: The Elderly, the Experts, and the State in American History*, ed. David Van Tassel and Peter N. Stearns (Westport, CT: Greenwood Press, 1986), esp. pp. 130–135; for other accounts of aging and the aging in traditional societies around the globe, see Erdman Palmore, *The Honorable Elders: A Cross–Cultural Analysis of Aging in Japan* (Durham, NC: Duke University Press, 1975); idem and Daisaku Maeda, *The Honorable Elders Revisited: A Revised Cross–Cultural Analysis of Aging in Japan* (Durham, NC: Duke University Press, 1985); Nancy Foner, "Age and Social Change," in *Age and Anthropological Theory*, ed. David I. Kertzer and Jennie Keith (Ithaca: Cornell University Press, 1984), pp. 195–216; Philip Silverman, "Comparative Studies," in *The Elderly as Modern Pioneers*, ed. idem (Bloomington: Indiana University Press, 1987), pp. 312–344; Colleen Leahy Johnson, "The Institutional Segregation of the Aged," pp. 375–388 in the same volume; Sylvia Vatuk, "Old Age in India," in *Old Age in Preindustrial Society*, ed. Peter N. Stearns (New York: Holmes & Meier, 1982), pp. 70–103.

4. The importance of asking "which aged" when questions of status arise was stressed by Leo Simmons in 1945, in *The Role of the Aged in Primitive Society* (New Haven, CT: Yale University Press, 1945), but has been overlooked in many accounts both before and since; Dorothy Ayers Counts and David R. Counts, "Linking Concepts: Aging and Gender, Aging and Death," in *Aging and Its Transformations*, ed. idem (Lanham, MD: University Press of America, 1985), p. 6; Anthony P. Glascock, "By Any Other Name, It Is Still Killing: A Comparison of the Treatment of the Elderly in America and Other Societies," in *The Cultural Context of Aging: Worldwide Perspectives*, ed. Jay Sokolovsky (New York: Bergin & Garvey, 1990), p. 51; Pamela T. Amoss and Stevan Harrell, "Introduction: An Anthropological Perspective on Aging," in *Other Ways of Growing Old: Anthropological Perspectives*, ed. idem (Stanford: Stanford University Press, 1981), p. 4; Robert J. Maxwell and Philip Silverman, "Information

and Esteem: Cultural Considerations in the Treatment of the Aged," in *In the Country of the Old*, ed. Jon Hendricks, (Farmingdale, NY: Baywood, 1980), p. 31; Charles Edward Fuller, "Aging Among Southern African Bantu," in *Aging and Modernization*, ed. Donald O. Cowgill and Lowell D. Holmes (New York: Appleton–Century–Crofts, 1972), pp. 67, 71; emphasis added.

5. Anthony P. Glascock and Susan L. Feinman, "Treatment of the Aged in Nonindustrial Societies," in *New Methods for Old Age Research: Strategies for Studying Diversity*, by Christine L. Fry, Jennie Keith, and contributors (South Hadley, MA: Bergin & Garvey, 1986), p. 286.

6. Dorothy Ayers Counts and David R. Counts, "I'm Not Dead Yet! Aging and Death: Process and Experience in Kaliai," in *Aging and Its Transformations*, ed. idem (Lanham, MD: University Press of America, 1985), pp. 146–147; William H. McKellin, "Passing Away and Loss of Life: Aging and Death Among the Managalese of Papua New Guinea," p. 199 in the same volume; David R. Counts and Dorothy A. Counts, "Conclusions: Coping with the Final Tragedy," in *Coping with the Final Tragedy: Cultural Variation in Dying and Grieving*, ed. idem (Amityville, NY: Baywood, 1991), pp. 280–283.

7. See Judith Treas and Barbara Logue, "Economic Development and the Older Population," *Population and Development Review* 12 (1986): 645–673; and Barbara J. Logue, "Modernization and the Status of the Frail Elderly: Perspectives on Continuity and Change," *Journal of Cross–Cultural Gerontology* 5 (1990): 345–374 for other uses of the four categories; Lawrence Stone, *The Past and the Present* (Boston: Routledge & Kegan Paul, 1981), p. 240.

8. Jay Sokolovsky (ed.), *Growing Old in Different Societies: Cross–Cultural Perspectives* (Belmont, CA: Wadsworth, 1983), p. 12; on "material resources of economic value" in particular, see Philip Silverman and Robert J. Maxwell, "Cross–Cultural Variation in the Status of Old People," in *Old Age in Preindustrial Society*, ed. Peter N. Stearns (New York: Holmes & Meier, 1982), p. 63; idem, "The Significance of Information and Power in the Comparative Study of the Aged," in *Growing Old in Different Societies: Cross–Cultural Perspectives*, ed. Jay Sokolovsky (Belmont, CA: Wadsworth, 1983), p. 51; William H. Harlan, "Social Status of the Aged in Three Indian Villages," in *Middle Age and Aging: A Reader in Social Psychology*, ed. Bernice L. Neugarten (Chicago: University of Chicago Press, 1968), p. 474; quote on seventeenth–century England is in Stone, *Past and Present*, p. 235; Quadagno, "Transformation," esp. pp. 130–133.

9. Achenbaum, *Old Age*; Donald O. Cowgill, *Aging Around the World* (Belmont, CA: Wadsworth, 1986), esp. p. 102; Jennie Keith, *Old People As People: Social and Cultural Influences on Aging and Old Age* (Boston: Little, Brown, 1982); Simmons, *Role of the Aged*; idem, "Attitudes Toward Aging and the Aged: Primitive Societies," *Journal of Gerontology* 1 (1946): 72–95; Nancy Foner, "Old and Frail and Everywhere Unequal,"

The Hastings Center Report 15 (1985): 27–31; Julianna Flinn, "Kinship, Gender, and Aging on Pulap, Caroline Islands," in *Aging and Its Transformations*, ed. Dorothy Ayers Counts and David R. Counts (Lanham, MD: University Press of America, 1985), p. 78.

10. Simmons, "Attitudes," p. 81; Maxwell and Silverman, "Information and Esteem," p. 18; Thomas R. Cole, "'Putting Off the Old': Middle–Class Morality, Antebellum Protestantism, and the Origins of Ageism," in *Old Age in a Bureaucratic Society: The Elderly, the Experts, and the State in American History*, ed. David Van Tassel and Peter N. Stearns (Westport, CT: Greenwood Press, 1986), p. 58; Achenbaum, *Old Age*, p. 33.

11. James D. Nason, "Respected Elder or Old Person: Aging in a Micronesian Community," in *Other Ways of Growing Old: Anthropological Perspectives*, ed. Pamela T. Amoss and Stevan Harrell (Stanford: Stanford University Press, 1981), p. 171; Foner, "Old and Frail," p. 28; Maria Lepowsky, "Gender, Aging, and Dying in an Egalitarian Society," in *Aging and Its Transformations*, ed. Dorothy Ayers Counts and David R. Counts (Lanham, MD: University Press of America, 1985), pp. 157–178; Silverman and Maxwell, "Significance of Information and Power"; Cowgill, *Aging Around the World*, p. 155; Nancy Foner, "Caring for the Elderly: A Cross–Cultural View," in *Growing Old in America: New Perspectives on Old Age* (3d ed.), ed. Beth B. Hess and Elizabeth W. Markson (New Brunswick, NJ: Transaction Books, 1985), p. 388; Fuller, "Southern African Bantu," p. 65; Eleanor Krassen Maxwell and Robert J. Maxwell, "Contempt for the Elderly: A Cross–Cultural Analysis," *Current Anthropology* 21 (1980): 570.

12. The death of the old woman in Kaliai is described in Counts and Counts, "I'm Not Dead Yet!" pp. 145–146; Foner, "Old and Frail," pp. 30–31; Frances McAleavey Adams, "The Role of Old People in Santo Tomás Mazaltepec," in *Aging and Modernization*, ed. Donald O. Cowgill and Lowell D. Holmes (New York: Appleton–Century–Crofts, 1972), p. 123.

13. Adams, "Role of Old People," p. 122.

14. Eleanor Krassen Maxwell, "Fading Out: Resource Control and Cross–Cultural Patterns of Deference," *Journal of Cross–Cultural Gerontology* 1 (1986): 81.

15. Harriet G. Rosenberg, "Complaint Discourse, Aging, and Caregiving Among the !Kung San of Botswana," in *The Cultural Context of Aging: Worldwide Perspectives*, ed. Jay Sokolovsky (New York: Bergin & Garvey, 1990), p. 28.

16. See, for example, Charlotte Ikels, "The Coming of Age in Chinese Society: Traditional Patterns and Contemporary Hong Kong," in *Aging in Culture and Society: Comparative Viewpoints and Strategies*, by Christine L. Fry and contributors (Brooklyn, NY: J. F. Bergin, 1980), p. 97.

17. Foner, "Old and Frail," p. 29; Barbara W. K. Yee, "Gender & Family Issues in Minority Groups," *Generations* 14 (1990): 39; quote is from Daniel Callahan, *Setting Limits: Medical Goals in an Aging Society* (New

York: Simon and Schuster, 1987), p. 154; Emily K. Abel, *Who Cares for the Elderly? Public Policy and the Experiences of Adult Daughters* (Philadelphia: Temple University Press, 1991), pp. 56–57.

18. For a survey of 3,000 years of negative attitudes towards aging and old people in the preindustrial Western world, see David H. Fowler, Lois Josephs Fowler, and Lois Lamdin, "Themes of Old Age in Preindustrial Western Literature," in *Old Age in Preindustrial Society*, ed. Peter N. Stearns (New York: Holmes & Meier, 1982), pp. 19–45; also see Nydegger, "Family Ties," p. 27; quote is from Stearns, *Old Age in European Society,* p.18; Adele Lindenmeyr, "Work, Charity, and the Elderly in Late–Nineteenth–Century Russia," in *Old Age in Preindustrial Society*, ed. Peter N. Stearns (New York: Holmes & Meier, 1982), esp. pp. 238, 243; Achenbaum, *Old Age*, esp. pp. 3, 25; Glascock, "By Any Other Name," pp. 52–53.

19. Simmons's quote is from "Attitudes," p. 74; on the importance of reciprocity, see Glascock, "By Any Other Name," p. 52; Margaret Clark, "Cultural Values and Dependency in Later Life," in *Aging and Modernization*, ed. Donald O. Cowgill and Lowell D. Holmes (New York: Appleton–Century–Crofts, 1972), pp. 263–274; and Foner, "Old and Frail," p. 28; Adams, "Role of Old People," pp. 112–113; Karen Jonas and Edward Wellin, "Dependency and Reciprocity: Home Health Aid in an Elderly Population," in *Aging in Culture and Society: Comparative Viewpoints and Strategies*, by Christine L. Fry and contributors (New York: Praeger, 1980), pp. 218–219; Anthony P. Glascock, "Decrepitude and Death–Hastening: The Nature of Old Age in Third World Societies," in *Aging and the Aged in the Third World*, Part I, Studies in Third World Societies, No. 22, pp. 43–66.

20. Harry D. Eastwell, "Voodoo Death and the Mechanism for Dispatch of the Dying in East Arnhem, Australia," *American Anthropologist* 84 (1982): 15; Glascock, "Decrepitude," p. 51; Leopold Rosenmayr, "The Elderly in Austrian Society," in *Aging and Modernization*, ed. Donald O. Cowgill and Lowell D. Holmes (New York: Appleton–Century–Crofts, 1972), p. 184; Christine L. Fry, "Theories of Age and Culture," in *Emergent Theories of Aging*, ed. James E. Birren and Vern L. Bengtson (New York: Springer, 1988), p. 450; Foner, "Old and Frail," p. 28; David W. Plath, "Japan: The After Years," in *Aging and Modernization*, ed. Donald O. Cowgill and Lowell D. Holmes (New York: Appleton–Century–Crofts, 1972), p. 138; for a suggestive portrayal of "passive" decision making, see Dorothy S. Mull and J. Dennis Mull, "Infanticide Among the Tarahumara of the Mexican Sierra Madre," in *Child Survival: Anthropological Perspectives on the Treatment and Maltreatment of Children*, ed. Nancy Scheper–Hughes (Dordrecht, The Netherlands: D. Reidel, 1987), pp. 113–132.

21. Counts and Counts, "I'm Not Dead Yet!" pp. 146–147; Foner, "Old and Frail," p. 31; Simmons, "Attitudes," p. 73; Judith Barker, "Between Humans and Ghosts: The Decrepit Elderly in a Polynesian Society," in *The*

Cultural Context of Aging: Worldwide Perspectives, ed. Jay Sokolovsky (New York: Bergin & Garvey, 1990), pp. 295–313, esp. p. 306; Adams, "Role of Old People," pp. 113–114; John Kirkpatrick, "Ko'oua: Aging in the Marquesas Islands," in *Aging and Its Transformations*, ed. Dorothy Ayers Counts and David R. Counts (Lanham, MD: University Press of America, 1985), p. 97.

22. Silverman and Maxwell, "Cross–Cultural Variation," pp. 66–67; Elizabeth Colson and Thayer Scudder, "Old Age in Gwembe District, Zambia," in *Other Ways of Growing Old: Anthropological Perspectives*, ed. Pamela T. Amoss and Stevan Harrell (Stanford, CA: Stanford University Press, 1981), p. 128; Nason, "Respected Elder," esp. pp. 164, 171.

23. Cowgill, *Aging Around the World*, p. 90; the Papua New Guinea incident is described by Dorothy A. Counts and David R. Counts, in "Loss and Anger: Death and the Expression of Grief in Kaliai," in *Coping with the Final Tragedy: Cultural Variation in Dying and Grieving*, ed. David R. Counts and Dorothy A. Counts (Amityville, NY: Baywood, 1991), pp. 197–198; Counts and Counts, "Introduction," pp. 19, 21.

24. Adams, "Role of Old People," pp. 112–113; Foner, "Old and Frail," p. 28; Harlan, "Social Status of Aged"; Quadagno, "Transformation."

25. Barker, "Humans and Ghosts," pp. 301, 311–312.

26. Haber, *Beyond Sixty–Five*; Quadagno, "Transformation"; Lindenmeyr, "Work, Charity," esp. pp. 239, 243; quoted material is from Charles E. Rosenberg, *The Care of Strangers: The Rise of America's Hospital System* (New York: Basic Books, 1987), p. 306.

27. Barker, "Humans and Ghosts," pp. 301, 305.

28. See, for example, Callahan, *Setting Limits*, p. 148; and Robert Kastenbaum and Brian L. Mishara, "Premature Death and Self–Injurious Behavior in Old Age," in *Old Age on the New Scene*, ed. Robert Kastenbaum (New York: Springer, 1981), pp. 269–282.

29. Counts and Counts, "Loss and Anger," p. 196.

30. Nancy Scheper–Hughes, "Deposed Kings: The Demise of the Rural Irish Gerontocracy," in *Growing Old in Different Societies: Cross–Cultural Perspectives*, ed. Jay Sokolovsky (Belmont, CA: Wadsworth, 1983), p. 140; Michael C. Kearl, *Endings: A Sociology of Death and Dying* (New York: Oxford University Press, 1989), pp. 121–122.

31. Glascock, "By Any Other Name," p. 48.

32. Robert Kastenbaum, "Death, Dying, and Bereavement in Old Age: New Developments and Their Possible Implications for Psychosocial Care," in *Aging* (5th ed.), ed. Harold Cox (Guilford, CT: Dushkin Publishing Group, 1987), p. 165; Eastwell, "Voodoo Death," pp. 12–14.

33. Anthony P. Glascock and Susan L. Feinman, "Social Asset or Social Burden: Treatment of the Aged in Non–Industrial Societies," in *Dimensions: Aging, Culture, and Health*, by Christine L. Fry and contributors (New York: Praeger, 1981), pp. 24–25; the 50 percent figure is from Glascock, "By Any Other Name," p. 51.

34. Simmons, "Attitudes," pp. 87–88.
35. Glascock and Feinman, "Social Asset," p. 28; Eastwell, "Voodoo Death," pp. 12–15; Glascock, "By Any Other Name," p. 47; Sokolovsky, "Introduction," pp. 3–5.
36. Lowell D. Holmes, "The Role and Status of the Aged in a Changing Samoa," in *Aging and Modernization*, ed. Donald O. Cowgill and Lowell D. Holmes (New York: Appleton–Century–Crofts, 1972), pp. 84–86; Eastwell, "Voodoo Death," pp. 15–16; Foner, "Old and Frail," p. 27; on death as a "sad and trying experience" for most elders, see Simmons, "Attitudes," p. 89.
37. Naomi M. Scaletta, "Death by Sorcery: The Social Dynamics of Dying in Bariai, West New Britain," in *Aging and Its Transformations*, ed. Dorothy Ayers Counts and David R. Counts (Lanham, MD: University Press of America, 1985), p. 241.

Chapter 3

1. The story of kuru is told by June Goodfield, *Quest for the Killers* (New York: Hill and Wang, 1985), pp. 1–49, esp. pp. 1–3, 11, 15, 32, 43.
2. Ibid., p. 15.
3. Quotes are from Goodfield, *Quest*, pp. 47, 49; Jersey Liang and Nancy Whitelaw, "Long–Term Care in the United States: Some Implications for China," in *Aging China: Family, Economics, and Government Policies in Transition*, ed. James H. Schulz and Deborah Davis–Friedmann (Washington, DC: Gerontological Society of America, 1987), p. 294; Robert N. Butler, "Overview on Aging: Some Biomedical, Social, and Behavioral Perspectives," in *Aging: Stability and Change in the Family*, ed. Robert W. Fogel, Elaine Hatfield, Sara B. Kiesler, and Ethel Shanas (New York: Academic Press, 1981), p. 2; and U.S. Congress, Office of Technology Assessment, *Losing a Million Minds: Confronting the Tragedy of Alzheimer's Disease and Other Dementias* (Washington, DC: U.S. Government Printing Office, 1987), pp. 14, 36; Michael C. Kearl, *Endings: A Sociology of Death and Dying* (New York: Oxford University Press, 1989), p. 126; Gloria Borger, "The Shadows Lurking behind Dr. Death," *U.S. News and World Report*, December 17, 1990, p. 31.
4. See, for example, Jan S. Greenberg and Marion Becker, "Aging Parents as Family Resources," *The Gerontologist* 28 (1988): 786–791, esp. 786.
5. Tish Sommers and Laurie Shields, with the Older Women's League Task Force on Caregivers and Judy MacLean, *Women Take Care: The Consequences of Caregiving in Today's Society* (Gainesville, FL: Triad, 1987), p. 19; Suzanne K. Steinmetz, *Duty Bound: Elder Abuse and Family Care* (Newbury Park, CA: Sage Publications, 1988), p. 227.
6. Nelson Wing–sun Chow, "The Chinese Family and Support of the Elderly in Hong Kong," *The Gerontologist* 23 (1983): 587; Nancy Guberman,

Pierre Maheu, and Chantal Maille, "Women as Family Caregivers: Why Do They Care?" *The Gerontologist* 32 (1992): 613.

7. Hilary Stout, "Soaring Health Costs Have a Silver Lining: A Host of New Jobs," *Wall Street Journal*, September 6, 1991; idem, "Godsend for Many, Home–Care Industry Also Has Potential for Fraud and Abuse," *Wall Street Journal*, November 21, 1991; Gabriella Stern, "Demographics Fuel Adult–Diaper Sales," *Wall Street Journal*, March 20, 1992; U.S. Congress, Office of Technology Assessment, *Life–Sustaining Technologies and the Elderly* (Washington, DC: U.S. Government Printing Office, 1987), p. 357.

8. On benefits to the young, see Daniel Callahan, *Setting Limits: Medical Goals in an Aging Society* (New York: Simon and Schuster, 1987), p. 129.

9. Derek Humphry and Ann Wickett, *The Right to Die: Understanding Euthanasia* (New York: Harper & Row, 1986), pp. 163, 165; for discussions of right–to–die issues around the globe, see Shi Da Pu, "Euthanasia in China: A Report," *Journal of Medicine and Philosophy* 16 (1991): 131–138; Jagdish Bhatia, "The New Code of Live and Let Die," *Far Eastern Economic Review* 134 (1986): 40–41; Maurice A. M. De Wachter, "Ethics and Health Policy in the Netherlands," in *Health Care Systems: Moral Conflicts in European and American Public Policy*, ed. Hans–Martin Sass and Robert U. Massey (Dordrecht, The Netherlands: Kluwer Academic Publishers, 1988), pp. 97–116; and Sol Levine, "The Changing Terrains in Medical Sociology: Emergent Concern With Quality of Life," *Journal of Health and Social Behavior* 28 (1987): 1–6.

10. Robert N. Butler, *Why Survive? Being Old in America* (New York: Harper & Row, 1975), p. xi.

11. Anthony P. Glascock, "By Any Other Name, It Is Still Killing: A Comparison of the Treatment of the Elderly in America and Other Societies," in *The Cultural Context of Aging: Worldwide Perspectives*, ed. Jay Sokolovsky (New York: Bergin & Garvey, 1990), p. 52; the respective quotes are from Erdman Palmore and Daisaku Maeda, *The Honorable Elders Revisited: A Revised Cross–Cultural Analysis of Aging in Japan* (Durham, NC: Duke University Press, 1985), p. 99; and David W. Plath, "Japan: The After Years," in *Aging and Modernization*, ed. Donald O. Cowgill and Lowell D. Holmes (New York: Appleton–Century–Crofts, 1972), p. 137; also see p. 138; Laurence J. Kotlikoff and John N. Morris, "How Much Care Do the Aged Receive from Their Children? A Bimodal Picture of Contact and Assistance," in *The Economics of Aging*, ed. David A. Wise (Chicago: University of Chicago Press, 1989), pp. 151–175.

12. Regarding lack of interaction among nursing home residents, see Andrea Fontana, "Growing Old Between Walls," in *Aging, the Individual and Society: Readings in Social Gerontology*, ed. Jill S. Quadagno (New York: St. Martin's Press, 1980), pp. 490–491; Congressional Budget Office, *Policy Choices for Long–Term Care* (Washington, DC: U.S. Government Printing Office, 1991), p. 5; Jaber F. Gubrium, *Living and Dying at Murray Manor* (New York: St. Martin's Press, 1975), esp. pp. 19, 26, 30,

111–113, 201; William L. Gekoski and V. Jane Knox, "Ageism or Healthism? Perceptions Based on Age and Health Status," *Journal of Aging and Health* 2 (1990): 15–27.

13. Nancy S. Jecker, "The Role of Intimate Others in Medical Decision Making," *The Gerontologist* 30 (1990): 69; Callahan, *Setting Limits*, pp. 20, 216; Jack D. McCue, ed., *The Medical Cost–Containment Crisis: Fears, Opinions, and Facts* (Ann Arbor, MI: Health Administration Press, 1989), p. 261; Phillip Longman, *Born to Pay: The New Politics of Aging in America* (Boston: Houghton Mifflin, 1987).

14. Isabel Moore, "The Nursing Home: Tender, Loving Care? Or Adult Orphanage?" *Nursing Homes and Senior Citizen Care* 35(6) (1986): 29.

15. Andrea Sankar, "The Living Dead: Cultural Constructions of the Oldest Old," in *The Elderly as Modern Pioneers*, ed. Philip Silverman (Bloomington: Indiana University Press, 1987), p. 345; Charles F. Longino, Jr., "Returning from the Sunbelt: Myths and Realities of Migratory Patterns among the Elderly," Symposium sponsored by the Brookdale Institute on Aging and Adult Human Development (Columbia University) and the International Exchange Center on Gerontology (University of South Florida), March 15, 1985, pp. 7–8; Palmore and Maeda, *Honorable Elders Revisited*, p. 94; Plath, "After Years," p. 137; Christie W. Kiefer, "Care of the Aged in Japan," in *Health, Illness, and Medical Care in Japan: Cultural and Social Dimensions*, ed. Edward Norbeck and Margaret Lock (Honolulu: University of Hawaii Press, 1987), pp. 89–90; survey results are reported by Takie Sugiyama Lebra, in "The Dilemma and Strategies of Aging Among Contemporary Japanese Women," *Ethnology* 18 (1979): 340, 344.

16. Elaine M. Brody, "Parent Care as a Normative Family Stress," *The Gerontologist* 25 (1985): 19–29; on growing skepticism about the medical system, see Hans–Martin Sass and Robert U. Massey, *Health Care Systems: Moral Conflicts in European and American Public Policy* (Dordrecht, The Netherlands: Kluwer Academic Publishers, 1988); Paul Starr, *The Social Transformation of American Medicine* (New York: Basic Books, 1982); and Kiefer, "Care of Aged."

17. Nancy Foner, *Ages in Conflict: A Cross–Cultural Perspective on Inequality between Old and Young* (New York: Columbia University Press, 1984); idem, "Caring for the Elderly: A Cross–Cultural View," in *Growing Old in America: New Perspectives on Old Age* (3d ed.), ed. Beth B. Hess and Elizabeth W. Markson (New Brunswick, NJ: Transaction Books, 1985), pp. 387–400; Linda K. George, "Caregiver Burden: Conflict Between Norms of Reciprocity and Solidarity," in *Elder Abuse: Conflict in the Family*, ed. Karl A. Pillemer and Rosalie S. Wolf (Dover, MA: Auburn House, 1986), pp. 67–92; Peter N. Stearns, "Old Age Family Conflict: The Perspective of the Past," pp. 3–24 in the same volume; Nancy J. Finley, M. Diane Roberts, and Benjamin F. Banahan, "Motivators and Inhibitors of Attitudes of Filial Obligation toward Aging Parents," *The Gerontologist*

28 (1988): 73–74; Plath, "After Years," p. 141; Sally Bould, Beverly Sanborn, and Laura Reif, *Eighty–Five Plus: The Oldest Old* (Belmont, CA: Wadsworth, 1989), p. 105.

18. Bould, Sanborn, and Reif, *Eighty–Five Plus*, pp. 4–5, 91–93; Candace Clark, "Sympathy Biography and Sympathy Margin," *American Journal of Sociology* 93 (1987): 290–321, esp. 316; Margaret Clark, "Cultural Values and Dependency in Later Life," in *Aging and Modernization*, ed. Donald O. Cowgill and Lowell D. Holmes (New York: Appleton–Century–Crofts, 1972), pp. 267, 270; Norman Daniels, *Am I My Parents' Keeper? An Essay on Justice between the Young and the Old* (New York: Oxford University Press, 1988), pp. 31, 34.

19. Jihui Yuan, "Developing Research on Aging in China," in *Chinese Perspectives on Aging in the People's Republic of China*, by Jersey Liang, Chu Chuanyi, and Jihui Yuan (Tampa, FL: International Exchange Center on Gerontology, 1985).

20. Rodney M. Coe, "Professional Perspectives on the Aged," in *Aging, the Individual and Society: Readings in Social Gerontology*, ed. Jill S. Quadagno (New York: St. Martin's Press, 1980), pp. 472–481; Samuel Shem, *The House of God* (New York: Dell, 1978), p. 424; idem, "The House of God... Revisited," *Journal of the American Medical Association* 264 (1990): 1743; on "gomerism," see also Deborah B. Leiderman and Jean–Anne Grisso, "The Gomer Phenomenon," *Journal of Health and Social Behavior* 26 (1985): 222–232; on nurses' attitudes and behaviors, see Ronald Philip Preston, *The Dilemmas of Care: Social and Nursing Adaptions to the Deformed, the Disabled, and the Aged* (New York: Elsevier North Holland, 1979), esp. pp. 139, 162.

21. Rosalie A. Kane and Robert L. Kane, with James Reinardy and Sharon Arnold, *Long–Term Care: Principles, Programs, and Policies* (New York: Springer, 1987), p. 89; U.S. Congress, Office of Technology Assessment, *Technology and Aging in America* (Washington, DC: U.S. Government Printing Office, 1985), p. 221; idem, *Life–Sustaining Technologies*, pp. 213–214, 297–298; Joseph A. Califano, *America's Health Care Revolution: Who Lives? Who Dies? Who Pays?* (New York: Random House, 1986), p. 172; Diana Crane, *The Sanctity of Social Life: Physicians' Treatment of Critically Ill Patients* (New York: Russell Sage Foundation, 1975); Colleen Leahy Johnson, "The Institutional Segregation of the Aged," in *The Elderly as Modern Pioneers*, ed. Philip Silverman (Bloomington: Indiana University Press, 1987), pp. 379; Charles I. Stannard, "Old Folks and Dirty Work: The Social Conditions for Patient Abuse in a Nursing Home," in *Aging, the Individual and Society: Readings in Social Gerontology*, ed. Jill S. Quadagno (New York: St. Martin's Press, 1980), pp. 500–515; Bruce C. Vladeck, *Unloving Care: The Nursing Home Tragedy* (New York: Basic Books, 1980); quote is from Philip W. Brickner, Anthony J. Lechich, Roberta Lipsman, and Linda K. Scharer, *Long Term Health Care: Providing a Spectrum of Services to the Aged* (New York:

Basic Books, 1987), pp. 30–31; Murray Feshbach, "Health in the U.S.S.R.: Organization, Trends, and Ethics," in *Health Care Systems: Moral Conflicts in European and American Public Policy*, ed. Hans–Martin Sass and Robert U. Massey (Dordrecht, The Netherlands: Kluwer Academic Publishers, 1988), pp. 117–132.

22. Alice M. Rivlin and Joshua M. Wiener, with Raymond J. Hanley and Denise A. Spence, *Caring for the Disabled Elderly: Who Will Pay?* (Washington, DC: The Brookings Institution, 1988), p. 61; Bould, Sanborn, and Reif, *Eighty–Five Plus*, pp. 190–192; Alan M. Garber, "Long–Term Care, Wealth, and Health of the Disabled Elderly Living in the Community," in *The Economics of Aging*, ed. David A. Wise (Chicago: University of Chicago Press, 1989), p. 260; National Research Council, Panel on Statistics for an Aging Population, *The Aging Population in the Twenty–First Century* (Washington, DC: National Academy Press, 1988), pp. 174–175; Vincent Mor and Susan Masterson–Allen, *Hospice Care Systems: Structure, Process, Costs, and Outcome* (New York: Springer, 1987), pp. 15, 33; U.S. Congress, *Life–Sustaining Technologies*, pp. 64–65; Betty H. Landsberger, *Long–Term Care for the Elderly: A Comparative View of Layers of Care* (New York: St. Martin's Press, 1985), p. 148; James H. Schulz, "Preface," in *The Situation of the Asian/Pacific Elderly*, ed. Charlotte Nusberg and Masako M. Osako (Washington, DC: International Federation on Ageing, 1981); Eileen J. Tell, Stanley S. Wallack, and Marc A. Cohen, "New Directions in Life Care: An Industry in Transition," *The Milbank Quarterly* 65 (1987): 551–574; John H. Skinner, "Federal Programs for the Vulnerable Aged," in *The Vulnerable Aged: People, Services, and Policies*, ed. Zev Harel, Phyllis Ehrlich, and Richard Hubbard (New York: Springer, 1990), p. 251.

23. Jeffrey C. Merrill and Alan B. Cohen, "Explicit Rationing of Medical Care: Is It Really Needed?" in *The Medical Cost–Containment Crisis: Fears, Opinions, and Facts*, ed. Jack D. McCue (Ann Arbor, MI: Health Administration Press, 1989), Editor's Note and p. 239.

24. Bernice L. Neugarten, "Older People: A Profile," in *Age or Need: Public Policies for Older People*, ed. Bernice L. Neugarten (Beverly Hills: Sage Publications, 1982), p. 43; Robert Kastenbaum, "Death, Dying, and Bereavement in Old Age: New Developments and Their Possible Implications for Psychosocial Care," in *Aging* (5th ed.), ed. Harold Cox (Guilford, CT: Dushkin Publishing Group, 1987), p. 165; on Britain's health care system, see Henry J. Aaron and William B. Schwartz, *The Painful Prescription: Rationing Hospital Care* (Washington, DC: The Brookings Institution, 1984), esp. pp. 96–97; Paul T. Menzel, *Strong Medicine: The Ethical Rationing of Health Care* (New York: Oxford University Press, 1990), pp. 191–192, 196, 200.

25. Goodfield, *Quest*, p. 32.

26. Califano, *America's Health Care Revolution*, pp. 172–173; Peter D. Fox and Steven B. Clauser, "Trends in Nursing Home Expenditures," *Health*

Care Financing Review 2 (1980): 65–70; Carole Haber, *Beyond Sixty–Five: The Dilemma of Old Age in America's Past* (Cambridge: Cambridge University Press, 1983); Johnson, "Institutional Segregation"; Kiefer, "Care of Aged"; Liang and Whitelaw, "Long–Term Care"; Jill S. Quadagno, "The Transformation of Old Age Security," in *Old Age in a Bureaucratic Society: The Elderly, the Experts, and the State in American History*, ed. David Van Tassel and Peter N. Stearns (Westport, CT: Greenwood Press, 1986), esp. pp. 131–137; Charles E. Rosenberg, "The Aged in a Structured Social Context: Medicine as a Case Study," pp. 231–245 in the same volume.

27. Rosenberg, "Aged in Structured Social Context," pp. 240–242; Frank J. Thompson, *Health Policy and the Bureaucracy: Politics and Implementation* (Cambridge, MA: MIT Press, 1981), p. 208; Daniels, *Parents' Keeper*, p. 105; Bruce A. Ferrell, "Pain Management in Elderly People," *Journal of the American Geriatrics Society* 39 (1991): 64–73; Neugarten, "Older People," pp. 49–51; Landsberger, *Long–Term Care*, esp. pp. 24, 148–149.

28. Vladeck, *Unloving Care*, p. 29; Robert Pear, "U.S. Agency Seeks Wide Rule Changes on Nursing Homes," *New York Times*, July 5, 1987; idem, "U.S. Laws Delayed by Complex Rules and Partisanship," *New York Times*, March 31, 1991.

29. Tell, Wallack, and Cohen, "New Directions," p. 551; Califano, *America's Health Care Revolution*, pp. 172–173.

30. Karen Davis, "Paying the Health–Care Bills of an Aging Population," in *Our Aging Society: Paradox and Promise*, ed. Alan Pifer and Lydia Bronte (New York: W. W. Norton, 1986), pp. 308–310; Tell, Wallack, and Cohen, "New Directions," p. 570; Stephen Crystal, *America's Old Age Crisis: Public Policy and the Two Worlds of Aging* (New York: Basic Books, 1982), p. 89; Frank Robinson's story is in Derek Humphry, *Let Me Die Before I Wake: Hemlock's Book of Self–Deliverance for the Dying* (Eugene OR: The Hemlock Society, 1986), esp. p. 37.

31. Terrie Wetle, Sue Levkoff, Julie Cwikel, and Amy Rosen, "Nursing Home Resident Participation in Medical Decisions: Perceptions and Preferences," *The Gerontologist* 28 (1988) (Supp.): 33; John E. Morley, Karen Vogel, and David H. Solomon, "Prevalence of Geriatric Articles in General Medical Journals," *Journal of the American Geriatrics Society* 38 (1990): 173: quote on futility of extensive care is from Carole Haber, "Geriatrics: A Specialty in Search of Specialists," in *Old Age in a Bureaucratic Society: The Elderly, the Experts, and the State in American History*, ed. David Van Tassel and Peter N. Stearns (Westport, CT: Greenwood Press, 1986), pp. 66–67; quote is on p. 80; Michael S. Wilkes and Miriam Shuchman, "What Is Too Old?" *New York Times Magazine*, June 4, 1989, p. 58.

32. Judith Treas and Barbara Logue, "Economic Development and the Older Population," *Population and Development Review* 12 (1986): 645–673; Linda G. Martin, "The Aging of Asia," *Journal of Gerontology* 43 (1988):

S99–113; Ken Tout, *Ageing in Developing Countries* (Oxford: Oxford University Press, 1989), p. 303; United Nations, *World Population Trends and Policies: 1987 Monitoring Report* (New York: United Nations, 1988), pp. 155–172, esp. 155–157; quote is from Brahm Prakash, "Some Development Implications of an Aging Population," in *Aging in India*, ed. K. G. Desai (Bombay: Tata Institute of Social Sciences, 1982), p. 22; also see J. D. Pathak, "Geriatrics in India: Some Suggestions," pp. 43–53 in the same volume; Walter Fernandez, "Aging in South Asia as Marginalisation in a Neo–Colonial Economy: An Introduction," in *Aging in South Asia: Theoretical Issues and Policy Implications*, ed. Alfred de Souza and Walter Fernandez (New Delhi: Indian Social Institute, 1982), pp. 1–23; Eli Ginzberg "The Elderly: An International Policy Perspective," *Milbank Memorial Fund Quarterly/Health and Society* 61 (1983): 473–488; Landsberger, *Long–Term Care*, pp. 41–52; Mary Fadel–Girgis, "Family Support for the Elderly in Egypt," *The Gerontologist* 23 (1983): 589–592; Melvyn C. Goldstein, Sidney Schuler, and James L. Ross, "Social and Economic Forces Affecting Intergenerational Relations in Extended Families in a Third World Country: A Cautionary Tale From South Asia," *Journal of Gerontology* 38 (1983): 716–724; Martin, "Aging of Asia"; Wu Yuanjin and Xu Qin, "The Impact of an Aging Population on Socio–Economic Development and Families in China," in *Aging China: Family, Economics, and Government Policies in Transition*, ed. James H. Schulz and Deborah Davis–Friedmann (Washington, DC: Gerontological Society of America, 1987), pp. 19–35; Chow, "Chinese Family"; Charlotte Nusberg and Masako M. Osako, eds., *The Situation of the Asian/Pacific Elderly* (Washington, DC: International Federation on Ageing, 1981); Sylvia Vatuk, "Old Age in India," in *Old Age in Preindustrial Society*, ed. Peter N. Stearns (New York: Holmes & Meier, 1982), pp. 70–103.

33. United Nations, *World Population Trends*, p. 159; Haber, "Geriatrics"; Kiefer, "Care of Aged"; statistics are from Edward F. Lawlor, "What Kind of Medicine?" *The Gerontologist* 32 (1992): 132; Bernice T. Halbur, *Turnover Among Nursing Personnel in Nursing Homes* (Ann Arbor, MI: UMI Research Press, 1980); U.S. Congress, *Technology and Aging*, pp. 216–217; idem, *Life–Sustaining Technologies*, pp. 362–366; on troubles in Sweden, see Harold J. Wershow, ed., *Controversial Issues in Gerontology* (New York: Springer, 1981), p. 132.

34. Crane, *Sanctity of Social Life*, pp. 11, 200; U.S. Congress, *Life–Sustaining Technologies*, pp. 18, 183–185, 263, 319, 346; De Wachter, "Ethics and Health Policy;" Feshbach, "Health in the U.S.S.R."; H. Gilbert Welch, "Comparing Apples and Oranges: Does Cost–Effectiveness Analysis Deal Fairly with the Old and Young?" *The Gerontologist* 31 (1991): 332–336.

35. Nancy J. Osgood and John L. McIntosh, "The Vulnerable Suicidal Elderly," in *The Vulnerable Aged: People, Services, and Policies*, ed. Zev Harel, Phyllis Ehrlich, and Richard Hubbard (New York: Springer, 1990), p. 181; respectives quotes are from Nancy J. Osgood, "Suicides," in

Handbook on the Aged in the United States, ed. Erdman B. Palmore (Westport, CT: Greenwood Press, 1984), p. 372; and idem, *Suicide in the Elderly: A Practitioner's Guide to Diagnosis and Mental Health Intervention* (Rockville, MD: Aspen Systems Corporation, 1985), p. xix.

36. Vladeck, *Unloving Care*, pp. 193, 264; Brickner et al., *Long Term Health Care*, p. 19; Steven K. Wisensale and Michael D. Allison, "An Analysis of 1987 State Family Leave Legislation: Implications for Caregivers of the Elderly," *The Gerontologist* 28 (1988): 782.

37. Johnson, "Institutional Segregation," p. 378; Gary M. Nelson, "Social Class and Public Policy for the Elderly," in *Age or Need: Public Policies for Older People*, ed. Bernice L. Neugarten (Beverly Hills, CA: Sage Publications, 1982), pp. 124–125; Crystal, *America's Old Age Crisis*, pp. 144–145, 158–160.

38. Brickner et al., *Long Term Health Care*, p. 29; quote on "program of last resort" is from David Wessell, "Medicaid is Beginning to Look More like Part of the Problem with the Health Care System," *Wall Street Journal*, August 8, 1991.

39. Carl Eisdorfer, "Foreword," in *Other Ways of Growing Old: Anthropological Perspectives*, ed. Pamela T. Amoss and Stevan Harrell (Stanford, CA: Stanford University Press, 1981), p. xix; William J. Winslade and Judith Wilson Ross, *Choosing Life or Death: A Guide for Patients, Families, and Professionals* (New York: Free Press, 1986), pp. 18–19; Robert Pear, "Medicare to Weigh Cost as a Factor in Reimbursement," *New York Times*, April 21, 1991; Pathak, "Geriatrics in India," p. 45.

40. Quote is from Jennie Keith, *Old People As People: Social and Cultural Influences on Aging and Old Age* (Boston: Little, Brown, 1982), p. 102; Bould, Sanborn, and Reif, *Eighty-Five Plus*, p. 26; Elias S. Cohen, "The Elderly Mystique: Constraints on the Autonomy of the Elderly With Disabilities," *The Gerontologist* 28 (1988) (Supp.): 24–31.

41. Henry Fairlie, "Greedy Geezers: Talkin' 'bout My Generation," *The New Republic*, March 28, 1988; Richard D. Lamm, "Again, Age Beats Youth," *New York Times*, December 2, 1990; Longman, *Born to Pay*; Samuel H. Preston, "Children and the Elderly: Divergent Paths for America's Dependents," *Demography* 21 (1984): 435–457; Walter A. Rosenbaum and James W. Button, "Is There a Gray Peril? Retirement Politics in Florida," *The Gerontologist* 29 (1989): 300–306; Steven K. Wisensale, "Generational Equity and Intergenerational Policies," *The Gerontologist* 28 (1988): 774; Harold A. Richman and Matthew W. Stagner, "Children: Treasured Resource or Forgotten Minority?" in *Our Aging Society: Paradox and Promise*, ed. Alan Pifer and Lydia Bronte (New York: W. W. Norton, 1986), pp. 161–179; Robert H. Binstock, "National Policies and the Vulnerable Aged: Present, Emerging, and Proposed," in *The Vulnerable Aged: People, Services, and Policies*, ed. Zev Harel, Phyllis Ehrlich, and Richard Hubbard (New York: Springer, 1990), pp. 235–247, esp. pp. 240–244.

42. Victor G. Cicirelli, "The Helping Relationship and Family Neglect in Later Life," in *Elder Abuse: Conflict in the Family*, ed. Karl A. Pillemer and Rosalie S. Wolf (Dover, MA: Auburn House, 1986), pp. 49–66; Karl Pillemer and David Finkelhor, "The Prevalence of Elder Abuse: A Random Sample Survey," *The Gerontologist* 28 (1988): 51–57; David E. Pitt, "The Elderly Often Find Crime a Family Matter," *New York Times*, September 27, 1987); Steinmetz, *Duty Bound*, passim.

43. Bould, Sanborn, and Reif, *Eighty–Five Plus*, p. 175; Brickner et al., *Long Term Health Care*, p. 40.

44. Wilkes and Shuchman, "What Is Too Old?"; John G. Francis and Leslie P. Francis, "Rationing of Health Care in Britain: An Ethical Critique of Public Policy–making," in *Should Medical Care Be Rationed by Age?* ed. Timothy Smeeding (Totowa, NJ: Rowman & Littlefield, 1987), pp. 119–134; Bould, Sanborn, and Reif, *Eighty–Five Plus*, pp. 176–177; Mor and Masterson–Allen, *Hospice Care Systems*, p. 15; Califano, *America's Health Care Revolution*, esp. pp. 172–173; Landsberger, *Long–Term Care*, p. 148; Tell, Wallack, and Cohen, "New Directions"; Binstock, "National Policies," p. 244.

45. Kris Bulcroft, Margaret R. Kielkopf, and Kevin Tripp, "Elderly Wards and Their Legal Guardians: Analysis of County Probate Records in Ohio and Washington," *The Gerontologist* 31 (1991): 156; Roger Peters, Winsor C. Schmidt, Jr., and Kent S. Miller, "Guardianship of the Elderly in Tallahassee, Florida," *The Gerontologist* 25 (1985): 536.

46. Peters, Schmidt, and Miller, "Guardianship of the Elderly, p. 533; quote is from Bulcroft, Kielkopf, and Tripp, "Elderly Wards," p. 157; also see pp. 160–161; Madelyn Anne Iris, "Guardianship and the Elderly. A Multi–Perspective View of the Decisionmaking Process," *The Gerontologist* 28 (1988) (Supp.): 42.

47. Rogers, Schmidt, and Miller, "Guardianship of the Elderly," pp. 537–538.

48. Kastenbaum, "Death, Dying," p. 165.

49. Robert Kastenbaum and Brian L. Mishara, "Premature Death and Self–Injurious Behavior in Old Age," in *Old Age on the New Scene*, ed. Robert Kastenbaum (New York: Springer, 1981), p. 272; Osgood, "Suicides," pp. 372, 380–381; Cheryl K. Smith, "Tragedy of Mis–diagnosed Woman Who Shot Herself," *Hemlock Quarterly*, No. 45, October, 1991, p. 2.

50. Osgood and McIntosh, "Vulnerable Suicidal Elderly," p. 178.

51. Andrew M. Kramer, Peter W. Shaughnessy, Marjorie K. Bauman, and Kathryn S. Crisler, "Assessing and Assuring the Quality of Home Health Care," *The Milbank Quarterly* 68 (1990): 413–414.

52. On premature institutionalization see, for example, Nancy Scheper–Hughes, "Deposed Kings: The Demise of the Rural Irish Gerontocracy," in *Growing Old in Different Societies: Cross–Cultural Perspectives*, ed. Jay Sokolovsky (Belmont, CA: Wadsworth, 1983), pp. 143–144; regarding the poor quality of many institutions and potential vic-

timization of clients, see Stannard, "Old Folks"; Vladeck, *Unloving Care*; Karl A. Pillemer, "Risk Factors in Elder Abuse: Results From a Case–Control Study," in *Elder Abuse: Conflict in the Family*, ed. idem and Rosalie S. Wolf (Dover, MA: Auburn House, 1986), pp. 239–263; idem, "Maltreatment of Patients in Nursing Homes: Overview and Research Agenda," *Journal of Health and Social Behavior* 29 (1988): 227–238; Judith Venglarik Braun, May H. Wykle, and W. Richard Cowling, III, "Failure to Thrive in Older Persons: A Concept Derived," *The Gerontologist* 28 (1988): 809–812; Ruth Campbell, "Nursing Homes and Long–Term Care in Japan," *Pacific Affairs* 57 (1984): 78–79; Johnson, "Institutional Segregation."

53. Vladeck, *Unloving Care*, pp. 175–177, 181; Stannard, "Old Folks," p. 504.

54. Cicirelli, "Helping Relationship," esp. p. 63; Maria Vesperi, "The Reluctant Consumer: Nursing Home Residents in the Post–Bergman Era," in *Growing Old in Different Societies: Cross–Cultural Perspectives*, ed. Jay Sokolovsky (Belmont, CA: Wadsworth, 1983), p. 236; other quotes are from Timothy Diamond, "Social Policy and Everyday Life in Nursing Homes: A Critical Ethnography," *Social Science and Medicine* 23 (1986): 1290 and Fontana, "Growing Old," p. 489.

55. Stannard, "Old Folks," p. 506.

56. J. Pierre Loebel, Justine S. Loebel, Stephen R. Dager, Brandon S. Centerwall, and Donald T. Reay, "Anticipation of Nursing Home Placement May Be a Precipitant of Suicide among the Elderly," *Journal of the American Geriatrics Society* 39 (1991): 407–408.

57. Donald E. Gibson, "Hospice: Morality and Economics," *The Gerontologist* 24 (1984): esp. 4–5.

58. Christine K. Cassel and Diane E. Meier, "Morals and Moralism in the Debate over Euthanasia and Assisted Suicide," *New England Journal of Medicine* 323 (1990): 751; quote is from C. G. Prado, *The Last Choice: Preemptive Suicide in Advanced Age* (Westport, CT: Greenwood Press, 1990), pp. 5, 44; Herbert S. Cohen, "Euthanasia as a Way of Life," *Hemlock Quarterly* No. 43, April 1991, pp. 7–8; Jerome A. Motto, "The Right to Suicide: A Psychiatrist's View," in *Death and Society*, ed. James P. Carse and Arlene B. Dallery (New York: Harcourt Brace Jovanovich, 1977), pp. 225–231.

59. Nancy R. Zweibel and Christine K. Cassel, "Treatment Choices at the End of Life: A Comparison of Decisions by Older Patients and Their Physician–Selected Proxies," *The Gerontologist* 29 (1989): 615–621; Eric L. Diamond, James A. Jernigan, Ray A. Moseley, Valerie Messina, and Robert A. McKeown, "Decision–Making Ability and Advance Directive Preferences in Nursing Home Patients and Proxies," *The Gerontologist* 29 (1989): 622–626.

60. See, for example, Callahan, *Setting Limits*, pp. 117, 119–121.

61. Marion Danis and Larry R. Churchill, "Autonomy and the Common

322 · *Last Rights*

Weal," *Hastings Center Report* 21 (1991): 27; Richard D. Lamm, "Euthanasia Should Be Based on Economic Factors," in *Euthanasia: Opposing Viewpoints*, ed. Neal Bernards (San Diego: Greenhaven Press, 1989), p. 132; B. P. Beckwith, "On the Right to Suicide by the Dying," *Dissent* 26 (1979): 231–233; Humphry and Wickett, *Right to Die*, p. 100; Winslade and Ross, *Choosing Life or Death*, esp. p. 84.

62. Robert S. Northrup, "Decision Making for Health Care in Developing Countries," in *Consequences of Mortality Trends and Differentials*, Population Studies No. 95 (New York: United Nations, 1986), pp. 142–143; Martin, "Aging of Asia," esp. pp. S107–108; quote is from Tout, *Ageing in Developing Countries*, p. 300.

63. Andrew H. Malcolm, "Many See Mercy in Ending Empty Lives," *New York Times*, September 23, 1984.

64. Haber, "Geriatrics," pp. 69–70; Peter N. Stearns, "The Modernization of Old Age in France: Approaches through History," *International Journal of Aging and Human Development* 13 (1981): 310.

65. On how America's system of medicine has changed over time, see Starr, *Social Transformation*, esp. p. 390; for the Robinsons' story, see Humphry, *Let Me Die*, p. 38; quote on "prolongation of suffering" is from Eliot Slater, "The Case for Voluntary Euthanasia," in *Death and Society*, ed. James P. Carse and Arlene B. Dallery (New York: Harcourt Brace Jovanovich, 1977), p. 90.

66. U.S. Congress, *Life-Sustaining Technologies*, p. 15; Kiefer, "Care of Aged"; Howard Levine, *Life Choices: Confronting the Life and Death Decisions Created by Modern Medicine* (New York: Simon and Schuster, 1986); Starr, *Social Transformation*; Ivan Illich, *Medical Nemesis: The Expropriation of Health* (New York: Pantheon, 1976), p. 34; Roger W. Evans, "Health Care Technology and the Inevitability of Resource Allocation and Rationing Decisions," *Journal of the American Medical Association* 249 (1983): 2049.

67. Margaret T. Loomis and T. Franklin Williams, "Evaluation of Care Provided to Terminally Ill Patients," *The Gerontologist* 23 (1983): 497.

68. Mor and Masterson–Allen, *Hospice Care Systems*, p. 7; Callahan, *Setting Limits*, pp. 196–197.

69. George Annas, "Into the Hands of Strangers," *Law, Medicine & Health Care* 13 (1985): 271; also see David Sudnow, "Dead on Arrival," in *Where Medicine Fails* (4th ed.), ed. Anselm L. Strauss (New Brunswick, NJ: Transaction Books, 1984), pp. 399–417; Elisabeth Rosenthal, "In Matters of Life and Death, the Dying Take Control," *New York Times*, August 18, 1991.

70. Humphry and Wickett, *Right to Die*, p. 215; Fenella Rouse, "Advance Directives: Where Are We Heading after *Cruzan*? *Law, Medicine & Health Care* 18 (1990): 355; Loomis and Williams, "Evaluation of Care," p. 497.

71. U.S. Congress, *Life-Sustaining Technologies*, p. 17; Goodfield, *Quest*, pp. 9, 15.

72. Alonzo L. Plough, *Borrowed Time: Artificial Organs and the Politics of Extending Lives* (Philadelphia: Temple University Press, 1986); Jerome L. Avorn, "Medicine: The Life and Death of Oliver Shay," in *Our Aging Society: Paradox and Promise*, ed. Alan Pifer and Lydia Bronte (New York: W. W. Norton, 1986), pp. 283–297; on the situation in the Netherlands, see De Wachter, "Ethics and Health Policy"; quote is from Kane et al., *Long–Term Care*, p. 371.

73. Janice Reid, "'Going Up' or 'Going Down': The Status of Old People in an Australian Aboriginal Society," *Ageing and Society* 5 (1985): 69–95; Alice Goldstein and Sidney Goldstein, "The Challenge of an Aging Population: The Case of the People's Republic of China," *Research on Aging* 8 (1986): 186; W. S. Chow, "The Urban Elderly in Developing East and Southeast Asian Countries," in *Aging China: Family, Economics and Government Policies in Transition*, ed. James H. Schulz and Deborah Davis–Friedmann (Washington, DC: Gerontological Society of America, 1987), pp. 93–103; Martin, "Aging of Asia"; Bhatia, "New Code"; Northrup, "Decision Making," p. 135; Chuanyi Chu, "The Reform of China's Social Security System for the Elderly," in *Chinese Perspectives on Aging in the People's Republic of China*, ed. Jersey Liang, Chuanyi Chu, and Yuan Jihui (Tampa, FL: International Exchange Center on Gerontology, 1985), pp. 22–30; Eisdorfer, "Foreword"; Ginzberg, "The Elderly"; Liang and Whitelaw, "Long–Term Care," p. 306; Pathak, "Geriatrics in India," p. 45; Shi Da Pu, "Euthanasia in China," p. 133.

74. U.S. Congress, *Losing a Million Minds*, pp. 3, 7, 14–15.

75. Glascock, "By Any Other Name," pp. 43, 56.

Chapter 4

1. S. Chandrasekhar, *"A Dirty, Filthy Book": The Writings of Charles Knowlton and Annie Besant on Reproductive Physiology and Birth Control and an Account of the Bradlaugh–Besant Trial* (Berkeley: University of California Press, 1981), pp. 23, 39, 67–68.

2. Ibid., p. 40.

3. Derek Humphry, *Let Me Die Before I Wake: Hemlock's Book of Self–Deliverance for the Dying* (Eugene, OR: The Hemlock Society, 1986), pp. 2–4.

4. Ansley J. Coale, "The Demographic Transition," in *The Population Debate: Dimensions and Perspectives* (New York: United Nations, 1975), p. 353; on the history of the birth control movement, see Linda Gordon, *Woman's Body, Woman's Right: A Social History of Birth Control in America* (New York: Grossman, 1976).

5. Gordon, *Woman's Body*, p. 189; on the hostility of churches and the medical profession toward birth control and the evolution in their attitudes over time, see Flann Campbell, "Birth Control and the Christian

Churches," in *Population, Evolution, and Birth Control: A Collage of Controversial Ideas*, assembled by Garrett Hardin (San Francisco: W. H. Freeman, 1964), pp. 211–232; and Garrett Hardin, "Resistance to Birth Control within the Medical Profession," pp. 232–235 in the same volume.

6. Elaine M. Brody, "Parent Care as a Normative Family Stress," *The Gerontologist* 25 (1985): 19–29.

7. David J. Rothman, *Strangers at the Bedside: A History of How Law and Bioethics Transformed Medical Decision Making* (New York: Basic Books, 1991), p. 107.

8. Quote is from Daniel Callahan, "Can We Return Death to Disease?" *Hastings Center Report* 19 (1989) (Special Supplement): 6; Paul Starr, *The Social Transformation of American Medicine* (New York: Basic Books, 1982), pp. 379–380, 390; Ivan Illich, *Medical Nemesis: The Expropriation of Health* (New York: Pantheon, 1976), p. 26.

9. Quote is from Gerald A. Larue, "Some Social Aspects of Terminal Illness," in *Let Me Die Before I Wake: Hemlock's Book of Self–Deliverance for the Dying*, by Derek Humphry (Eugene, OR: The Hemlock Society, 1986), p. 87. For more information on the Quinlan case, see Derek Humphry and Ann Wickett, *The Right to Die: Understanding Euthanasia* (New York: Harper & Row, 1986), passim.

10. For more background on the *Cruzan* case and its significance, see Fenella Rouse, "The Role of State Legislatures after Cruzan: What Can—and Should—State Legislatures Do?" *Law, Medicine & Health Care* 19 (1991): 83–90; and Dallas M. High, "A New Myth About Families of Older People?" *The Gerontologist* 31 (1991): esp. 614–615.

11. Andrew Malcolm, "Death, Ethics, and Choice," in *Aging & Health: Linking Research and Public Policy*, ed. Steven Lewis (Chelsea, MI: Lewis Publishers, 1989), p. 176; quote on payment refusals is from William J. Winslade and Judith Wilson Ross, *Choosing Life or Death: A Guide for Patients, Families, and Professionals* (New York: Free Press, 1986), pp. 257–258; Bernard M. Dickens, "Medico–Legal Issues Concerning the Elderly—An Overview," in *An Aging World: Dilemmas and Challenges for Law and Social Policy*, ed. John Eekelaar and David Pearl (Oxford: Clarendon Press, 1989), esp. pp. 503, 506; Linda L. Emanuel, Michael J. Barry, John D. Stoeckle, Lucy M. Ettelson, and Ezekiel J. Emanuel, "Advance Directives for Medical Care—A Case for Greater Use," *New England Journal of Medicine* 324 (1991): esp. 889–891; quote on treatment refusals is on p. 889; Callahan, *Setting Limits*, pp. 178–180; Diana Crane, *The Sanctity of Social Life: Physicians' Treatment of Critically Ill Patients* (New York: Russell Sage Foundation, 1975), esp. pp. 11, 13, 206; Sol Levine, "The Changing Terrains in Medical Sociology: Emergent Concern with Quality of Life," *Journal of Health and Social Behavior* 28 (1987): 1–6.

12. Dickens, "Medico–Legal Issues," p. 506; Emanuel et al., "Advance Directives," p. 894; Lisa Belkin, "Choosing to Die at Home: Dignity Has

Its Burdens," *New York Times*, March 2, 1992.

13. Lou Glasse and David R. Murray, "Limiting Life–Sustaining Medical Care for the Terminally Ill," in *The Life–Threatened Elderly*, ed. Margot Tallmer, Elizabeth R. Prichard, Austin H. Kutscher, Robert DeBellis, Mahlon S. Hale and Ivan K. Goldberg (New York: Columbia University Press, 1984), pp. 324–340; John M. Ostheimer, "The Polls: Changing Attitudes Toward Euthanasia," *Public Opinion Quarterly* 44 (1980): 123–128, esp. p. 124; Russell A. Ward, "Age and Acceptance of Euthanasia," *Journal of Gerontology* 35 (1980): 421–431; James Allan Davis and Tom W. Smith, *General Social Surveys, 1972–1988: Cumulative Codebook* (Chicago: National Opinion Research Center, 1988), pp. 246–247; Bernice A. Pescosolido and Sharon Georgianna, "Durkheim, Suicide, and Religion: Toward a Network Theory of Suicide," *American Sociological Review* 54 (1989): 33–48; William T. Martin, "Religiosity and United States Suicide Rates, 1972–1978," *Journal of Clinical Psychology* 40 (1984): 1166–1169; David E. Jorgenson and Ron C. Neubecker, "Euthanasia: A National Survey of Attitudes Toward Voluntary Termination of Life," *Omega* 11 (1981): 281–291.

14. Humphry and Wickett, *Right to Die*, pp. 66–67; the California survey results are in Bernard Lo, Gary A. McLeod, and Glenn Saika, "Patient Attitudes to Discussing Life–Sustaining Treatment," *Archives of Internal Medicine* 146 (1986): 1614; Carole Michelson, Michael Mulvihill, Ming–Ann Hsu, and Ellen Olson, "Eliciting Medical Care Preferences from Nursing Home Residents," *The Gerontologist* 31 (1991): 358–363.

15. Winslade and Ross, *Choosing Life or Death*, p. 84; American Association of Retired Persons, *Tomorrow's Choices: Preparing Now for Future Legal, Financial, and Health Care Decisions* (Washington, DC: AARP, 1988), pp. 48–49, 53; Gerald A. Larue, *Euthanasia and Religion: A Survey of the Attitudes of World Religions to the Right–to–Die* (Los Angeles: The Hemlock Society, 1985), p. 83.

16. American Association of Retired Persons, *Tomorrow's Choices*, pp. 5, 50; The Hastings Center, *Guidelines on the Termination of Life–Sustaining Treatment and Care of the Dying* (Bloomington: Indiana University Press, 1987), p. 121.

17. Pam Lambert, Joan McIver Gibson, and Paul Nathanson, "The Values History: An Innovation in Surrogate Medical Decision–Making," *Law, Medicine & Health Care* 18 (1990): 202–212; Emanuel et al., "Advance Directives," p. 893; Humphry and Wickett, *Right to Die*, p. 312; Paul T. Menzel, *Strong Medicine: The Ethical Rationing of Health Care* (New York: Oxford University Press, 1990), p. 195; Evans, "Health Care Technology," pp. 2047, 2208; quote is from Jeffrey C. Merrill and Alan B. Cohen, "Explicit Rationing of Medical Care: Is It Really Needed?" in *The Medical Cost–Containment Crisis: Fears, Opinions, and Facts*, ed. Jack D. McCue (Ann Arbor, MI: Health Administration Press, 1989), p. 237.

18. Humphry and Wickett, *Right to Die*, p. 92; Cheryl K. Smith, "70 Chapters

Give Life to Hemlock," *Hemlock Quarterly*, No. 42, January, 1991, p. 4; "Hemlock Membership Composition," *Hemlock Quarterly*, No. 47, April, 1992, p. 1.

19. Chandrasekhar, *"Dirty, Filthy Book,"* pp. 23–25, 42, 45; Gordon, *Woman's Body*, pp. 206, 228; on Sanger's efforts, see Ellen Chesler, *Woman of Valor: Margaret Sanger and the Birth Control Movement in America* (New York: Simon and Schuster, 1992).

20. Humphry and Wickett, *Right to Die*, passim.

21. Quote is from Humphry and Wickett, *Right to Die*, p. 91; Andrew Malcolm, *This Far And No More* (New York: Times Books, 1987); Betty Rollin, *Last Wish* (New York: Linden Press/Simon and Schuster, 1985); Philip Roth, *Patrimony* (New York: Simon and Schuster, 1991); Malcolm's quote is from "Death, Ethics, and Choice," p. 173; the account of his mother's death appears in "The Ultimate Decision," *New York Times Magazine*, December 3, 1989.

22. Winslade and Ross, *Choosing Life or Death*, pp. 73–84; *Newsweek*, August 26, 1991; Dallas M. High, "All in the Family: Extended Autonomy and Expectations in Surrogate Health Care Decision–Making," *The Gerontologist* 28 (1988) (Supp.): 48.

23. Derek Humphry, *"Final Exit* Bombshell," *Hemlock Quarterly*, No. 45, October, 1991, pp. 1, 12.

24. V. V. Prakasa Rao, Frances Staten, and V. Nandini Rao, "Racial Differences in Attitudes toward Euthanasia," *The Euthanasia Review* 2 (1988): 260–261; Humphry and Wickett, *Right to Die*, p. 114; George J. Annas, "The Health Care Proxy and the Living Will," *New England Journal of Medicine* 324 (1991): 1211; Emanuel et al., "Advance Directives," esp. p. 892.

25. James Reed, "Doctors, Birth Control, and Social Values, 1830–1970," in *Women and Health in America: Historical Readings*, ed. Judith Walzer Leavitt (Madison: University of Wisconsin Press, 1984), pp. 124–125; Gordon, *Woman's Body*, pp. 170, 254, 261, 321; Carl N. Degler, *At Odds: Women and the Family in America from the Revolution to the Present* (Oxford: Oxford University Press, 1980), p. 199.

26. Humphry and Wickett, *Right to Die*, pp. 64–65; Emanuel et al., "Advance Directives," p. 895; Levine, "Changing Terrains," esp. pp. 3–4; Bebe Lavin, Marie Haug, Linda Liska Belgrave, and Naomi Breslau, "Change in Student Physicians' Views on Authority Relationships with Patients," *Journal of Health and Social Behavior* 28 (1987): 258, 268.

27. Quote on "leaders of medicine" is from Rothman, *Strangers at the Bedside*, p. 169; also see p. 170; Malcolm, "Ultimate Decision," p. 40.

28. Humphry and Wickett, *Right to Die*, pp. 99–101, 126–127.

29. Elisabeth Rosenthal, "In Matters of Death and Dying, the Dying Take Control," *New York Times*, August 18, 1991.

30. Quote is from Robert N. Butler, *Why Survive? Being Old in America* (New York: Harper & Row, 1975), p. 376; Humphry and Wickett, *Right to Die*,

pp. 125, 203, 306; Winslade and Ross, *Choosing Life or Death*, pp. 69–70; on the emotional significance of food and water to some people, see Peter Steinfels, "Counting Food and Water as Extraordinary Support," *New York Times*, April 30, 1989; on why the argument is fallacious, see R. J. Connelly, "The Sentiment Argument for Artificial Feeding of the Dying," *Omega* 20 (1989): 229–237; the AMA poll results are reported in U.S. Congress, Office of Technology Assessment, *Life–Sustaining Technologies and the Elderly* (Washington, DC: U.S. Government Printing Office, 1987), p. 48.

31. Richard Doerflinger, "Assisted Suicide: Pro–Choice or Anti–Life?" *Hastings Center Report* 19 (1989) (Special Supplement): 18; Robert F. Weir, "The Morality of Physician–Assisted Suicide," *Law, Medicine & Health Care* 20 (1992): 122; Timothy E. Quill, "Death and Dignity: A Case of Individualized Decision Making," *New England Journal of Medicine* 324 (1991): 691–694; "Dealing Death, or Mercy?" *New York Times*, March 17, 1991; Ralph Mero, "Doctor Assisted Death Initiative Qualifies," *Hemlock Quarterly*, No. 42, January, 1991, p. 1.

32. Rothman, *Strangers at the Bedside*, p. 228; quote is from Malcolm, "Ultimate Decision," p. 40.

33. Nicola Clark, "The High Costs of Dying," *Wall Street Journal*, February 26, 1992; quotes are from Sarah D. Cohn, "The Living Will From the Nurse's Perspective," *Law, Medicine & Health Care* 11 (1983): 122; Andrew H. Malcolm, "Many See Mercy in Ending Empty Lives," *New York Times*, September 23, 1984.

34. Annas, "Health Care Proxy," p. 1211; Larry Gostin and Robert F. Weir, "Life and Death Choices after *Cruzan*: Case Law and Standards of Professional Conduct," *The Milbank Quarterly* 69 (1991): 167.

35. Andrew H. Malcolm, "A Judicial Sanction for Death by Assent," *New York Times*, June 28, 1987.

36. American Nurses' Association, *Code for Nurses, with Interpretive Statements* (Kansas City, MO: American Nurses' Association, 1985), pp. 2–3.

37. The nurse is Barbara Huttman, in "A Crime of Compassion," *Newsweek*, August 8, 1983; other quotes are from Winslade and Ross, *Choosing Life or Death*, p. 68.

38. Gordon, *Woman's Body*, pp. 47, 230–233, 321; Rothman, *Strangers at the Bedside*, pp. 240–241.

39. Rothman, *Strangers at the Bedside*, p. 224; Chandrasekhar, *"Dirty, Filthy Book,"* pp. 38, 40.

40. Malcolm, "Judicial Sanction"; Humphry and Wickett, *Right to Die*, pp. 133, 135; Eleanor Garner Hannah, "Judge Tries to Soften Ordeal for Aged Mercy–Killing Suspect," *Sacramento Bee*, December 6, 1981.

41. Quote is from Humphry and Wickett, *Right to Die*, p. 138; also see pp. 41, 44, 60, 172–173, 225; U.S. Congress, *Life–Sustaining Technologies*, p. 192.

42. Fenella Rouse, "Advance Directives: Where Are We Heading after *Cruzan*?

Law, Medicine & Heath Care 18 (1990): 356.

43. Malcolm, "Judicial Sanction"; "U.S. Court, in Precedent, Says Feeding of Ill Woman May End," *New York Times*, October 23, 1988.

44. Stuart J. Eisendrath and Albert R. Jonsen, "The Living Will: Help or Hindrance?" *Journal of the American Medical Association* 249 (1983): 2054; Humphry and Wickett, *Right to Die*, pp. 86–87, 99, 108–109; Emanuel et al., "Advance Directives," p. 889.

45. Annas, "Health Care Proxy," p. 1210; Emanuel et al., "Advance Directives," p. 889.

46. Rothman, *Strangers at the Bedside*, pp. 232–233, Humphry and Wickett, *Right to Die*, p. 276; Rouse, "Advance Directives," p. 356; quotes are from Gostin and Weir, "Life and Death Choices," pp. 147, 168.

47. "Doctor Assisted Death Initiative Qualifies," *Hemlock Quarterly*, No. 42, January, 1991, p. 1; Abigail Gleicher, "Four New Bills Demand Physician Assisted Dying," *Hemlock Quarterly*, No. 47, April, 1992, p. 3.

48. On euthanasia in the Netherlands and the influence of Dutch practices on other nations, see Marvin E. Newman, "Voluntary Active Euthanasia: An Individual's Right to Determine the Time and Manner of Death," in *Perspectives on Death and Dying: Cross-Cultural and Multi-Disciplinary Views*, ed. Arthur Berger et al. (Philadelphia: Charles Press, 1989), esp. pp. 179, 181, 184.

49. "Kevorkian Ban Made Permanent," *Hemlock Quarterly*, No. 43, April, 1991, p. 2; "Murder Charges against Kevorkian Are Dismissed," *New York Times*, July 22, 1992; Derek Humphry, "Dr. Kevorkian's Assisted Suicide Tactics Could Derail Law Reform," *Hemlock Quarterly*, No. 47, April, 1992, pp. 4–5.

50. For the Dutch definition, see Carlos F. Gomez, *Regulating Death: Euthanasia and the Case of the Netherlands* (New York: Free Press, 1991), pp. 16–17; Newman, "Voluntary Active Euthanasia," pp. 178–179, 182; Humphry and Wickett, *Right to Die*, pp. 178–179.

51. See Gomez, *Regulating Death*, p. 58.

52. Ibid., p. 118.

53. Ibid., pp. 55, 117.

54. Rothman, *Strangers at the Bedside*, pp. 168, 247–250.

55. Karen Davis, "Paying the Health-Care Bills of an Aging Population," in *Our Aging Society: Paradox and Promise*, ed. Alan Pifer and Lydia Bronte (New York: W. W. Norton, 1986), p. 300.

56. Rothman, *Strangers at the Bedside*, pp. 256–257; U.S. Congress, *Life-Sustaining Technologies*, p. 40.

57. Robert H. Binstock, "National Policies and the Vulnerable Aged: Present, Emerging, and Proposed," in *The Vulnerable Aged: People, Services, and Policies*, ed. Zev Harel, Phyllis Ehrlich, and Richard Hubbard (New York: Springer, 1990), pp. 241–242; Callahan, *Setting Limits*, esp. pp. 115–116, 171–172.

58. Congressional Budget Office, *Rising Health Care Costs: Causes,*

Implications, and Strategies (Washington, DC: U.S. Government Printing Office, 1991), pp. 1–2; idem, *Policy Choices for Long–Term Care* (Washington, DC: U.S. Government Printing Office, 1991), pp. 31–32.

59. President's Commission for the Study of Ethical Problems in Medicine and Biomedical and Behavioral Research, *Deciding to Forego Life–Sustaining Treatment* (Washington, DC: U.S. Government Printing Office, 1983), p. 25n; Donald E. Gibson, "Hospice: Morality and Economics," *The Gerontologist* 24 (1984): 4–8; Jill Rhymes, "Hospice Care in America," *Journal of the American Medical Association* 264 (1990): 369–372.

60. Lisa Belkin, "Hospitals Will Now Ask Patients if They Wish to Make Death Plan," *New York Times*, December 1, 1991; Winslade and Ross, *Choosing Life or Death*, p. 72.

61. Renée C. Fox, "Advanced Medical Technology—Social and Ethical Implications," *Annual Review of Sociology* 2 (1976): esp. 231–235; R. R. Faden and N. E. Kass, "Bioethics and Public Health in the 1980s: Resource Allocation and AIDS," *Annual Review of Public Health* 12 (1991): 335–336; Rothman, *Strangers at the Bedside*, pp. 241–246.

62. Callahan, *Setting Limits*, passim; also see Norman Daniels, *Am I My Parents' Keeper? An Essay on Justice Between the Young and the Old* (New York: Oxford University Press, 1988); Phillip Longman, *Born to Pay: The New Politics of Aging in America* (Boston: Houghton Mifflin, 1987); Gerontological Society of America, *The Common Stake: The Interdependence of Generations* (Washington, DC: Gerontological Society of America); Humphry and Wickett, *Right to Die*, p. 48.

63. This discussion draws on the work of James Rachels, "Active and Passive Euthanasia," in *Death and Society*, ed. James P. Carse and Arlene B. Dallery (New York: Harcourt Brace Jovanovich, 1977), p. 116.

64. Arthur L. Caplan, "Is Medical Care the Right Prescription for Chronic Illness?" in *The Economics and Ethics of Long–Term Care and Disability*, ed. Sean Sullivan and Marion Ein Lewin (Washington, DC: American Enterprise Institute for Public Policy Research, 1988), pp. 83, 85.

65. Menzel, *Strong Medicine*, pp. 192–195; Callahan, *Setting Limits*, esp. pp. 49, 126; Binstock, "National Policies," pp. 241–243.

66. U.S. Congress, *Life–Sustaining Technologies*, p. 63; Humphry and Wickett, *Right to Die*, p. 275n.

67. H. Tristram Engelhardt, Jr., "Fashioning an Ethic for Life and Death in a Post–Modern Society," *Hastings Center Report* 19 (1989) (Special Supplement): 7–9; Gomez, *Regulating Death*, pp. 127–128; also see the special issue on comparative medical ethics in *Journal of Medicine and Philosophy* 13 (1988).

68. Jiska Cohen–Mansfield, Janet A. Droge, and Nathan Billig, "Factors Influencing Hospital Patients' Preferences in the Utilization of Life–Sustaining Treatments," *The Gerontologist* 32 (1992): 92; Nancy J. Osgood, *Suicide in the Elderly: A Practitioner's Guide to Diagnosis and Mental Health Intervention* (Rockville, MD: Aspen Systems Corporation, 1985), pp. 3–4.

69. Evans, "Health Care Technology," p. 2213; Ralph Mero, "Fear Campaign Beat the Washington Initiative," *Hemlock Quarterly*, No. 46, January, 1992, p. 5; the priest is quoted in Lawrence Maloney, "A New Understanding about Death," *U.S. News and World Report*, July 11, 1983; the bishop is quoted in James Rachels, *The End of Life: Euthanasia and Morality* (Oxford: Oxford University Press, 1986), p. 164.

70. Barbara Finlay, "Right to Life vs. The Right to Die: Some Correlates of Euthanasia Attitudes," *Sociology and Social Research* 69 (1985): 548–560; Humphry and Wickett, *Right to Die*, p. 294.

71. Humphry, *Let Me Die*, p. 5; Humphry and Wickett, *Right to Die*, pp. 71, 73.

72. Note that distinctions between "ordinary" and "extraordinary" treatments are inherently arbitrary, and that what is "extraordinary" in one era may become quite "ordinary" in the next; on this point and religious aspects generally, see Humphry and Wickett, esp. pp. 71–73, 78–82, 169, from which this summation is drawn; also see pp. 288–294; quotes appear on pp. 78–79, 82.

73. Ibid., pp. 168–169; Derek Humphry, ed., *Compassionate Crimes, Broken Taboos* (Los Angeles: The Hemlock Society, 1986), p. 79; Robert H. Weller and Leon F. Bouvier, *Population: Demography and Policy* (New York: St. Martin's Press, 1981), pp. 131–133.

74. Humphry and Wickett, *Right to Die*, pp. 288–290; Rosenthal, "Matters of Life and Death"; "Washington Ballot on November 5," *Hemlock Quarterly*, No. 43, April, 1991, p. 6; Ralph Mero, "Strong Clergy Support for 119," *Hemlock Quarterly*, No. 44, July, 1991, p. 3; for a survey of the attitudes of specific religions, see Larue, *Euthanasia and Religion*.

75. William Bole, "Suicide Beliefs Examined: Ethicists, Theologians Rethinking Traditional Views," *United Methodist Reporter*, May 9, 1986; Larue, *Euthanasia and Religion*, p. 3; Rachels, *End of Life*, pp. 161–162; Humphry and Wickett, *Right to Die*, pp. 291, 293–294; Bennett is quoted in Larue, *Euthanasia and Religion*, p. 85.

76. Hadley Arkes, Matthew Berke, Midge Decter et al., "'Always to Care, Never to Kill,'" *Wall Street Journal*, November 27, 1991.

77. U.S. Congress, *Life-Sustaining Technologies*, pp. 48, 52; C. Everett Koop, "The Challenge of Definition," *Hastings Center Report* 19 (1989) (Special Supplement): 2–3; Doerflinger, "Assisted Suicide," pp. 17–18; Patricia Blake, "Going Gentle Into That Good Night: Do Suicide Manuals Help Create a Bias toward Death?" in *Compassionate Crimes, Broken Taboos*, ed. Derek Humphry (Eugene, OR: The Hemlock Society, 1986), p. 27.

78. Callahan, *Setting Limits*, pp. 217–219.

79. Sheryl A. Russ, "Euthanasia Should Not Be Based on Quality of Life," in *Euthanasia: Opposing Viewpoints*, ed. Neal Bernards (San Diego: Greenhaven Press, 1989), p. 116; also see Larue, *Euthanasia and Religion*, p. 38.

80. The court is quoted in Rouse, "Advance Directives," p. 354; Koop, "Challenge of Definition"; quote on euthanasia for the aged in particular is from Callahan, *Setting Limits*, p. 197.

81. Finlay, "Right to Life," p. 550; Gordon, *Woman's Body*, pp. 415–416; Koop, "Challenge of Definition"; Tamar Lewin, "Despite Daughter's Death, Parents Pursue Right–to–Die Case," *New York Times*, July 28, 1991.

82. Sue Fisher, *In the Patient's Best Interest: Women and the Politics of Medical Decisions* (New Brunswick, NJ: Rutgers University Press, 1986), p. 18; Russell J. Ohta and Brenda M. Ohta, "Special Units for Alzheimer's Disease Patients: A Critical Look," *The Gerontologist* 28 (1988): 803–808.

83. Quote on "absolute importance" is from Finlay, "Right to Life," p. 549; Koop, "Challenge of Definition"; other quotes are from Susan M. Wolf, "Holding the Line on Euthanasia," *Hastings Center Report* 19 (1989) (Special Supplement): 13, 15.

84. Leon R. Kass, *Toward a More Natural Science: Biology and Human Affairs* (New York: Free Press, 1985), p. 159.

85. Humphry and Wickett, *Right to Die*, pp. 100, 117.

86. Ibid., pp. 163–164; "Bomb Threat Fails to Cancel Meeting," *Hemlock Quarterly*, No. 42, January, 1991, p. 3.

87. Rosenthal, "Matters of Life and Death."

Chapter 5

1. The respective statements are (1) from the suicide note of Dr. Paul Lafargue in 1911, as quoted in Nancy J. Osgood, *Suicide in the Elderly: A Practitioner's Guide to Diagnosis and Mental Health Intervention* (Rockville, MD: Aspen Systems Corporation, 1985), p. 3; (2) Sonia Hertz, following her seven–year battle with cancer, as recounted by Derek Humphry, in *Let Me Die Before I Wake: Hemlock's Book of Self–Deliverance for the Dying* (Eugene, OR: The Hemlock Society, 1986), p. 10; (3) Manley Tyler's experiences, as described by his wife, Jean Tyler, in *The Diminished Mind: One Family's Extraordinary Battle with Alzheimer's: The Jean Tyler Story* (told by Harry Anifantakis) (Blue Ridge Summit, PA: TAB Books/McGraw–Hill, 1991); (4) Alan L. Otten, "Can't We Put My Mother to Sleep?" *Wall Street Journal*, June 5, 1985.

2. Judith Walzer Leavitt, *Brought to Bed: Childbearing in America, 1750–1950* (New York: Oxford University Press, 1986), pp. 14, 20, 28.

3. Carolyn Wiener, Shizuko Fagerhaugh, Anselm Strauss, and Barbara Suczek, "What Price Chronic Illness?" in *Where Medicine Fails* (4th ed.), ed. Anselm L. Strauss (New Brunswick, NJ: Transaction Books, 1984), p. 15.

4. "Elderly Couple Commits Suicide to Avoid Separate Deaths, Nursing Home," *Houston Post*, July 28, 1986; for a vivid description of a "good"

home, see Jaber F. Gubrium, *Living and Dying at Murray Manor* (New York: St. Martin's Press, 1975). A nonprofit, church–related facility praised by a variety of observers, Murray Manor still had serious short-comings, as Gubrium shows in his admirably detailed account of its daily workings.

5. Gubrium, *Living and Dying*, pp. 89, 113.

6. B. P. Beckwith, "On the Right to Suicide by the Dying," *Dissent* 26 (1979): 231–233; Daniel Callahan, "Health Care in the Aging Society: A Moral Dilemma," in *Our Aging Society: Paradox and Promise*, ed. Alan Pifer and Lydia Bronte (New York: W. W. Norton, 1986), p. 320; quote is from Nancy J. Osgood and John L. McIntosh, "The Vulnerable Suicidal Elderly," in *The Vulnerable Aged: People, Services, and Policies*, ed. Zev Harel, Phyllis Ehrlich, and Richard Hubbard (New York: Springer, 1990), p. 171.

7. Margaret Pabst Battin, "Euthanasia is Ethical," in *Euthanasia: Opposing Viewpoints*, ed. Neal Bernards (San Diego: Greenhaven Press, 1989), pp. 22–23; President's Commission for the Study of Ethical Problems in Medicine and Biomedical and Behavioral Research, *Deciding to Forego Life–Sustaining Treatment* (Washington, DC: U.S. Government Printing Office, 1983), p. 25; Marvin E. Newman, "Voluntary Active Euthanasia: An Individual's Right to Determine the Time and Manner of Death," in *Perspectives on Death and Dying: Cross–Cultural and Multi–Disciplinary Views*, ed. Arthur Berger et al. (Philadelphia: Charles Press, 1989), p. 178.

8. Beckwith, "Right to Suicide," pp. 231–232; Robert F. Weir, "The Morality of Physician–Assisted Suicide," *Law, Medicine & Health Care* 20 (1992): 123; Anna Quindlen, "Seeking a Sense of Control," *New York Times*, December 9, 1990.

9. Stephen Crystal, *America's Old Age Crisis: Public Policy and the Two Worlds of Aging* (New York: Basic Books, 1982), pp. 49–51; Karen Jonas and Edward Wellin, "Dependency and Reciprocity: Home Health Aid in an Elderly Population," in *Aging in Culture and Society: Comparative Viewpoints and Strategies*, by Christine L. Fry and contributors (New York: Praeger, 1980), p. 217; Judith Treas, "Aging and the Family," in *Aging: Scientific Perspectives and Social Issues* (2d ed.), ed. Diana S. Woodruff and James E. Birren (Monterey, CA: Brooks/Cole, 1983), p. 96; Maria M. Talbott, "The Negative Side of the Relationship between Older Widows and Their Adult Children: The Mothers' Perspective," *The Gerontologist* 30 (1990): 595–603; Gary R. Lee, "Kinship and Social Support of the Elderly: The Case of the United States," *Ageing and Society* 5 (1985): 19, 33; Neal Krause, "Perceived Health Problems, Formal/Informal Support, and Life Satisfaction among Older Adults," *Journal of Gerontology* 45 (1990): S193–205.

10. The daughter is quoted in Elaine M. Brody, *Women in the Middle: Their Parent–Care Years* (New York: Springer, 1990), p. 238; Steven Long, *Death Without Dignity: The Story of the First Nursing Home Corporation*

Indicted for Murder (Austin: Texas Monthly Press, 1987); Crystal, *America's Old Age Crisis*, p. 92; Bruce C. Vladeck, *Unloving Care: The Nursing Home Tragedy* (New York: Basic Books, 1980), pp. 29, 215.

11. "Iron hand" quote is from Andrea Fontana, "Growing Old between Walls," in *Aging, the Individual and Society: Readings in Social Gerontology*, ed. Jill S. Quadagno (New York: St. Martin's Press, 1980), p. 496; Renée Rose Shield, "Liminality in an American Nursing Home: The Endless Transition," in *The Cultural Context of Aging: Worldwide Perspectives*, ed. Jay Sokolovsky (New York: Bergin & Garvey, 1990), pp. 341–342; Lore K. Wright, "A Reconceptualization of the 'Negative Staff Attitudes and Poor Care in Nursing Homes' Assumption," *The Gerontologist* 28 (1988): 817. The nurse is quoted in Ronald Philip Preston, *The Dilemmas of Care: Social and Nursing Adaptions to the Deformed, the Disabled, and the Aged* (New York: Elsevier North Holland, 1979), p. 132.

12. Rosalie A. Kane, "Everyday Life in Nursing Homes: 'The Way Things Are,'" in *Everyday Ethics: Resolving Dilemmas in Nursing Home Life*, ed. idem and Arthur L. Caplan (New York: Springer, 1990), p. 14; Linda Teri and Rebecca G. Logsdon, "Identifying Pleasant Activities for Alzheimer's Disease Patients: The Pleasant Events Schedule–AD," *The Gerontologist* 31 (1991): 124–127; Debra L. Cherry and Marilyn J. Rafkin, "Adapting Day Care to the Needs of Adults with Dementia," *The Gerontologist* 28 (1988): 118.

13. Lynn Ritter, "Developing a Therapeutic Activities Program in a Dementia Unit," in *Dementia Units in Long–Term Care*, ed. Philip D. Sloane and Laura J. Mathew (Baltimore: Johns Hopkins University Press, 1991), esp. p. 242.

14. Ibid., p. 245.

15. Congressional Budget Office, *Policy Choices for Long–Term Care* (Washington, DC: U.S. Government Printing Office, 1991), p. 7; Berkeley Rice, "Death by Design: A Case in Point," in *Compassionate Crimes, Broken Taboos*, ed. Derek Humphry (Los Angeles: The Hemlock Society, 1986), p. 9.

16. Quote on uncertainty is from C. G. Prado, *The Last Choice: Preemptive Suicide in Advanced Age* (Westport, CT: Greenwood Press, 1990), p. 147; Bridgman is quoted in Osgood, *Suicide in the Elderly*, p. xxxix.

17. Dan W. Brock, "Justice and the Severely Demented Elderly," *Journal of Medicine and Philosophy* 13 (1988): 93.

18. On opting out, see Anselm L. Strauss, "Chronic Illness," in *Where Medicine Fails* (4th ed.), ed. idem (New Brunswick, NJ: Transaction Books, 1984), p. 156; also see Betty Pelletz, "Suicide at 88 Ends 'Pointless Life,'" *Hemlock Quarterly*, No. 43, April, 1991, pp. 4–6; for arguments in favor of preemptive suicide for those *not* yet terminally ill, see Prado, *Last Choice*; Steven C. Neu and Carl M. Kjellstrand, "Stopping Long–Term Dialysis: An Empirical Study of Withdrawal of Life–Supporting

Treatment," *New England Journal of Medicine* 314 (1986): 14–20.

19. Barbara A. Brant and Nancy J. Osgood, "The Suicidal Patient in Long–Term Care Institutions," *Journal of Gerontological Nursing* 16 (1990): 15, 17–18; Maria Vesperi, "The Reluctant Consumer: Nursing Home Residents in the Post–Bergman Era," in *Growing Old in Different Societies: Cross–Cultural Perspectives*, ed. Jay Sokolovsky (Belmont, CA: Wadsworth, 1983), pp. 225–237; Osgood and McIntosh, "Vulnerable Suicidal Elderly," p. 178; Franklyn L. Nelson and Norman L. Farberow, "Indirect Self–destructive Behavior in the Elderly Nursing Home Patient," *Journal of Gerontology* 35 (1980): 949, 956.

20. Dallas M. High, "All in the Family: Extended Autonomy and Expectations in Surrogate Health Care Decision–Making," *The Gerontologist* 28 (1988) (Supp.): 46–51.

21. The daughter is quoted in Humphry, *Let Me Die*, p. 54; the husband is quoted in Clara Pratt, Vicki Schmall, and Scott Wright, "Ethical Concerns of Family Caregivers to Dementia Patients," *The Gerontologist* 27 (1987): 636.

22. The Hastings Center, *Guidelines on the Termination of Life–Sustaining Treatment and Care of the Dying* (Bloomington: Indiana University Press, 1987), p. 121.

23. On the hospice patient and others like her, see Anne Munley, *The Hospice Alternative: A New Context for Death and Dying* (New York: Basic Books, 1983), pp. 143, 166, and passim; also see Ronald E. Cranford, "Going Out in Style, the American Way, 1987," *Law, Medicine & Health Care* 17 (1989): 208; Stephen A. Moses, "The Fallacy of Impoverishment," *The Gerontologist* 30 (1990): 21–25.

24. Michael C. Kearl, *Endings: A Sociology of Death and Dying* (New York: Oxford University Press, 1989), pp. 120–123.

25. Beckwith, "Right to Suicide," pp. 231–232; Paul Menzel, *Strong Medicine: The Ethical Rationing of Health Care* (New York: Oxford University Press, 1990), p. 194.

26. Beckwith, "Right to Suicide," p. 233; on preferences for decisions by relatives, see High, "All in the Family"; that relatives may not want such responsibility is shown in poll results reported by Steven R. Steiber, "Right to Die: Public Balks at Deciding for Others," *Hospitals* 61 (1987): 72; Andrew Malcolm, "The Ultimate Decision," *New York Times Magazine*, December 3, 1989, p. 54.

27. Gloria Moorer, "Obtaining Drugs Is the Hassle," *Hemlock Quarterly*, No. 46, January, 1992, p. 9; Carlos F. Gomez, *Regulating Death: Euthanasia and the Case of the Netherlands* (New York: Free Press, 1991), pp. 73–77; David Margolick, "Patient's Lawsuit Says Saving Life Ruined It," *New York Times*, March 18, 1990.

28. Suzanne K. Steinmetz, *Duty Bound: Elder Abuse and Family Care* (Newbury Park, CA: Sage Publications, 1988), p. 227; Emily K. Abel, *Who Cares for the Elderly? Public Policy and the Experiences of Adult*

Daughters (Philadelphia: Temple University Press, 1991), p. 92; the daughter is quoted in Brody, *Women in the Middle*, p. 158; the son's experiences are described in Tyler, *Diminished Mind*, esp. p. 126.

29. Dorothy P. Rice, "Long–Term Care for the Elderly," in *Women's Life Cycle and Economic Insecurity: Problems and Proposals*, ed. Martha N. Ozawa (New York: Praeger, 1989), p. 179; U.S. Congress, Office of Technology Assessment, *Losing a Million Minds: Confronting the Tragedy of Alzheimer's Disease and Other Dementias* (Washington, DC: U.S. Government Printing Office, 1987), p. 3; Nancy R. Zweibel and Christine K. Cassel, "Treatment Choices at the End of Life: A Comparison of Decisions by Older Patients and Their Physician–Selected Proxies," *The Gerontologist* 29 (1989): 619; quote is from Humphry, *Let Me Die*, p. 7.

30. Nancy Neveloff Dubler, "Refusals of Medical Care in the Home Setting," *Law, Medicine & Health Care* 18 (1990): 229; President's Commission, *Deciding to Forego*, pp. 46–47; quote is from Bryan S. Turner, *Medical Power and Social Knowledge* (Beverly Hills, CA: Sage Publications, 1987), p. 126.

31. Vladeck, *Unloving Care*, p. 176.

32. Robyn Stone, Gail Lee Cafferata, and Judith Sangl, "Caregivers of the Frail Elderly: A National Profile," *The Gerontologist* 27 (1987): 616–626.

33. Renée C. Fox, "Advanced Medical Technology—Social and Ethical Implications," *Annual Review of Sociology* 2 (1976): 253.

34. Lucy Rose Fischer and Nancy N. Eustis, "DRGs and Family Care for the Elderly: A Case Study," *The Gerontologist*, 28 (1988): 383–389.

35. Marjorie Cantor and Virginia Little, "Aging and Social Care," in *Handbook of Aging and the Social Sciences* (2d ed.), ed. Robert H. Binstock and Ethel Shanas (New York: Van Nostrand Reinhold, 1985), p. 758; on "protective caregiving," see Barbara Bowers, "Family Perceptions of Care in a Nursing Home," in *Circles of Care: Work and Identity in Women's Lives*, ed. Emily K. Abel and Margaret K. Nelson (Albany: State University of New York Press, 1990), pp. 281–283; also see Steven H. Zarit and Carol J. Whitlatch, "Institutional Placement: Phases of the Transition," *The Gerontologist* 32 (1992): 665; Barbara Bowers and Marion Becker, "Nurse's Aides in Nursing Homes: The Relationship between Organization and Quality," *The Gerontologist* 32 (1992): 364–365.

36. Humphry, *Let Me Die*, esp. pp. 37–39.

37. Preston, *Dilemmas of Care*, pp. 5–7.

38. Alice T. Day, "Who Cares? Demographic Trends Challenge Family Care for the Elderly," *Population Trends and Public Policy*, Number 9 (Washington, DC: Population Reference Bureau, 1985), p. 10; Victor G. Cicirelli, "A Comparison of Helping Behavior to Elderly Parents of Adult Children with Intact and Disrupted Marriages," *The Gerontologist* 23 (1983): 619–625.

39. Pamela Doty, "Family Care of the Elderly: The Role of Public Policy," *The Milbank Quarterly* 64 (1986): 61; Candace Clark, "Sympathy Biography and Sympathy Margin," *American Journal of Sociology* 93 (1987): 316; the wife is quoted in Pratt, Schmall, and Wright, "Ethical Concerns," p. 634; see the same article, passim, on the moral dilemmas for families; on caregiver stress and burden, see Linda S. Noelker, "Family Caregivers: A Valuable but Vulnerable Resource," in *The Vulnerable Aged: People, Services, and Policies*, ed. Zev Harel, Phyllis Ehrlich, and Richard Hubbard (New York: Springer, 1990), pp. 189–204.

40. U.S. Congress, Office of Technology Assessment, *Technology and Aging in America* (Washington, DC: U.S. Government Printing Office, 1985), pp. 201–202; on gray areas generally, see Greg Arling and William J. McAuley, "The Feasibility of Public Payments to Family Caregiving," *The Gerontologist* 23 (1983): 300–306; Stone, Cafferata, and Sangl, "Caregivers of Frail Elderly"; the daughter is quoted in Pratt, Schmall, and Wright, "Ethical Concerns," p. 634.

41. Emily K. Abel, "Family Care of the Frail Elderly," in *Circles of Care: Work and Identity in Women's Lives*, ed. idem and Margaret K. Nelson (Albany: State University of New York Press, 1990), p. 69; Sheldon S. Tobin, "A Structural Approach to Families," in *Aging, Health, and Family: Long–Term Care*, ed. Timothy H. Brubaker (Newbury Park, CA: Sage Publications, pp. 45, 50.

42. William J. Winslade and Judith Wilson Ross, *Choosing Life or Death: A Guide for Patients, Families, and Professionals* (New York: Free Press, 1986), p. 83; Philip Roth, "The Last Days of Herman Roth," *New York Times Magazine*, December 30, 1990, p. 22; Cranford, "Going Out in Style," p. 208.

43. Quote is from Tish Sommers and Laurie Shields, with the Older Women's League Task Force on Caregivers and Judy MacLean, *Women Take Care: The Consequences of Caregiving in Today's Society* (Gainesville, FL: Triad, 1987), p. 59; the survey results are reported by Paul Starr, in *The Social Transformation of American Medicine* (New York: Basic Books, 1982), pp. 381–382.

44. Norman Daniels, *Am I My Parents' Keeper? An Essay on Justice between the Young and the Old* (New York: Oxford University Press, 1988), p. 104; Abel, "Family Care," p. 68; for the priest's statement, see Frank E. Moss and Val J. Halamandaris, *Too Old, Too Sick, Too Bad: Nursing Homes in America* (Germantown, MD: Aspen Systems Corporation, 1977), pp. 23–24; Teri and Logsdon, "Identifying Pleasant Activities."

45. Sommers et al., *Women Take Care*, p. 50; Robert P. Hey and Elliot Carlson, "'Granny Dumping:' New Pain for U.S. Elders," *AARP Bulletin* 32, No. 8 (1991), pp. 1, 16; "Granny Dumping by the Thousands," *New York Times*, March 29, 1992; Frank Robinson's story is told in Humphry, *Let Me Die*, pp. 34–44.

46. Humphry, *Let Me Die,* passim; idem, ed., *Compassionate Crimes, Broken Taboos* (Los Angeles: The Hemlock Society, 1986), passim; Pelletz, "Suicide at 88."

47. Peter N. Stearns, "Old Age Family Conflict: The Perspective of the Past," in *Elder Abuse: Conflict in the Family,* ed. Karl A. Pillemer and Rosalie S. Wolf (Dover, MA: Auburn House, 1986), pp. 3–24; Corinne N. Nydegger, "Family Ties of the Aged in Cross–Cultural Perspective," *The Gerontologist* 23 (1983): 26–32; Lillian E. Troll, ed., *Family Issues in Current Gerontology* (New York: Springer, 1986), p. 141.

48. Karl Pillemer and David Finkelhor, "The Prevalence of Elder Abuse: A Random Sample Survey," *The Gerontologist* 28 (1988): 51, 54; Suzanne K. Steinmetz and Deborah J. Amsden, "Dependent Elders, Family Stress, and Abuse," in *Family Relationships in Later Life,* ed. Timothy H. Brubaker (Beverly Hills, CA: Sage Publications, 1983), pp. 185–186; Mary Joy Quinn and Susan K. Tomita, *Elder Abuse and Neglect: Causes, Diagnosis, and Intervention Strategies* (New York: Springer, 1986), pp. 40–41; Victor G. Cicirelli, "The Helping Relationship and Family Neglect in Later Life," in *Elder Abuse: Conflict in the Family,* ed. Karl A. Pillemer and Rosalie S. Wolf (Dover, MA: Auburn House, 1986), pp. 51, 63; Rosalie S. Wolf, "Major Findings from Three Model Projects of Elderly Abuse," esp. p. 234, in the same volume.

49. Elaine M. Brody, "Parent Care as a Normative Family Stress," in *Family Issues in Current Gerontology,* ed. Lillian E. Troll (New York: Springer, 1986), p. 108; also see Suzanne Selig, Tom Tomlinson, and Tom Hickey, "Ethical Dimensions of Intergenerational Reciprocity: Implications for Practice," *The Gerontologist* 31 (1991): 624–630; AARP, *Tomorrow's Choices,* p. 55; Daniel Callahan, "What Do Children Owe Elderly Parents?" *The Hastings Center Report* 15 (1985): 33; Arling and McAuley, "Feasibility of Public Payments," pp. 301, 304.

50. Moses, "Fallacy of Impoverishment," p. 23; Marjorie Abend–Wein, "Medicaid's Effect on the Elderly: How Reimbursement Policy Affects Priorities in the Nursing Home," *Journal of Applied Gerontology* 10 (1991): 71–87; David E. Pitt, "The Elderly Often Find Crime a Family Matter," *New York Times,* September 27, 1987.

51. Colleen Leahy Johnson and Donald J. Catalano, "A Longitudinal Study of Family Supports to Impaired Elderly," in *Family Issues in Current Gerontology,* ed. Lillian E. Troll (New York: Springer, 1986), pp. 32–48; the caregiver ia quoted in Nancy Guberman, Pierre Maheu, and Chantal Maille, "Women as Family Caregivers: Why Do They Care?" *The Gerontologist* 32 (1992): 611; Pratt, Schmall, and Wright, "Ethical Concerns"; Strauss, "Chronic Illness," esp. pp. 151, 154; quote on feeling trapped is from Abel, "Family Care," p. 68; Quinn and Tomita, *Elder Abuse and Neglect,* p. 65; Derek Humphry and Ann Wickett, *The Right to Die: Understanding Euthanasia* (New York: Harper & Row, 1986), p.138.

52. Edgar F. Borgatta and Rhonda J. V. Montgomery, "Aging Policy and Societal Values," in *Critical Issues in Aging Policy: Linking Research and Values*, ed. idem (Newbury Park, CA: Sage Publications, 1987), p. 22; the survey results are reported in Arling and McAuley, "Feasibility of Public Payments," p. 303 (Table 3).

53. See *Hemlock Quarterly*, No. 43, April, 1991, p. 6 for the Gallup Poll results; the "good death" quote is from Gerald A. Larue, "Some Social Aspects of Terminal Illness," in *Let Me Die Before I Wake: Hemlock's Book of Self-Deliverance for the Dying*, by Derek Humphry (Eugene, OR: The Hemlock Society, 1986), p. 93; the phrase "stopping behavior" is often used in the literature on birth control. In that context, it refers to couples who stop having children (or attempted to stop when known methods of control were less efficacious), after achieving their desired family size.

54. Myrna Lewis, "Older Women and Health: An Overview," *Women & Health* 10 (1985): 9.

55. Timothy E. Quill, "Death and Dignity: A Case of Individualized Decision Making," *New England Journal of Medicine* 324 (1991): 691–694; M. Powell Lawton, Elaine M. Brody, and Avalie R. Saperstein, *Respite for Caregivers of Alzheimer Patients: Research and Practice* (New York: Springer, 1991), p. 135.

56. On "actions" versus "omissions," see Joseph Fletcher, "Ethics and Euthanasia," in *Death and Society*, ed. James P. Carse and Arlene B. Dallery (New York: Harcourt Brace Jovanovich, 1977), pp. 163–174; and President's Commission, *Deciding to Forego*, esp. pp. 63–67.

57. Richard W. Besdine, "Decisions to Withhold Treatment from Nursing Home Residents," in *Legal and Ethical Aspects of Health Care for the Elderly*, ed. Marshall B. Kapp, Harvey E. Pies, Jr., and A. Edward Doudera (Ann Arbor, MI: Health Administration Press, 1985), pp. 272–273.

58. U.S. Congress, Office of Technology Assessment, *Life-Sustaining Technologies and the Elderly* (Washington, DC: U.S. Government Printing Office, 1987), p. 9.

59. David J. Rothman, *Strangers at the Bedside: A History of How Law and Bioethics Transformed Medical Decision Making* (New York: Basic Books, 1991), p. 131; Nathan E. Martin, "A Doctor's Regrets, "*Hemlock Quarterly*, No. 46, January, 1992, p. 8.

60. Karen Davis, "Paying the Health-Care Bills of an Aging Population," in *Our Aging Society: Paradox and Promise*, ed. Alan Pifer and Lydia Bronte (New York: W. W. Norton, 1986), pp. 301–302.

61. U.S. Congress, *Life-Sustaining Technologies*, pp. 12–13, 15; Congressional Budget Office, *Policy Choices for Long-Term Care*, pp. x–xi; William B. Schwartz, "Cutting Costs Means Painful Choices," *New York Times*, May 8, 1988; Daniel Callahan, *Setting Limits: Medical Goals in an Aging Society* (New York: Simon and Schuster, 1987), pp. 121, 123–126; Roger

W. Evans, "Health Care Technology and the Inevitability of Resource Allocation and Rationing Decisions," *Journal of the American Medical Association* 249 (1983): 2047–2053, 2208–2219, esp. 2047; William B. Schwartz and Daniel N. Mendelson, "Hospital Cost Containment in the 1980s: Hard Lessons Learned and Prospects for the 1990s," *New England Journal of Medicine* 324 (1991): 1037–1042.

62. R. J. Blendon, "Health Policy Choices for the 1990s," *Issues in Science and Technology* 2 (1986): 67; Robert Pear, "Medicare to Weigh Cost as a Factor in Reimbursement," *New York Times*, April 21, 1991; Martin Tolchin, "Proposals to Avoid Insolvency in Medicare Trust Fund Bring Sharp Debate," *New York Times*, January 22, 1989; James F. Fries and Lawrence M. Crapo, *Vitality and Aging: Implications of the Rectangular Curve* (San Francisco: W. H. Freeman, 1981); Davis, "Paying Health–Care Bills"; Dorothy P. Rice and Jacob J. Feldman, "Living Longer in the United States: Demographic Changes and Health Needs of the Elderly," *Milbank Memorial Fund Quarterly/Health and Society* 61 (1983): 362–396.

63. S. J. Olshansky, Mark A. Rudberg, Bruce A. Carnes, Christine K. Cassel, and Jacob A. Brody, "Trading Off Longer Life for Worsening Health: The Expansion of Morbidity Hypothesis," *Journal of Aging and Health* 3 (1991): 207; Eileen J. Tell, Stanley S. Wallack, and Marc A. Cohen, "New Directions in Life Care: An Industry in Transition," *The Milbank Quarterly* 65 (1987): 551.

64. Ernest M. Gruenberg, "The Failures of Success," *Milbank Memorial Fund Quarterly/Health and Society* 55 (1977): 3–24; Lois M. Verbrugge, "Longer Life but Worsening Health? Trends in Health and Mortality of Middle–aged and Older Persons," *Milbank Memorial Fund Quarterly/Health and Society* 62 (1984): 475–519; Rice and Feldman, "Living Longer," p. 393; Wiener et al., "What Price Chronic Illness?" esp. p. 20.

65. Alice M. Rivlin and Joshua M. Wiener, with Raymond J. Hanley and Denise A. Spence, *Caring for the Disabled Elderly: Who Will Pay?* (Washington, DC: The Brookings Institution, 1988), p. 12; Callahan, "What Do Children Owe?" p. 32.

66. John H. Skinner, "Federal Programs for the Vulnerable Aged," in *The Vulnerable Aged: People, Services, and Policies*, ed. Zev Harel, Phyllis Ehrlich, and Richard Hubbard (New York: Springer, 1990), p. 251; Moses, "Fallacy of Impoverishment," p. 22.

67. Callahan, *Setting Limits*, esp. p. 116; idem, "Health Care in the Aging Society"; Harold A. Richman and Matthew W. Stagner, "Children: Treasured Resource or Forgotten Minority?" in *Our Aging Society: Paradox and Promise*, ed. Alan Pifer and Lydia Bronte (New York: W. W. Norton, 1986), pp. 161–179; Edward A. Wynne, "Will the Young Support the Old?" pp. 243–261 in the same volume; Samuel H. Preston, "Children and the Elderly: Divergent Paths for America's Dependents," *Demography*

21 (1984): 435–457; Marilyn Waring, *If Women Counted: A New Feminist Economics* (San Francisco: Harper & Row, 1988), p. 9.

68. Philip J. Hilts, "Say Ouch: Demands to Fix U.S. Health Care Reach a Crescendo," *New York Times*, May 19, 1991; Steve Early, "Yes to a National Health Care Plan," *New York Times*, June 2, 1991; "Letting Very Ill Patients Decide Their Fate," *Wall Street Journal*, January 14, 1992.

69. Hastings Center, *Guidelines on the Termination of Life–Sustaining Treatment*, pp. 119–121.

Chapter 6

1. Elizabeth Ogg, "Euthanasia Should Be Legalized," in *Euthanasia: Opposing Viewpoints*, ed. Neal Bernards (San Diego: Greenhaven Press, 1989), pp. 63–64.

2. Eric L. Diamond, James A. Jernigan, Ray A. Moseley, Valerie Messina, and Robert A. McKeown, "Decision–Making Ability and Advance Directive Preferences in Nursing Home Patients and Proxies," *The Gerontologist* 29 (1989): 622.

3. Linda L. Emanuel, Michael J. Barry, John D. Stoeckle, Lucy M. Ettelson, and Ezekiel J. Emanuel, "Advance Directives for Medical Care—A Case for Greater Use," *New England Journal of Medicine* 324 (1991): 894–895.

4. Emanuel et al., "Advance Directives"; Carole Michelson, Michael Mulvihill, Ming–Ann Hsu, and Ellen Olson, "Eliciting Medical Care Preferences from Nursing Home Residents," *The Gerontologist* 31 (1991): 358–363.

5. Joanne Lynn, "Why I Don't Have a Living Will," *Law, Medicine & Health Care* 19 (1991): 102.

6. George J. Annas, "The Health Care Proxy and the Living Will," *New England Journal of Medicine* 324 (1991): 1210; Lynn, "Why I Don't Have Living Will," p. 102.

7. Engelbert L. Schucking, "Death at a New York Hospital," *Law, Medicine & Health Care* 13 (1985): 261–268.

8. Lauraine Thomas, "Living Will Could Let You Down," *Hemlock Quarterly*, No. 46, January, 1992, pp. 10–11; Judith Areen, "Advance Directives Under State Law and Judicial Decisions," *Law, Medicine & Health Care* 19 (1991): 91–100. Concern for Dying and the Society for the Right to Die recently merged as Choice in Dying.

9. Ronald E. Cranford, "Going Out in Style, the American Way, 1987," *Law, Medicine & Health Care* 17 (1987): 210.

10. George J. Annas, "Into the Hands of Strangers," *Law, Medicine & Health Care* 13 (1985): 271; Norman Paradis, "Making a Living off the Dying," *New York Times*, April 25, 1992.

11. Daniel Callahan, *What Kind of Life: The Limits of Medical Progress* (New

York: Simon and Schuster, 1990), pp. 224–225; Anne Alexis Coté, "The Hospital Perspective," *Law, Medicine & Health Care* 13 (1985): 270; Emanuel et al., "Advance Directives," p. 889.

12. Marion Danis, Leslie I. Southerland, Joanne M. Garrett, Janet L. Smith, Frank Hielema, C. Glenn Pickard, David M. Egner, and Donald L. Patrick, "A Prospective Study of Advance Directives for Life–Sustaining Care," *New England Journal of Medicine* 324 (1991): 882–888.

13. Ibid., passim.

14. Annas, "Health Care Proxy," p. 1211; Thomas, "Living Will," p. 10.

15. John Collette and Peter Y. Windt, "Medical Decision–Making, Dying, and Quality of Life Among the Elderly," in *Should Medical Care Be Rationed by Age?* ed. Timothy Smeeding (Totowa, NJ: Rowman & Littlefield, 1987), pp. 99–118.

16. Richard F. Uhlman, Robert A. Pearlman, and Kevin C. Cain, "Physicians' and Spouses' Predictions of Elderly Patients' Resuscitation Preferences," *Journal of Gerontology* 43 (1988): esp. pp. M119–120.

17. Steven R. Steiber, "Right to Die: Public Balks at Deciding for Others," *Hospitals* 61 (1987): 72; Annas, "Health Care Proxy," p. 1212.

18. Cheryl K. Smith, "Some Tattoo a Message to Doctors," *Hemlock Quarterly*, No. 43, April, 1991, p. 3; "D.N.R. Bracelets Now Available," *Hemlock Quarterly*, No. 45, October, 1991, p. 6.

19. Dallas M. High, "All in the Family: Extended Autonomy and Expectations in Surrogate Health Care Decision–Making," *The Gerontologist* 28 (1988) (Supp.): 49.

20. Terrie Wetle, Sue Levkoff, Julie Cwikel, and Amy Rosen, "Nursing Home Resident Participation in Medical Decisions: Perceptions and Preferences," *The Gerontologist* 28 (1988) (Supp.): 32–38; Michelson, Mulvihill, Hsu, and Olson, "Eliciting Medical Care Preferences," p. 358; Richard W. Besdine, "Decisions to Withhold Treatment from Nursing Home Residents," in *Legal and Ethical Aspects of Health Care for the Elderly*, ed. Marshall B. Kapp, Harvey E. Pies, Jr., and A. Edward Doudera (Ann Arbor, MI: Health Administration Press, 1985), p. 269.

21. Susan M. Wolf, "Conflict between Doctor and Patient," *Law, Medicine & Health Care* 16 (1988): 201.

22. "Fairy tale" quote is from Troyen A. Brennan, "Silent Decisions: Limits of Consent and the Terminally Ill Patient," *Law, Medicine & Health Care* 16 (1988): 204; second quote is from Wolf, "Conflict Between Doctor and Patient," p. 198; also see p. 199.

23. Michelson, Mulvihill, Hsu, and Olson, "Eliciting Medical Care Preferences," p. 362.

24. On the problems of suicide and assisted suicide without physician involvement, see Derek Humphry, *Let Me Die Before I Wake: Hemlock's Book of Self–Deliverance for the Dying* (Eugene, OR: The Hemlock Society, 1986), passim; on the thwarted attempt, see Richard Selzer, "A Question of Mercy," *New York Times Magazine*, September 22, 1991.

25. Selzer, "Question of Mercy"; Betty Hosmer Mawardi, "Aspects of the Impaired Physician," in *Stress and Burnout in the Human Services Professions*, ed. Barry A. Farber (New York: Pergamon Press, 1983), p. 122.

26. Angus McLaren, *A History of Contraception: From Antiquity to the Present Day* (Oxford: Basil Blackwell, 1990), p. 196; Linda Gordon, *Woman's Body, Woman's Right: A Social History of Birth Control in America* (New York: Grossman, 1976), p. 170; on the history of euthanasia, see Margaret P. Battin, "Age Rationing and the Just Distribution of Health Care: Is There a Duty to Die?" in *Should Medical Care Be Rationed by Age?* ed. Timothy Smeeding (Totowa, NJ: Rowman & Littlefield, 1987), pp. 69–94; and Derek Humphry and Ann Wickett, *The Right to Die: Understanding Euthanasia* (New York: Harper & Row, 1986); W. Bruce Fye, "Active Euthanasia: An Historical Survey of Its Conceptual Origins and Introduction into Medical Thought," *Bulletin of the History of Medicine* 52 (1978): 496.

27. A variety of means are described in Humphry, *Let Me Die*, pp. 56–59.

28. McLaren, *History of Contraception*, esp. p. 27; Larry L. Bumpass and Harriet B. Presser, "The Increasing Acceptance of Sterilization and Abortion," in *Toward the End of Growth: Population in America*, ed. Charles F. Westoff et al. (Englewood Cliffs, NJ: Prentice–Hall, Inc., 1973), pp. 34–35.

29. Newman, "Voluntary Active Euthanasia," p. 181.

30. Bernard M. Dickens, "Medico–Legal Issues Concerning the Elderly—An Overview," in *An Aging World: Dilemmas and Challenges for Law and Social Policy*, ed. John Eekelaar and David Pearl (Oxford: Clarendon Press, 1989), p. 502; Besdine, "Decisions to Withhold Treatment," p. 273; Anne Munley, *The Hospice Alternative: A New Context for Death and Dying* (New York: Basic Books, 1983), pp. 204–206.

31. Besdine, "Decisions to Withhold Treatment, pp. 273–274; Jack McKay Zimmerman, *Hospice: Complete Care for the Terminally Ill* (Baltimore: Urban & Schwarzenberg, 1986), pp. 54–55, 282; Ralph Mero, "Doctor Assisted Death Initiative Qualifies," *Hemlock Quarterly*, No. 42, January, 1991, p. 1; "Washington Ballot on November 5," *Hemlock Quarterly*, No. 43, April, 1991, pp. 1, 6; and "Law Reforms Sought in Three States," *Hemlock Quarterly*, No. 44, July, 1991, p. 1.

32. The wife's story is told in Humphry, *Let Me Die*, p. 25; Jaber F. Gubrium, *Living and Dying at Murray Manor* (New York: St. Martin's Press, 1975), pp. 203, 205; the hospice patient is quoted in Munley, *The Hospice Alternative*, p. 145; also see pp. 142, 204–206.

33. Robert J. Miller, "Hospice Care as an Alternative to Euthanasia," *Law, Medicine & Health Care* 20 (1992): 129–130.

34. Sandra Harris, "'Final Exit' Provides Control," *Hemlock Quarterly*, No. 47, April, 1992, p. 10; "Sad Farewells for Young Woman Starting on Road to Death," *New York Times*, December 16, 1990; Roth, "Last Days of Herman Roth," p. 22.

35. Quill, "Death and Dignity," p. 694.

Chapter 7

1. "Jury Refuses to Indict Man in Mercy Killing of Wife," in *Compassionate Crimes, Broken Taboos*, ed. Derek Humphry (Los Angeles: The Hemlock Society, 1986), p. 4.
2. Esther Hing, "Use of Nursing Homes by the Elderly: Preliminary Data from the 1985 National Nursing Home Survey," *Advance Data From Vital and Health Statistics*, No. 135 (Hyattsville, MD: Public Health Service, 1987), p. 7; Martha Baum and Mary Page, "Caregiving and Multigenerational Families," *The Gerontologist* 31 (1991): 768; Colleen L. Johnson and Lillian Troll, "Family Functioning in Late Late Life," *Journal of Gerontology* 47 (1992): S66–72.
3. Susan Sheehan, *Kate Quinton's Days* (New York: Mentor, 1984), passim.
4. Rhonda J. V. Montgomery, Laurie Russell Hatch, Thomas Pullum, Donald E. Stull, and Edgar F. Borgatta, "Dependency, Family Extension, and Long–Term Care Policy," in *Critical Issues in Aging Policy: Linking Research and Values*, ed. Edgar F. Borgatta and Rhonda J. V. Montgomery (Newbury Park: Sage Publications, 1987), p. 162.
5. Nancy Guberman, Pierre Maheu, and Chantal Maille, "Women as Family Caregivers: Why Do They Care?" *The Gerontologist* 32 (1992): 611; Pamela Doty, "Family Care of the Elderly: The Role of Public Policy," *The Milbank Quarterly* 64 (1986): 68.
6. Jonathan L. York and Robert J. Calsyn, "Family Involvement in Nursing Homes," in *Family Issues in Current Gerontology*, ed. Lillian E. Troll (New York: Springer, 1986), esp. pp. 179, 181–184.
7. Edgar F. Borgatta and Rhonda J. V. Montgomery, "Aging Policy and Societal Values," in *Critical Issues in Aging Policy: Linking Research and Values*, ed. idem (Newbury Park, CA: Sage Publications, 1987), p. 22.
8. Robyn Stone, Gail Lee Cafferata, and Judith Sangl, "Caregivers of the Frail Elderly: A National Profile," *The Gerontologist* 27 (1987): 616–626, esp. p. 620; Colleen Leahy Johnson and Donald J. Catalano, "A Longitudinal Study of Family Supports to Impaired Elderly," in *Family Issues in Current Gerontology*, ed. Lillian E. Troll (New York: Springer, 1986), p. 37.
9. Eleanor Palo Stoller and Karen L. Pugliesi, "Other Roles of Caregivers: Competing Responsibilities or Supportive Resources," *Journal of Gerontology* 44 (1989): S235, S237; on the problems associated with mental deterioration, see Tish Sommers and Laurie Shields, with the Older Women's League Task Force on Caregivers and Judy MacLean, *Women Take Care: The Consequences of Caregiving in Today's Society* (Gainesville, FL: Triad, 1987), passim.

10. Quote is from Elaine M. Brody, "Parent Care as a Normative Family Stress," in *Family Issues in Current Gerontology*, ed. Lillian E. Troll (New York: Springer, 1986), p. 108; Johnson and Catalano, "Longitudinal Study of Family Supports," pp. 44–45.

11. Mary Joy Quinn and Susan K. Tomita, *Elder Abuse and Neglect: Causes, Diagnosis, and Intervention Strategies* (New York: Springer, 1986), passim; Jordan I. Kosberg, "Preventing Elder Abuse: Identification of High Risk Factors Prior to Placement Decisions," *The Gerontologist* 28 (1988): 43–50.

12. Suzanne K. Steinmetz, *Duty Bound: Elder Abuse and Family Care* (Newbury Park, CA: Sage Publications, 1988), pp. 12, 210–211; the story of the sons and their mother appears in Ruth Macklin, *Mortal Choices: Bioethics in Today's World* (New York: Pantheon Books, 1987), p. 140.

13. Owen T. Thornberry, Ronald W. Wilson, and Patricia M. Golden, "Health Promotion Data for the 1990 Objectives: Estimates from the National Health Interview Survey of Health Promotion and Disease Prevention, United States, 1985," *Advance Data from Vital and Health Statistics*, No. 126 (Hyattsville, MD: Public Health Service, 1986), p. 7; Linda S. Noelker, "Family Caregivers: A Valuable but Vulnerable Resource," in *The Vulnerable Aged: People, Services, and Policies*, ed. Zev Harel, Phyllis Ehrlich, and Richard Hubbard (New York: Springer, 1990), pp. 191–192.

14. Victor G. Cicirelli, "A Comparison of Helping Behavior to Elderly Parents of Adult Children with Intact and Disrupted Marriages," *The Gerontologist* 23 (1983): 619–625.

15. Rosalie A. Kane and Arthur L. Caplan, eds., *Everyday Ethics: Resolving Dilemmas in Nursing Home Life* (New York: Springer, 1990), pp. 138, 148; Quinn and Tomita, *Elder Abuse and Neglect*, pp. 50–51.

16. Gregory C. Smith, Mary F. Smith, and Ronald W. Toseland, "Problems Identified by Family Caregivers in Counseling," *The Gerontologist* 31(1991): 20.

17. Quote is from Smith, Smith, and Toseland, "Problems Identified by Family Caregivers," p. 18; Steinmetz, *Duty Bound*, p. 12; on family caregiving potential, see Stephen Crystal, *America's Old Age Crisis: Public Policy and the Two Worlds of Aging* (New York: Basic Books, 1982), p. 12.

18. Maria M. Talbott, "The Negative Side of the Relationship between Older Widows and Their Adult Children: The Mothers' Perspective," *The Gerontologist* 30 (1990): 595; quotes are from Gary R. Lee, "Kinship and Social Support of the Elderly: The Case of the United States," *Ageing and Society* 5 (1985): 25, 29.

19. The Robinsons' story is told by Derek Humphry in *Let Me Die Before I Wake: Hemlock's Book of Self–Deliverance for the Dying* (Eugene, OR: The Hemlock Society, 1986), esp. pp. 40, 42.

20. Emily K. Abel, "Family Care of the Frail Elderly," in *Circles of Care: Work*

and Identity in Women's Lives, ed. idem and Margaret K. Nelson (Albany: State University of New York Press, 1990), pp. 79–80; Dolores Gallagher, Steven Lovett, and Antonette Zeiss, "Interventions with Caregivers of Frail Elderly Persons," in *Aging and Health Care: Social Science and Policy Perspectives*, ed. Marcia G. Ory and Kathleen Bond (London: Routledge, 1989), p. 181.

21. Abel, "Family Care," p. 77.
22. U.S. Congress, Office of Technology Assessment, *Life–Sustaining Technologies and the Elderly* (Washington, DC: U.S. Government Printing Office, 1987), pp. 14–15; Debra L. Cherry and Marilyn J. Rafkin, "Adapting Day Care to the Needs of Adults with Dementia," *The Gerontologist* 28 (1988): 116–117; Burton V. Reifler, "Making Something Good Out of Something Bad," *Respite Report*, Spring, 1992, p. 3; Congressional Budget Office, *Policy Choices for Long–Term Care* (Washington, DC: U.S. Government Printing Office, 1991), p. 9; Rona Smyth Henry, ""Financial Lessons to be Applied to New Program," *Respite Report*, Winter, 1992, p. 3.
23. Abel, "Family Care," pp. 75–76; Doty, "Family Care," p. 68.
24. Abel, "Family Care," p. 76; the daughter-in-law is quoted in Elaine M. Brody, *Women in the Middle: Their Parent–Care Years* (New York: Springer, 1990), pp. ix–x; Emily K. Abel, *Who Cares for the Elderly? Public Policy and the Experiences of Adult Daughters* (Philadelphia: Temple University Press, 1991), p. 124.
25. Steven K. Wisensale and Michael D. Allison, "An Analysis of 1987 State Family Leave Legislation: Implications for Caregivers of the Elderly," *The Gerontologist* 28 (1988): 779–785; quote is on p. 785; Sue Shellenbarger, "Workers Slow to Accept Support on Elder Care," *Wall Street Journal*, November 1, 1991; Brody, *Women in the Middle*, p. 229; "Caregivers and Their Companies, *Aging Today*, July/August 1992, pp. 9, 12.
26. Wisensale and Allison, "Family Leave Legislation," pp. 782, 785.
27. Ibid., pp. 782, 784; Clifford Krauss, "House Sees Uphill Fight on Parental–Leave Bill," *New York Times*, October 6, 1991; Judith David, "Family Leave: A Trend, Not a Fad," *Aging Today*, July/August 1992, pp. 11–12.
28. Abel, "Family Care," p. 75; Merl C. Hokenstad and Lennarth Johansson, "Swedish Policy Initiatives to Support Family Caregiving for the Elderly," *Ageing International* 17 (1990): 33–34.
29. Abel, "Family Care," pp. 80–83; Janice Gibeau, "Working Caregivers: Family Conflicts and Adaptations of Older Workers," in *Retirement Reconsidered: Economic and Social Roles for Old People*, ed. Robert Morris and Scott A. Bass (New York: Springer, 1988), p. 197.
30. Stephen Berman, Nancy Delaney, Dolores Gallagher, Phyllis Atkins, and Mark P. Graeber, "Respite Care: A Partnership Between a Veterans Administration Nursing Home and Families to Care for Frail Elders at Home," *The Gerontologist* 27 (1987): 581.

31. Quote is from Jill Quadagno, Cebra Sims, D. Ann Squier, and Georgia Walker, "Long–Term Care Community Services and Family Caregiving," in *Aging, Health, and Family: Long–Term Care*, ed. Timothy H. Brubaker (Newbury Park, CA: Sage Publications, 1987), p. 127; Clara Pratt, Vicki Schmall, Scott Wright, and Jan Hare, "The Forgotten Client: Family Caregivers to Institutionalized Dementia Patients," in *Aging, Health, and Family: Long–Term Care*, ed. Timothy H. Brubaker, (Newbury Park, CA: Sage Publications, 1987), pp. 197–213; Kathleen Coen Buckwalter and Geri Richards Hall, "Families of the Institutionalized Older Adult: A Neglected Resource," p. 181 in the same volume.

32. Brody, "Parent Care," p. 117.

33. Noelker, "Family Caregivers," p. 192.

34. Borgatta and Montgomery, "Aging Policy," pp. 20–21.

35. Marjorie Cantor and Virginia Little, "Aging and Social Care," in *Handbook of Aging and the Social Sciences* (2d ed.), ed. Robert H. Binstock and Ethel Shanas (New York: Van Nostrand Reinhold, 1985), p. 758; Rhonda J. V. Montgomery and Mary McGlinn Datwyler, "Women & Men in the Caregiving Role," *Generations* 14 (1990): 36; Janet Finch and Dulcie Groves, eds., *A Labour of Love: Women, Work, and Caring* (London: Routledge & Kegan Paul, 1983), p. 73.

36. Nancy J. Finley, M. Diane Roberts, and Benjamin F. Banahan, III, "Motivators and Inhibitors of Attitudes of Filial Obligation toward Aging Parents," *The Gerontologist* 28 (1988): 73–74; Rhonda J. V. Montgomery and Laurie Russell Hatch, "The Feasibility of Volunteers and Families Forming a Partnership for Caregiving," in *Aging, Health, and Family: Long–Term Care*, ed. Timothy H. Brubaker (Newbury Park, CA: Sage Publications, 1987), p. 158.

37. On violent outcomes, see Derek Humphry, ed., *Compassionate Crimes, Broken Taboos* (Los Angeles: The Hemlock Society, 1986) and idem and Ann Wickett, *The Right to Die: Understanding Euthanasia* (New York: Harper & Row, 1986), passim; less measurable problems are evident from accounts in Sommers et al., *Women Take Care*, for example; M. Powell Lawton, Elaine M. Brody, and Avalie R. Saperstein, *Respite for Caregivers of Alzheimer Patients: Research and Practice* (New York: Springer, 1991), esp. p. 136; Gregory J. Paveza, Donna Cohen, Carl Eisdorfer, Sally Freels, Todd Semla, J. Wesson Ashford, Philip Gorelick, Robert Hirschman, Daniel Luchins, and Paul Levy, "Severe Family Violence and Alzheimer's Disease: Prevalence and Risk Factors," *The Gerontologist* 32 (1992): 495.

38. Brody, *Women in the Middle*, p. 239; idem, "Parent Care," p. 104.

39. Crystal, *America's Old Age Crisis*, p. 65; Gibeau, "Working Caregivers," pp. 185–186.

40. Abel, "Family Care," pp. 73–75; Sommers et al., *Women Take Care*, pp. 116–120.

41. Margaret Adams, "The Compassion Trap," in *Woman in Sexist Society: Studies in Power and Powerlessness*, ed. Vivian Gornick and Barbara K.

Moran (New York: Basic Books, 1971), p. 402; David S. Greer and Vincent Mor, "How Medicare Is Altering the Hospice Movement," *Hastings Center Report* 15 (1985): 7–8.

42. Stone, Cafferata, and Sangl, "Caregivers of Frail Elderly," p. 620; quote is from Cantor and Little, "Aging and Social Care," p. 759; Abel, "Family Care," pp. 71–72; Montgomery and Datwyler, "Women & Men," p. 38.

43. Stone, Cafferata, and Sangl, "Caregivers of Frail Elderly"; Montgomery and Datwyler, "Women & Men," p. 37.

44. Abel, "Family Care," pp. 70–72.

45. Gibeau, "Working Caregivers," p. 189.

46. Brody, *Women in the Middle*, p. 38; Sandra L. Boyd and Judith Treas, "Family Care of the Frail Elderly: A New Look at 'Women in the Middle,'" *Women's Studies Quarterly* 17 (1989): 66–74.

47. Baila Miller and Andrew Montgomery, "Family Caregivers and Limitations in Social Activities," *Research on Aging* 12 (1990): 75; Baila Miller, "Gender Differences in Spouse Management of the Caregiver Role," in *Circles of Care: Work and Identity in Women's Lives*," ed. Emily K. Abel and Margaret K. Nelson (Albany: State University of New York Press, 1990), p. 98; Rachel A. Pruchno and Nancy L. Resch, "Husbands and Wives as Caregivers: Antecedents of Depression and Burden," *The Gerontologist* 29 (1989): 164.

48. Quadagno et al., "Long–Term Care Community Services," pp. 127–128.

49. Borgatta and Montgomery, "Aging Policy," p. 20.

50. Robyn I. Stone, "The Feminization of Poverty among the Elderly," *Women's Studies Quarterly* 17 (1989): 28; Korbin Liu, Pamela Doty, and Kenneth Manton, "Medicaid Spenddown in Nursing Homes," *The Gerontologist* 30 (1990): 12–13; Korbin Liu and Kenneth Manton, "Nursing Home Length of Stay and Spenddown in Connecticut, 1977–1986," *The Gerontologist* 31 (1991): 172; Timothy Diamond, "Social Policy and Everyday Life in Nursing Homes: A Critical Ethnography," *Social Science and Medicine* 23 (1986): 1289.

51. Amy Horowitz, "Sons and Daughters as Caregivers to Older Parents: Differences in Role Performance and Consequences," *The Gerontologist* 25 (1985): 615–616.

52. Laurie Russell Hatch, "Effects of Work and Family on Women's Later–Life Resources," *Research on Aging* 12 (1990): 311–338, esp. 321–322.

53. Abel, "Family Care," p. 75; Robert B. Enright, Jr., "Time Spent Caregiving and Help Received by Spouses and Adult Children of Brain–Impaired Adults," *The Gerontologist* (1991): 380; Brody, "Parent Care," p. 112.

54. Quote is from Gibeau, "Working Caregivers," p. 189; Stone, "Feminization of Poverty," p. 22.

55. Robyn I. Stone and Peter Kemper, "Spouses and Children of Disabled Elders: How Large a Constituency for Long–Term Care Reform?" *The Milbank Quarterly* 67 (1989): 497; Jean Tyler, *The Diminished Mind: One Family's Extraordinary Battle with Alzheimer's: The Jean Tyler Story*

(Told by Harry Anifantakis) (Blue Ridge Summit, PA: TAB Books/McGraw–Hill, 1991), pp. 147, 149.

56. Andrew E. Scharlach and Sandra L. Boyd, "Caregiving and Employment: Results of an Employee Survey," *The Gerontologist* 29 (1989): 382–387; Barbara J. Logue, "Women at Risk: Predictors of Financial Stress for Retired Women Workers," *The Gerontologist* 31 (1991): 657–665; quote is from Beth B. Hess and Joan Waring, "Family Relationships of Older Women: A Women's Issue," in *Older Women: Issues and Prospects,* ed. Elizabeth W. Markson (Lexington, MA: Lexington Books, 1983), p. 229.

57. Marilyn J. Bonjean, "Psychotherapy with Families Caring for a Mentally Impaired Elderly Member," in *Chronic Illness and Disability,* ed. Catherine S. Chilman, Elam W. Nunnally, and Fred M. Cox (Newbury Park, CA: Sage Publications, 1988), pp. 148–149.

58. Emily K. Abel, "Informal Care for the Disabled Elderly: A Critique of Recent Literature," *Research on Aging* 12 (1990): 148.

59. Ibid., pp. 146–147.

60. Sheryl Ruzek, "Feminist Visions of Health: An International Perspective," in *Perspectives in Medical Sociology,* ed. Phil Brown (Belmont, CA: Wadsworth, 1989), p. 563.

61. Allen Buchanan and Dan W. Brock, "Deciding for Others," *The Milbank Quarterly* 64 (1986): 17–18; President's Commission for the Study of Ethical Problems in Medicine and Biomedical and Behavioral Research, *Deciding to Forego Life–Sustaining Treatment* (Washington, DC: U.S. Government Printing Office, 1983), p. 127; Nancy R. Zweibel and Christine K. Cassel, "Treatment Choices at the End of Life: A Comparison of Decisions by Older Patients and Their Physician–Selected Proxies," *The Gerontologist* 29 (1989): 615.

62. Quote is from Clara Pratt, Vicki Schmall, and Scott Wright, "Ethical Concerns of Family Caregivers to Dementia Patients," *The Gerontologist* 27 (1987): 632–638; Linda K. George, "Caregiver Burden: Conflict between Norms of Reciprocity and Solidarity," in *Elder Abuse: Conflict in the Family,* ed. Karl A. Pillemer and Rosalie S. Wolf (Dover, MA: Auburn House, 1986), pp. 67–92; Brody, "Parent Care," p. 100; York and Calsyn, "Family Involvement."

63. President's Commission, *Deciding to Forego,*" p. 46.

64. David E. Jorgenson and Ron C. Neubecker, "Euthanasia: A National Survey of Attitudes toward Voluntary Termination of Life," *Omega* 11 (1981): 281–291; Richard G. Niemi, John Mueller, and Tom W. Smith, *Trends in Public Opinion: A Compendium of Survey Data* (Westport, CT: Greenwood Press, 1989), pp. 215–216; Russell A. Ward, "Age and Acceptance of Euthanasia," *Journal of Gerontology* 35 (1980): 428; Cheryl Brown Travis, *Women and Health Psychology: Biomedical Issues* (Hillsdale, NJ: Lawrence Erlbaum Associates, 1988), esp. pp. 26–27, 29.

65. President's Commission, *Deciding to Forego,* p. 23; Linda L. Emanuel, Michael J. Barry, John D. Stoeckle, Lucy M. Ettelson, and Ezekiel J.

Emanuel, "Advance Directives for Medical Care—A Case for Greater Use," *New England Journal of Medicine* 324 (1991): 892; Stoller and Pugliesi, "Other Roles of Caregivers," p. S231.

Chapter 8

1. "Voluntary Active Euthanasia," *Journal of the American Geriatrics Society* 39 (1991): 826; Dame Cicely Saunders, "Foreword," in Jack McKay Zimmerman, *Hospice: Complete Care for the Terminally Ill* (Baltimore: Urban & Schwarzenberg, 1986).
2. Daniel Callahan, *What Kind of Life: The Limits of Medical Progress* (New York: Simon and Schuster, 1990), pp. 66–67; Hadley Arkes, Matthew Berke, Midge Decter et al., "'Always to Care, Never to Kill,'" *Wall Street Journal*, November 27, 1991.
3. Penny Hollander Feldman, with Alice M. Sapienza and Nancy M. Kane, *Who Cares for Them? Workers in the Home Care Industry* (Westport, CT: Greenwood Press, 1990), p. 66; Charlene Harrington, Leslie A. Grant, Stanley R. Ingman, and Sherry A. Hobson, "The Regulation of Home Health Care Quality," *Journal of Applied Gerontology* 10 (1991): 54.
4. Nancy M. Kane, "The Home Care Crisis of the Nineties," *The Gerontologist* 29 (1989): 30; Andrew M. Kramer, Peter W. Shaughnessy, Marjorie K. Bauman, and Kathryn S. Crisler, "Assessing and Assuring the Quality of Home Health Care," *The Milbank Quarterly* 68 (1990): 413–414; Feldman, Sapienza, and Kane, *Who Cares for Them?* pp. 9, 29.
5. Hilary Stout, "Godsend for Many, Home–Care Industry Also Has Potential for Fraud and Abuse," *Wall Street Journal*, November 21, 1991.
6. Ibid.; Harrington et al., "Regulation of Home Health Care," pp. 53–54, 64–65; U.S. Congress, Office of Technology Assessment, *Losing a Million Minds: Confronting the Tragedy of Alzheimer's Disease and Other Dementias* (Washington, DC: U.S. Government Printing Office, 1987), p. 369.
7. Harrington et al., "Regulation of Home Health Care," esp. pp. 64–65; *Kate Quinton's Days* (New York: Mentor, 1984), passim; quotes are on p. 55.
8. U.S. Congress, Office of Technology Assessment, *Life–Sustaining Technologies and the Elderly* (Washington, DC: U.S. Government Printing Office, 1987), pp. 14–15; Congressional Budget Office, *Policy Choices for Long–Term Care* (Washington, DC: U.S. Government Printing Office, 1991), pp. 44–45; Charles Jannings, "Mom Did It Her Way," *Hemlock Quarterly*, No. 46, January, 1992, p. 8.
9. Linda S. Noelker, "Family Caregivers: A Valuable but Vulnerable Resource," in *The Vulnerable Aged: People, Services, and Policies*, ed. Zev Harel, Phyllis Ehrlich, and Richard Hubbard (New York: Springer, 1990), p. 200; Debra L. Cherry and Marilyn J. Rafkin, "Adapting Day Care to

the Needs of Adults with Dementia," *The Gerontologist* 28 (1988): 116–120.

10. Noelker, "Family Caregivers," p. 199; Rona Smyth Henry, "Financial Lessons to be Applied to New Program," *Respite Report*, Winter, 1992, p. 3; quote is from M. Powell Lawton, Elaine M. Brody, and Avalie R. Saperstein, *Respite for Caregivers of Alzheimer Patients: Research and Practice* (New York: Springer, 1991), p. 136; also see p. 140.

11. Lawton et al., *Respite for Caregivers*, pp. 137, 140–141, 143; quote is from p. 138; idem, "A Controlled Study of Respite Service for Caregivers of Alzheimer's Patients," *The Gerontologist* 29 (1989): 8–16.

12. Joseph A. Califano, *America's Health Care Revolution: Who Lives? Who Dies? Who Pays?* (New York: Random House, 1986), pp. 172–173.

13. Karl Pillemer, "Maltreatment of Patients in Nursing Homes: Overview and Research Agenda," *Journal of Health and Social Behavior* 29 (1988): 233; Mary Joy Quinn and Susan K. Tomita, *Elder Abuse and Neglect: Causes, Diagnosis, and Intervention Strategies* (New York: Springer, 1986), p. 42.

14. Jonathan L. York and Robert J. Calsyn, "Family Involvement in Nursing Homes," in *Family Issues in Current Gerontology*, ed. Lillian E. Troll (New York: Springer, 1986), pp. 178–188; Bernice T. Halbur, *Turnover among Nursing Personnel in Nursing Homes* (Ann Arbor, MI: UMI Research Press, 1980); Bruce C. Vladeck, *Unloving Care: The Nursing Home Tragedy* (New York: Basic Books, 1980); Robert Pear, "U.S. Agency Seeks Wide Rule Changes on Nursing Homes," *New York Times*, July 5, 1987.

15. Scott Miyake Geron, "Regulating the Behavior of Nursing Homes through Positive Incentives: An Analysis of Illinois' Quality Incentive Program (QUIP)," *The Gerontologist* 31 (1991): 292–301.

16. Ralph L. Cherry, "Agents of Nursing Home Quality of Care: Omsbudsmen and Staff Ratios Revisited," *The Gerontologist* 31 (1991): 302–308.

17. Linda K. George, "The Institutionalized," in *Handbook on the Aged in the United States*, ed. Erdman B. Palmore (Westport, CT: Greenwood Press, 1984), pp. 339–354; Charles I. Stannard, "Old Folks and Dirty Work: The Social Conditions for Patient Abuse in a Nursing Home," in *Aging, the Individual and Society: Readings in Social Gerontology*, ed. Jill S. Quadagno (New York: St. Martin's Press, 1980), pp. 500–515; Seymour Spilerman and Eugene Litwak, "Reward Structures and Organizational Design: An Analysis of Institutions for the Elderly," *Research on Aging* 4 (1982): 43–70; Vladeck, *Unloving Care*, esp. p. 193; quote is on p. 264.

18. President's Commission for the Study of Ethical Problems in Medicine and Biomedical and Behavioral Research, *Deciding to Forego Life–Sustaining Treatment* (Washington, DC: U.S. Government Printing Office, 1983), pp. 110–111; Richard W. Besdine, "Decisions to Withhold Treatment from Nursing Home Residents," in *Legal and Ethical Aspects of Health Care for the Elderly*, ed. Marshall B. Kapp, Harvey E. Pies, Jr., and A. Edward Doudera (Ann Arbor, MI: Health Administration Press, 1985), p. 271.

19. Robert N. Butler, *Why Survive? Being Old in America* (New York: Harper & Row, 1975), p. 260; Philip W. Brickner, Anthony J. Lechich, Roberta Lipsman, and Linda K. Scharer, *Long Term Health Care: Providing a Spectrum of Services to the Aged* (New York: Basic Books, 1987), pp. 18–19.

20. Vladeck, *Unloving Care*, pp. 29, 206, 215; Emily B. Campbell, Mary Knight, Marlene Benson, and Joyce Colling, "Effect of an Incontinence Training Program on Nursing Home Staff's Knowledge, Attitudes, and Behavior," *The Gerontologist* 31 (1991): 791.

21. Jaber F. Gubrium, *Living and Dying at Murray Manor* (New York: St. Martin's Press, 1975), pp. 123–124; quote is from Stannard, "Old Folks," p. 500.

22. Stephen Crystal, *America's Old Age Crisis: Public Policy and the Two Worlds of Aging* (New York: Basic Books, 1982), p. 90.

23. U.S. Congress, *Life-Sustaining Technologies*, pp. 64–65; for a glowing report on the potential of hospice care to alleviate suffering for some patients, see Cicely Saunders, "Dying They Live: St. Christopher's Hospice," in *Aging, the Individual and Society: Readings in Social Gerontology*, ed. Jill S. Quadagno (New York: St. Martin's Press, 1980), pp. 554–568; on transferring the hospice concept to long–term care, see Tish Sommers and Laurie Shields, with the Older Women's League Task Force on Caregivers and Judy MacLean, *Women Take Care: The Consequences of Caregiving in Today's Society* (Gainesville, FL: Triad, 1987), pp. 167–169.

24. "Most Die Free of Pain, Says Survey," *Hemlock Quarterly*, No. 42, January, 1991, p. 2; Eliot Slater, "The Case for Voluntary Euthanasia," in *Death and Society*, ed. James P. Carse and Arlene B. Dallery (New York: Harcourt Brace Jovanovich, 1977), p. 90; Jill Rhymes, "Hospice Care in America," *Journal of the American Medical Association* 264 (1990): 371; Judith A. Levy and Audrey K. Gordon, "Stress and Burnout in the Social World of Hospice," in *Stress and Burnout Among Providers Caring for the Terminally Ill and Their Families*, ed. Lenora Finn Paradis (New York: The Haworth Press, 1987), p. 37; "Montana's Hospice Six Raise Issue of 'Compassion,'" *American Journal of Nursing* 91(8) (1991): 65, 71.

25. Slater, "Case for Voluntary Euthanasia," p. 90; Callahan, *What Kind of Life*, p. 254.

26. Robert J. Miller, "Hospice Care as an Alternative to Euthanasia," *Law, Medicine & Health Care* 20 (1992): 128.

27. Lenora Finn Paradis, "An Assessment of Sociology's Contributions to Hospice: Priorities for Future Research," *The Hospice Journal* 4 (1988): 64.

28. David W. Rehm, "Hospice Care of Rhode Island: Past, Present and Future," *Rhode Island Medical Journal* 72 (1989): 233; quote is from Levy and Gordon, "Stress and Burnout," p. 43.

29. Rehm, "Hospice Care," p. 235; John N. Morris, Sylvia Sherwood, Susan M. Wright, and Claire E. Gutkin, "The Last Weeks of Life: Does Hospice Care

Make a Difference?" in *The Hospice Experiment*, ed. Vincent Mor, David Greer, and Robert Kastenbaum (Baltimore: Johns Hopkins University Press, 1988), pp. 109–110.

30. National Institute on Aging, *Personnel for Health Needs of the Elderly through the Year 2020* (Washington, DC: U.S. Government Printing Office, 1987), p. 2.

31. U.S. Congress, Office of Technology Assesssment, *Life–Sustaining Technologies*, pp. 362–366; David A. Peterson and Pamela F. Wendt, "Employment in the Field of Aging: A Survey of Professionals in Four Fields," *The Gerontologist* 30 (1990): 679–684.

32. David A. Peterson, *Career Paths in the Field of Aging: Professional Gerontology* (Lexington, MA: Lexington Books/D. C. Heath, 1987).

33. Karen Brodkin Sacks, "Does It Pay to Care?" in *Circles of Care: Work and Identity in Women's Lives*, ed. Emily K. Abel and Margaret K. Nelson (Albany: State University of New York Press, 1990), p. 188; Feldman, Sapienza, and Kane, *Who Cares for Them?* p. 21; Helen Evers, "Care or Custody? The Experiences of Women Patients in Long–Stay Geriatric Wards," in *Controlling Women: The Normal and the Deviant*, ed. Bridget Hutter and Gillian Williams (London: Croom Helm, 1981), p. 112; Frederic W. Hafferty, *Into the Valley: Death and the Socialization of Medical Students* (New Haven, CT: Yale University Press, 1991), p. 198; quote is from Andrea Fontana, "Growing Old Between Walls," in *Aging, the Individual and Society: Readings in Social Gerontology*, ed. Jill S. Quadagno (New York: St. Martin's Press, 1980), p. 485.

34. Jacquelyn H. Flaskerud, Edward J. Halloran, Janice Janken, Mary Lund, and Joan Zetterlund, "Avoidance and Distancing: A Descriptive View of Nursing," in *Burnout in the Nursing Profession: Coping Strategies, Causes, and Costs*, ed. Edwina A. McConnell (St. Louis: C. V. Mosby, 1982), pp. 124–130, esp. p. 129.

35. Michael Smyer, Diane Brannon, and Margaret Cohn, "Improving Nursing Home Care through Training and Job Redesign," *The Gerontologist* 32 (1992): 327, 332; Campbell et al., "Incontinence Training Program," pp. 792–793.

36. Stannard, "Old Folks," p. 501.

37. Vladeck, *Unloving Care*, p. 22; Katsuya Kanda and Mathy Mezey, "Registered Nurse Staffing in Pennsylvania Nursing Homes: Comparison before and after Implementation of Medicare's Prospective Payment System," *The Gerontologist* 31 (1991): 318; U.S. Congress, Office of Technology Assessment, *Technology and Aging in America* (Washington, DC: U.S. Government Printing Office, 1985), p. 53.

38. Jeffrey H. Horen, "The Labor Supply Question," in *Long–Term Care: Perspectives From Research and Demonstrations*, ed. Ronald J. Vogel and Hans C. Palmer (Rockville, MD: Aspen Systems Corporation, 1985), p. 735.

39. Stannard, "Old Folks," esp. pp. 501–502, 505.

40. Rebecca Donovan, "'We Care for the Most Important People in Your

Life': Home Care Workers in New York City," *Women's Studies Quarterly* 17 (1989): 58.

41. Jordan I. Kosberg, "Preventing Elder Abuse: Identification of High Risk Factors prior to Placement Decisions," *The Gerontologist* 28 (1988): 43–50; Quinn and Tomita, *Elder Abuse and Neglect*, p. 42.

42. "Pinched and hardened" quote is from Sharon R. Curtin, "Social Death and Aging," in *Death and Society*, ed. James P. Carse and Arlene B. Dallery (New York: Harcourt, Brace, Jovanovich, 1977), p. 346; Myrna Lewis, "Older Women and Health: An Overview," *Women & Health* 10 (1985): 13; Donovan, "'We Care for the Most Important People,'" p. 61; Feldman, Sapienza, and Kane, *Who Cares for Them?* pp. 26, 57; "two parties" quote is from V. Tellis–Nayak and Mary Tellis–Nayak, "Quality of Care and the Burden of Two Cultures: When the World of the Nurse's Aide Enters the World of the Nursing Home," *The Gerontologist* 29 (1989): 312.

43. Terrie Wetle, Sue Levkoff, Julie Cwikel, and Amy Rosen, "Nursing Home Resident Participation in Medical Decisions: Perceptions and Preferences," *The Gerontologist* 28 (1988) (Supp.): passim; President's Commission, *Deciding to Forego*, p. 58; David J. Rothman, *Strangers at the Bedside: A History of How Law and Bioethics Transformed Medical Decision Making* (New York: Basic Books, 1991), pp. 134–135; Peter Conrad, "Learning to Doctor: Reflections on Recent Accounts of the Medical School Years," *Journal of Health and Social Behavior* 29 (1988): 323–325, 329.

44. Conrad, "Learning to Doctor," pp. 328–329; Edward F. Lawlor, "What Kind of Medicine?" *The Gerontologist* 32 (1992): 132; Hafferty, *Into the Valley*, p. 198.

45. Jerome L. Avorn, "Medicine: The Life and Death of Oliver Shay," in *Our Aging Society: Paradox and Promise*, ed. Alan Pifer and Lydia Bronte (New York: W. W. Norton, 1986), p. 291; Conrad, "Learning to Doctor," p. 329; Susan K. Green, Karla J. Keith, and L. Gregory Pawlson, "Medical Students' Attitudes toward the Elderly," *Journal of the American Geriatrics Society* 31 (1983): 305–309; the report on medical education is quoted in Donald W. Light, "Toward a New Sociology of Medical Education," *Journal of Health and Social Behavior* 29 (1988): 309; quote on survey results is from Alan C. Mermann, Darlene B. Gunn, and George E. Dickinson, "Learning to Care for the Dying: A Survey of Medical Schools and a Model Course," *Academic Medicine* 66 (1991): 35–36; David B. Reuben, Thomas B. Bradley, Jack Zwanziger, Susan Vivell, Arlene Fink, Susan H. Hirsch, and John C. Beck, "Geriatrics Faculty in the United States: Who Are They and What Are They Doing?" *Journal of the American Geriatrics Society* 39 (1991): 804.

46. Conrad, "Learning to Doctor," p. 328; Light, "Toward a New Sociology," p. 317; Carole Haber, "Geriatrics: A Specialty in Search of Specialists," in *Old Age in a Bureaucratic Society: The Elderly, the Experts, and the State in American History*, ed. David Van Tassel and Peter N. Stearns (Westport,

CT: Greenwood Press, 1986), p. 66.

47. Quote is from Samuel W. Bloom, "Structure and Ideology in Medical Education: An Analysis of Resistance to Change," *Journal of Health and Social Behavior* 29 (1988): 294; Light, "Toward a New Sociology," p. 312; Rothman, *Strangers at the Bedside*, p. 128.

48. William J. Kassler, Steven A. Wartman, and Rebecca A. Silliman, "Why Medical Students Choose Primary Care Careers," *Academic Medicine* 66 (1991): 41; quote on "talking to patients" is from Daniel J. McCarty, "Why Are Today's Medical Students Choosing High–Technology Specialties Over Internal Medicine?" *New England Journal of Medicine* 317 (1987): 568; Milt Freudenheim, "Doctors Dropping Medicare Patients," *New York Times*, April 12, 1992.

49. Quotes on "Tender Loving Care" and "the ambitions of nursing leaders" are from Ronald Philip Preston, *The Dilemmas of Care: Social and Nursing Adaptions to the Deformed, the Disabled, and the Aged* (New York: Elsevier North Holland, 1979), p. 206; Flaskerud et al., "Avoidance and Distancing," p. 126; the nurse's words are from Alice Lind, "Hospitals and Hospices: Feminist Decisions about Care for the Dying," in *Healing Technology: Feminist Perspectives*, ed. Kathryn Strother Ratcliff, Myra Marx Ferree, Gail O. Mellow et al. (Ann Arbor, MI: University of Michigan Press, 1989), p. 268.

50. Flaskerud et al., "Avoidance and Distancing," esp. pp. 125–127; quotes are from Lind, "Hospitals and Hospices," pp. 265–266.

51. Flaskerud et al., "Avoidance and Distancing," passim.

52. Lucy Rose Fischer, Daniel P. Mueller, and Philip W. Cooper, "Older Volunteers: A Discussion of the Minnesota Senior Study," *The Gerontologist* 31 (1991): 183–194.

53. U.S. Senate Special Committee on Aging, American Association of Retired Persons, Federal Council on the Aging, and U.S. Administration on Aging, *Aging America: Trends and Projections* (1991 ed.) (Washington, DC: U.S. Government Printing Office, n.d.), p. 204; Fischer, Mueller, and Cooper, "Older Volunteers," p. 186.

54. Rhonda J. V. Montgomery and Laurie Russell Hatch, "The Feasibility of Volunteers and Families Forming a Partnership for Caregiving," in *Aging, Health, and Family: Long–Term Care*, ed. Timothy H. Brubaker (Newbury Park, CA: Sage Publications, 1987).

55. Ibid.; Linda S. Noelker, "Family Caregivers: A Valuable but Vulnerable Resource," in *The Vulnerable Aged: People, Services, and Policies*, ed. Zev Harel, Phyllis Ehrlich, and Richard Hubbard (New York: Springer, 1990), p. 200.

56. Lenora Finn Paradis, Beverly Miller, and Vicki M. Runnion, "Volunteer Stress and Burnout: Issues for Administrators," in *Stress and Burnout among Providers Caring for the Terminally Ill and Their Families*, ed. Lenora Finn Paradis (New York: The Haworth Press, 1987), pp. 166–168, 175, 178; Vincent Mor and Susan Masterson–Allen, *Hospice Care*

Systems: Structure, Process, Costs, and Outcome (New York: Springer, 1987), pp. 19, 224–225.

57. Lenora Finn Paradis, ed., *Stress and Burnout among Providers Caring for the Terminally Ill and Their Families* (New York: The Haworth Press, 1987); D. T. Wessells, Jr., Austin H. Kutscher, Irene B. Seeland, Florence E. Selder, Daniel J. Cherico, and Elizabeth J. Clark, eds., *Professional Burnout in Medicine and the Helping Professions* (New York: The Haworth Press, 1988); Edwina A. McConnell, ed., *Burnout in the Nursing Profession: Coping Strategies, Causes, and Costs* (St. Louis: C. V. Mosby, 1982), p. 74.

58. On satisfactions of caregiving see, for example, Marjorie H. Cantor, "Family and Community: Changing Roles in an Aging Society," *The Gerontologist* 31 (1991): 343; Thomas W. Muldary, *Burnout and Health Professionals: Manifestations and Management* (Norwalk, CT: Appleton–Century–Crofts, 1983), p. 103; quote is from Christina Maslach, "Job Burnout: How People Cope," in *Burnout in the Nursing Profession: Coping Strategies, Causes, and Costs*, ed. Edwina A. McConnell (St. Louis: C. V. Mosby, 1982), p. 76.

59. J. Neil Henderson, "Mental Disorders among the Elderly: Dementia and Its Sociocultural Correlates," in *The Elderly as Modern Pioneers*, ed. Philip Silverman (Bloomington: Indiana University Press, 1987), pp. 366–367; for definition of burnout, see Eileen Berlin Ray, Michael R. Nichols, and Lea J. Perritt, "A Model of Job Stress and Burnout," in *Stress and Burnout Among Providers Caring for the Terminally Ill and Their Families*, ed. Lenora Finn Paradis (New York: The Haworth Press, 1987), pp. 6–7; also see p. 3; quote on medical textbooks is from James H. Humphrey, *Stress in the Nursing Profession* (Springfield, IL: Charles C Thomas Publisher, 1988), p. 28; Sommers et al., *Women Take Care*, pp. 54–55.

60. Julie Fisher Robertson and Corenna C. Cummings, "What Makes Long–Term Care Nursing Attractive?" *American Journal of Nursing* 91(11) (1991): 43; Cantor, "Family and Community," p. 343.

61. "Staff Feels Stress of Participants' Declining Health," *Respite Report*, Spring, 1992, pp. 4–5; Humphrey, *Stress in Nursing Profession*, pp. 47–49.

62. Nancy L. Marshall, Rosalind C. Barnett, Grace K. Baruch, and Joseph H. Pleck, "Double Jeopardy: The Costs of Caring at Work and at Home," in *Circles of Care: Work and Identity in Women's Lives*, ed. Emily K. Abel and Margaret K. Nelson (Albany: State University of New York Press, 1990), p. 273.

63. Terry Heiselman and Linda S. Noelker, "Enhancing Mutual Respect among Nursing Assistants, Residents, and Residents' Families," *The Gerontologist* 31 (1991): 552–555; Sacks, "Does It Pay to Care?"; respective quotes are from Vladeck, *Unloving Care*, p. 20 and Barbara Bowers and Marion Becker, "Nurse's Aides in Nursing Homes: The Relationship Between Organization and Quality," *The Gerontologist* 32 (1992): 365.

64. Daniel E. Everitt, David R. Fields, Stephen S. Soumerai, and Jerry Avorn,

"Resident Behavior and Staff Distress in the Nursing Home," *Journal of the American Geriatrics Society* 39 (1991): 792–798; Gubrium, *Living and Dying*, pp. 122–157, passim; Karl Pillemer and Ronet Bachman–Prehn, "Helping and Hurting: Predictors of Maltreatment of Patients in Nursing Homes," *Research on Aging* 13 (1991): 79, 85.

65. Ray, Nichols, and Perritt, "Model of Job Stress," pp. 5–7, 16; Levy and Gordon, "Stress and Burnout," pp. 42–43; Finn Paradis, ed., *Stress and Burnout*, p. 1; Anne Munley, *The Hospice Alternative: A New Context for Death and Dying* (New York: Basic Books, 1983), pp. 202–203.

66. "Staff Feels Stress of Participants' Declining Health," *Respite Report*, Spring, 1992, pp. 4–5; Finn Paradis, Miller, and Runnion, "Volunteer Stress and Burnout," esp. pp. 175, 178; Catherine A. Martin and Rachel A. Julian, "Causes of Stress and Burnout in Physicians Caring for the Chronically and Terminally Ill," in *Stress and Burnout among Providers Caring for the Terminally Ill and Their Families*, ed. Lenora Finn Paradis (New York: The Haworth Press, 1987), pp. 136–138; Halbur, *Turnover among Nursing Personnel*, p. 53; Amy Horowitz and Lois W. Shindelman, "Social and Economic Incentives for Family Caregivers," *Health Care Financing Review* 5 (1983): 25; York and Calsyn, "Family Involvement in Nursing Homes"; Lawton, Brody, and Saperstein, *Respite for Caregivers*, pp. 135–136.

67. Maria Vesperi, "The Reluctant Consumer: Nursing Home Residents in the Post–Bergman Era," in *Growing Old in Different Societies: Cross–Cultural Perspectives*, ed. Jay Sokolovsky (Belmont, CA: Wadsworth, 1983), p. 236; quotes are from Preston, *Dilemmas of Care*, pp. 123, 129.

68. Sharon R. Kaufman and Gaylene Becker, "Content and Boundaries of Medicine in Long–Term Care: Physicians Talk About Stroke," *The Gerontologist* 31 (1991): 244; quotes are from Lind, "Hospitals and Hospices," pp. 266–267; on overlap between hospice staff and Hemlock membership, see Derek Humphry and Ann Wickett, *The Right to Die: Understanding Euthanasia* (New York: Harper & Row, 1986), pp. 185–186.

69. On marketing mentality, see Paul Starr, *The Social Transformation of American Medicine* (New York: Basic Books, 1982), p. 448; U.S. Congress, *Life–Sustaining Technologies*, p. 9; Freudenheim, "Doctors Dropping Medicare Patients"; David Haber, *Health Care for an Aging Society: Cost-Conscious Community Care and Self–Care Approaches* (New York: Hemisphere Publishing Corporation, 1989), pp. 24–25; Brickner et al., *Long Term Health Care*, p. 40; Joan Retsinas, "Crowding Under the Medicaid Tent," *Aging Today*, July/August 1992, p. 8.

70. Nancy M. Kane, "The Home Care Crisis of the Nineties," *The Gerontologist* 29 (1989): 28–29; James J. Callahan, Jr., "Play It Again Sam—There Is No Impact," *The Gerontologist* 29 (1989): 5; quote is from Vladeck, *Unloving Care*, p. 211; also see pp. 217–218; Milt Freudenheim, "The Elderly and the Politics of Health Care," *New York Times*, May 22,

1988; Kane et al., *Long–Term Care*, p. 95; "Project ONE–AGE Recruits Older Nurses for LTC," *Gerontology News*, November, 1991, p. 3.

71. Dorothy P. Rice and Jacob J. Feldman, "Living Longer in the United States: Demographic Changes and Health Needs of the Elderly," *Milbank Memorial Fund Quarterly/Health and Society* 61 (1983): 380.

72. Quote is from Claire Tehan, "Has Success Spoiled Hospice?" *Hastings Center Report* 15 (1985): 11–12; also see p. 13; Rehm, "Hospice Care, p. 234; David S. Greer and Vincent Mor, "How Medicare Is Altering the Hospice Movement," *Hastings Center Report* 15 (1985): 5; Donald E. Gibson, "Hospice: Morality and Economics," *The Gerontologist* 24 (1984): 4–8.

73. Greer and Mor, "How Medicare Is Altering Hospice Movement," esp. p. 7; Ray, Nichols, and Perritt, "Model of Job Stress," p. 18.

74. U.S. Congress, *Technology and Aging*, p. 203; Rhymes, "Hospice Care," pp. 370–371.

75. Alice M. Rivlin and Joshua M. Wiener, with Raymond J. Hanley and Denise A. Spence, *Caring for the Disabled Elderly: Who Will Pay?* (Washington, DC: The Brookings Institution, 1988), pp. 21–23.

76. Greg Arling, Harald Buhaug, Shelley Hagan, and David Zimmerman, "Medicaid Spenddown among Nursing Home Residents in Wisconsin," *The Gerontologist* 31 (1991): 181.

77. Rivlin et al., *Caring for Disabled Elderly*, pp. 24–27.

78. Kevin Sack, "New York Medicaid Strained by Newly Poor," *New York Times*, March 22, 1992; Stephen A. Moses, "The Fallacy of Impoverishment," *The Gerontologist* 30 (1990): 24–25.

79. Elinor Lenz and Barbara Myerhoff, *The Feminization of America: How Women's Values Are Changing Our Public and Private Lives* (Los Angeles: Jeremy P. Tarcher, 1985), pp. 119, 121.

80. Tamar Lewin, "Day Care Becomes a Growing Burden," *New York Times*, June 5, 1988; Robyn I. Stone and Peter Kemper, "Spouses and Children of Disabled Elders: How Large a Constituency for Long–Term Care Reform?" *The Milbank Quarterly* 67 (1989): 485–506; Haber, *Health Care for an Aging Society*, p. 35.

81. Lenz and Myerhoff, *Feminization of America*, p. 2.

82. Cindy J. Smith, Paul Rodenhauser, and Ronald J. Markert, "Gender Bias of Ohio Physicians in the Evaluation of the Personal Statements of Residency Applicants," *Academic Medicine* 66 (1991): 479; Hafferty, *Into the Valley*, pp. 198–199.

83. Steven C. Martin, Robert M. Arnold, and Ruth M. Parker, "Gender and Medical Socialization," *Journal of Health and Social Behavior* 29 (1988): 334, 336, 340; Nancy G. Kutner and Donna Brogan, "Gender Roles, Medical Practice Roles, and Ob–Gyn Career Choice: A Longitudinal Study," *Women & Health* 16: 103–104.

84. S. J. Olshansky, Mark A. Rudberg, Bruce A. Carnes, Christine K. Cassel, and Jacob A. Brody, "Trading off Longer Life for Worsening Health: The

Expansion of Morbidity Hypothesis," *Journal of Aging and Health* 3 (1991): esp. 207–208, 211; Jack M. Guralnik, "Prospects for the Compression of Morbidity: The Challenge Posed by Increasing Disability in the Years Prior to Death," *Journal of Aging and Health* 3 (1991): 150.

85. Guralnik, "Prospects for Compression," p. 139; Olshansky et al., "Trading Off Longer Life."
86. Lois M. Verbrugge, "The Dynamics of Population Aging and Health," in *Aging & Health: Linking Research and Public Policy*, ed. Steven Lewis (Chelsea, MI: Lewis Publishers, 1989), pp. 36–37.
87. Dorothy P. Rice, "Long–Term Care for the Elderly," in *Women's Life Cycle and Economic Insecurity*, ed. Martha N. Ozawa (New York: Praeger, 1989), p. 185.
88. Howard Caplan, "Doctors Should Support Euthanasia Decisions," in *Euthanasia: Opposing Viewpoints*, ed. Neal Bernards (San Diego: Greenhaven Press, 1989), p. 91; emphasis in original.
89. Lawlor, "What Kind of Medicine?" p. 133.

Chapter 9

1. Carlos F. Gomez, *Regulating Death: Euthanasia and the Case of the Netherlands* (New York: Free Press, 1991), pp. 50–51.
2. David Sudnow, "Dead on Arrival," in *Where Medicine Fails* (4th ed.), ed. Anselm L. Strauss (New Brunswick, NJ: Transaction Books, 1984), pp. 399–417; Anselm L. Strauss, "Medical Ghettos," pp. 55–72 in the same volume; Sue Fisher, *In the Patient's Best Interest: Women and the Politics of Medical Decisions* (New Brunswick, NJ: Rutgers University Press, 1986); Marti Loring and Brian Powell, "Gender, Race, and DSM–III: A Study of the Objectivity of Psychiatric Behavior," *Journal of Health and Social Behavior* 29 (1988): 1–22; Deborah B. Leiderman and Jean–Anne Grisso, "The Gomer Phenomenon," *Journal of Health and Social Behavior* 26 (1985): 222–232; quote is from Renée R. Anspach, "Notes on the Sociology of Medical Discourse: The Language of Case Presentation," *Journal of Health and Social Behavior* 29 (1988): 359; Irving Kenneth Zola, "Bringing Our Bodies and Ourselves Back In: Reflections on a Past, Present, and Future 'Medical Sociology,'" *Journal of Health and Social Behavior* 32 (1991): 7.
3. Virginia L. Olesen, "Caregiving, Ethical and Informal: Emerging Challenges in the Sociology of Health and Illness," *Journal of Health and Social Behavior* 30 (1989): 2; Barbara Ehrenreich and John Ehrenreich, "Health Care and Social Control," *Social Policy* 51 (1974): 34.
4. Lois M. Verbrugge and Richard P. Steiner, "Physician Treatment of Men and Women Patients: Sex Bias or Appropriate Care?" *Medical Care* 19 (1981): 630–631.
5. Myrna Lewis, "Older Women and Health: An Overview," *Women &*

Health 10 (1985): 12–13; for dramatic examples of disdain for older women in particular, see Pat Moore, with Charles Paul Conn, *Disguised* (Waco, TX: Word Books, 1985), passim; on male gynecologists' views, see John M. Smith, *Women and Doctors* (New York: Atlantic Monthly Press, 1992), esp. pp. 25–27; Joellen W. Hawkins and Cynthia S. Haber, "The Content of Advertisements in Medical Journals: Distorting the Image of Women," *Women & Health* 14 (1988): 52, 56–57; Council on Ethical and Judicial Affairs, American Medical Association, "Gender Disparities in Clinical Decision Making," *Journal of the American Medical Association* 266 (1991): 560–561.

6. Barbara Bernstein and Robert Kane, "Physicians' Attitudes toward Female Patients," *Medical Care* 19 (1981): 600, 607.

7. Dorothy P. Rice, "Long–Term Care for the Elderly," in *Women's Life Cycle and Economic Insecurity: Problems and Prospects*, ed. Martha N. Ozawa (New York: Praeger, 1989), p. 173; Lewis, "Older Women and Health"; Lois M. Verbrugge, "Longer Life but Worsening Health? Trends in Health and Mortality of Middle–aged and Older Persons," *Milbank Memorial Fund Quarterly/Health and Society* 62 (1984): 475–519, esp. 509; idem, "A Health Profile of Older Women with Comparisons to Older Men," *Research on Aging* 6 (1984): 291–322, esp. 314; U.S. Congress, Office of Technology Assessment, *Losing a Million Minds: Confronting the Tragedy of Alzheimer's Disease and Other Dementias* (Washington, DC: U.S. Government Printing Office, 1987), p. 7.

8. Robyn Stone, Gail Lee Cafferata, and Judith Sangl, "Caregivers of the Frail Elderly: A National Profile," *The Gerontologist* 27 (1987): 619; Council on Ethical and Judicial Affairs, American Medical Association, "Gender Disparities"; Roma S. Hanks and Barbara H. Settles, "Theoretical Questions and Ethical Issues in a Family Caregiving Relationship," in *Aging and Caregiving: Theory, Research, and Policy*, ed. David E. Biegel and Arthur Blum (Newbury Park, CA: Sage Publications, 1990), pp. 98–118; Hawkins and Haber, "Content of Advertisements"; Barbara J. Logue, "Taking Charge: Death Control as an Emergent Women's Issue," *Women & Health* 17 (1991): 97–121.

9. Colleen Leahy Johnson and Donald J. Catalano, "A Longitudinal Study of Family Supports to Impaired Elderly," in *Family Issues in Current Gerontology*, ed. Lillian E. Troll (New York: Springer, 1986), pp. 33, 43–44.

10. Quote is from Beth B. Hess and Joan Waring, "Family Relationships of Older Women: A Women's Issue," in *Older Women: Issues and Prospects*, ed. Elizabeth W. Markson (Lexington, MA: Lexington Books., 1983), p. 227; Karl Pillemer and David Finkelhor, "The Prevalence of Elder Abuse: A Random Sample Survey," *The Gerontologist* 28 (1988): 54–55; Karl Pillemer, "Maltreatment of Patients in Nursing Homes: Overview and Research Agenda," *Journal of Health and Social Behavior* 29 (1988): 233; Lewis, "Older Women and Health," p. 14.

11. Sheila Leader, "The Treatment of Women under Medicare," in *The Economics and Ethics of Long–Term Care and Disability*, ed. Sean Sullivan and Marion Ein Lewin (Washington, DC: American Enterprise Institute for Public Policy Research, 1988), pp. 138–139; Don McLeod, "At Long Last, Congress Turns to Long–Term Care," *AARP Bulletin* 33(8) (1992): 5–6, 17.

12. Nancy J. Osgood and John L. McIntosh, "The Vulnerable Suicidal Elderly," in *The Vulnerable Aged: People, Services, and Policies*, ed. Zev Harel, Phyllis Ehrlich, and Richard Hubbard (New York: Springer, 1990), pp. 169, 176; K. Warner Schaie and Sherry L. Willis, *Adult Development and Aging* (2d ed.) (Boston: Little, Brown, 1986), pp. 426–428; Nancy J. Osgood, Barbara A. Brant, and Aaron A. Lipman, "Patterns of Suicidal Behavior in Long–Term Care Facilities: A Preliminary Report on an Ongoing Study," *Omega* 19 (1988–1989): 74.

13. Michael S. Wilkes and Miriam Shuchman, "What Is Too Old?" *New York Times Magazine*, June 4, 1989.

14. R. J. Havlik, B. M. Liu, M. G. Kovar et al., "Health Statistics on Older Persons, United States, 1986," *Vital and Health Statistics*, Series 3, No. 25 (Washington, DC: U.S. Government Printing Office, 1987), p. 73 (derived from data in Table 57); Esther Hing, "Use of Nursing Homes by the Elderly: Preliminary Data from the 1985 National Nursing Home Survey," *Advance Data From Vital and Health Statistics*, No. 135 (Hyattsville, MD: Public Health Service, 1987, p. 2.

15. Hing, "Use of Nursing Homes," p. 6; U.S. Congress, Office of Technology Assessment, *Life–Sustaining Technologies and the Elderly* (Washington, DC: U.S. Government Printing Office, 1987), pp. 18, 46. Helen Evers's work on gender differences in geriatric care in British institutions is suggestive of worse treatment for women. She found that they were "subjected to particular forms of oppression," such as depersonalization and negative labelling. See her "Care or Custody? The Experiences of Women Patients in Long–Stay Geriatric Wards," in *Controlling Women: The Normal and the Deviant*, ed. Bridget Hutter and Gillian Williams (London: Croom Helm, 1981), esp. pp. 108–109.

16. President's Commission for the Study of Ethical Problems in Medicine and Biomedical and Behavioral Research, *Deciding to Forego Life–Sustaining Treatment* (Washington, DC: U.S. Government Printing Office, 1983), p. 115.

17. Nancy S. Jecker, "Age–Based Rationing and Women," *Journal of the American Medical Association* 266 (1991): 3012.

18. Lois Grau, "Illness–Engendered Poverty among the Elderly," *Women & Health* 12 (1987): 103–118; Timothy Diamond, "Social Policy and Everyday Life in Nursing Homes: A Critical Ethnography," *Social Science and Medicine* 23 (1986): 1289; Isabel Moore, "The Nursing Home: Tender, Loving Care? Or Adult Orphanage?" *Nursing Homes and Senior Citizen Care* 35(6) (1986): 28–29.

19. William B. Schwartz, "Cutting Costs Means Painful Choices," *New York Times*, May 8, 1988; Daniel Callahan, *Setting Limits: Medical Goals in an Aging Society* (New York: Simon and Schuster, 1987), pp. 123–126; Roger W. Evans, "Health Care Technology and the Inevitability of Resource Allocation and Rationing Decisions," *Journal of the American Medical Association* 249 (1983): 2047–2053, 2208–2219; Jecker, "Age–Based Rationing and Women," p. 3012.

20. Madelyn Anne Iris, "Guardianship and the Elderly. A Multi–Perspective View of the Decisionmaking Process," *The Gerontologist* 28 (1988) (Supp.): 42; Nancy R. Zweibel and Christine K. Cassel, "Treatment Choices at the End of Life: A Comparison of Decisions by Older Patients and Their Physician–Selected Proxies," *The Gerontologist* 29 (1989): 615–621.

21. Mary K. Zimmerman, "The Women's Health Movement: A Critique of Medical Enterprise and the Position of Women," in *Analyzing Gender: A Handbook of Social Science Research*," ed. Beth B. Hess and Myra Marx Ferree (Newbury Park, CA: Sage Publications, 1987), p. 443; Council on Ethical and Judicial Affairs, American Medical Association, "Gender Disparities"; quote is from Robert B. Hudson and Judith G. Gonyea, "Political Mobilization & Older Women: A Perspective on Women in Politics," *Generations* 14 (1990): 69.

22. Callahan, *Setting Limits*, p. 176.

23. David E. Jorgenson and Ron C. Neubecker, "Euthanasia: A National Survey of Attitudes toward Voluntary Termination of Life," *Omega* 11 (1981): 290; Derek Humphry and Ann Wickett, *The Right to Die: Understanding Euthanasia* (New York: Harper & Row, 1986), p. 133; Leonard H. Glantz, "Withholding and Withdrawing Treatment: The Role of the Criminal Law," *Law, Medicine & Health Care* 15 (1987): 231–241; Derek Humphry, with Ann Wickett, *Jean's Way* (London: Quartet Books, 1978), esp. pp. 21, 31, 108.

24. Pauline Boss, Wayne Caron, and Joan Horbal, "Alzheimer's Disease and Ambiguous Loss," in *Chronic Illness and Disability*, ed. Catherine S. Chilman, Elam W. Nunnally, and Fred M. Cox (Newbury Park, CA: Sage Publications, 1988), p. 131.

25. Steven H. Miles and Allison August, "Courts, Gender and 'The Right to Die,'" *Law, Medicine & Health Care* 18 (1990): 87–88, 90, 92.

26. Elinor Lenz and Barbara Myerhoff, *The Feminization of America: How Women's Values Are Changing Our Public and Private Lives* (Los Angeles: Jeremy P. Tarcher, 1985), pp. 115–121.

27. Cheryl Brown Travis, *Women and Health Psychology: Biomedical Issues* (Hillsdale, NJ: Lawrence Erlbaum Associates, 1988), pp. 26–27.

28. Sheryl Ruzek, "Feminist Visions of Health: An International Perspective," in *Perspectives in Medical Sociology*, ed. Phil Brown (Belmont, CA: Wadsworth, 1989), pp. 565, 571.

29. Linda Gordon, *Woman's Body, Woman's Right: A Social History of Birth*

Control in America (New York: Grossman, 1976), pp. 67, 288–289, 320, 417.

30. Linda Evers Cool, "The Effects of Social Class and Ethnicity on the Aging Process," in *The Elderly as Modern Pioneers*, ed. Philip Silverman (Bloomington: Indiana University Press, 1987), p. 264.

31. Ibid., p. 275; James J. Dowd and Vern L. Bengtson, "Aging in Minority Populations: An Examination of the Double Jeopardy Hypothesis," in *Aging, the Individual, and Society: Readings in Social Gerontology*, ed. Jill S. Quadagno (New York: St. Martin's Press, 1980, pp. 338–355.

32. John F. Kilner, *Who Lives? Who Dies? Ethical Criteria in Patient Selection* (New Haven, CT: Yale University Press, 1990), esp. pp. 27, 39; Kenneth C. Goldberg, Arthur J. Hartz, Steven J. Jacobsen, Henry Krakauer, and Alfred A. Rimm, "Racial and Community Factors Influencing Coronary Artery Bypass Graft Surgery Rates for All 1986 Medicare Patients," *Journal of the American Medical Association* 267 (1992): 1473–1477.

33. Gary M. Nelson, "Tax Expenditures for the Elderly," *The Gerontologist* 23 (1983): 473; Carroll L. Estes, Lenore E. Gerard, Jane Sprague Zones, and James H. Swan, *Political Economy, Health, and Aging* (Boston: Little, Brown, 1984), p. 101.

34. Robert H. Binstock, "National Policies and the Vulnerable Aged: Present, Emerging, and Proposed," in *The Vulnerable Aged: People, Services, and Policies*, ed. Zev Harel, Phyllis Ehrlich, and Richard Hubbard (New York: Springer, 1990), p. 236; Stephen Crystal, *America's Old Age Crisis: Public Policy and the Two Worlds of Aging* (New York: Basic Books, 1982), p. 160; Henry Fairlie, "Greedy Geezers: Talkin' 'bout My Generation," *The New Republic*, March 28, 1988.

35. Linda S. Noelker, "Family Caregivers: A Valuable but Vulnerable Resource," in *The Vulnerable Aged: People, Services, and Policies*, ed. Zev Harel, Phyllis Ehrlich, and Richard Hubbard (New York: Springer, 1990), p. 199.

36. Paul Starr, *The Social Transformation of American Medicine* (New York: Basic Books, 1982), pp. 435–436.

37. U.S. Senate Special Committee on Aging, American Association of Retired Persons, Federal Council on the Aging, and U.S. Administration on Aging, *Aging America: Trends and Projections* (1991 ed.) (Washington, DC: U.S. Government Printing Office, n.d.), pp. 109, 142; Evans, "Health Care Technology," p. 2217; Congressional Budget Office, *Policy Choices for Long-Term Care* (Washington, DC: U.S. Government Printing Office, 1991), p. 47; idem, *Rising Health Care Costs: Causes, Implications, and Strategies* (Washington, DC: U.S. Government Printing Office, 1991), p. 42.

38. U.S. Senate Special Committee on Aging et al., *Aging America* (1991 ed.), p. 142; Jill Quadagno, Madonna Harrington Meyer, and J. Blake Turner, "Falling into the Medicaid Gap: The Hidden Long-Term Care Dilemma," *The Gerontologist* 31 (1991): 521–526.

39. President's Commission, *Deciding to Forego*, p. 46.

40. Howard Waitzkin, "Information Giving in Medical Care," *Journal of Health and Social Behavior* 26 (1985): 81–101; Ruth Macklin, *Mortal Choices: Bioethics in Today's World* (New York: Pantheon Books, 1987), p. 44; Bebe Lavin, Marie Haug, Linda Liska Belgrave, and Naomi Breslau, "Change in Student Physicians' Views on Authority Relationships with Patients," *Journal of Health and Social Behavior* 28 (1987): 259; Sue Fisher, "Doctor Talk/Patient Talk: How Treatment Decisions Are Negotiated in Doctor–Patient Communication," in *The Social Organization of Doctor–Patient Communication*, ed. idem and Alexandra Dundas Todd (Washington, DC: Center for Applied Linguistics, 1983), esp. pp. 137–138, 153; Sue V. Rosser, "Is There Androcentric Bias in Psychiatric Diagnosis?" *Journal of Medicine and Philosophy* 17 (1992): 223–225.

41. Barbara Finlay, "Right to Life vs. the Right to Die: Some Correlates of Euthanasia Attitudes," *Sociology and Social Research* 69 (1985): 550; Jiska Cohen–Mansfield, Janet A. Droge, and Nathan Billig, "Factors Influencing Hospital Patients' Preferences in the Utilization of Life–Sustaining Treatments," *The Gerontologist* 32 (1992): 93–94; Bernard M. Dickens, "Medico–Legal Issues Concerning the Elderly—An Overview," in *An Aging World: Dilemmas and Challenges for Law and Social Policy*, ed. John Eekelaar and David Pearl (Oxford: Clarendon Press, 1989), p. 505.

42. Arthur L. Caplan, "One Law Does Not Make a Right," *The Gerontologist* 31 (1991): 583.

43. U.S. Senate Special Committee on Aging, American Association of Retired Persons, Federal Council on the Aging, and U.S. Administration on Aging, *Aging America: Trends and Projections* (1987–1988 ed.) (Washington, DC: U.S. Government Printing Office, n.d.), p. 19. Hispanics may be of any race. In the 24 percent example, minorities include white Hispanics, blacks (both Hispanic and non–Hispanic), and all other nonwhites.

44. Dale E. Yeatts, Thomas Crow, and Edward Folts, "Service Use among Low–Income Minority Elderly: Strategies for Overcoming Barriers," *The Gerontologist* 32 (1992): 26.

45. Jay Sokolovsky, "Bringing Culture Back Home: Aging, Ethnicity, and Family Support," in *The Cultural Context of Aging: Worldwide Perspectives*, ed. idem (New York: Bergin & Garvey, 1990), pp. 202–203; Binstock, "National Policies," p. 236; Crystal, *America's Old Age Crisis*, p. 154; Rose C. Gibson, "Outlook for the Black Family," in *Our Aging Society: Paradox and Promise*, ed. Alan Pifer and Lydia Bronte (New York: W. W. Norton, 1986), pp. 181–197; Fernando Torres–Gil, "Hispanics: A Special Challenge," pp. 219–242 in the same volume.

46. Richard G. Rogers, "Living and Dying in the U.S.A.: Sociodemographic Determinants of Death among Blacks and Whites," *Demography* 29 (1992): 290; Eli Ginzberg, "Access to Health Care for Hispanics," *Journal of the*

American Medical Association 265 (1991): 238–241; Richard B. Rothenberg and Jeffrey P. Koplan, "Chronic Disease in the 1990s," *Annual Review of Public Health* 11 (1990): 283.

47. David Barton Smith, "Population Ecology and the Racial Integration of Hospitals and Nursing Homes in the United States," *The Milbank Quarterly* 68 (1990): 585; Spero M. Manson, "Long–Term Care in American Indian Communities: Issues for Planning and Research," *The Gerontologist* 29 (1989): 39; J. Neil Henderson, "Mental Disorders among the Elderly: Dementia and its Sociocultural Correlates," in *The Elderly as Modern Pioneers*, ed. Philip Silverman (Bloomington: Indiana University Press, 1987), p. 369; Gibson, "Outlook for Black Family," p. 181.

48. Manson, "Long–Term Care in American Indian Communities," p. 39; Smith, "Population Ecology," p. 586; Torres–Gil, "Hispanics," pp. 230–231.

49. Crystal, *America's Old Age Crisis*, pp. 75, 89, 156.

50. Manson, "Long–Term Care in American Indian Communities," p. 41.

51. Tish Sommers and Laurie Shields, with the Older Women's League Task Force on Caregivers and Judy MacLean, *Women Take Care: The Consequences of Caregiving in Today's Society* (Gainesville, FL: Triad, 1987), pp. 116–123; Nancy L. Marshall, Rosalind C. Barnett, Grace K. Baruch, and Joseph H. Pleck, "Double Jeopardy: The Costs of Caring at Work and at Home," in *Circles of Care: Work and Identity in Women's Lives*, ed. Emily K. Abel and Margaret K. Nelson (Albany: State University of New York Press, 1990), pp. 266–277; Jordan I. Kosberg, "Preventing Elder Abuse: Identification of High Risk Factors Prior to Placement Decisions," *The Gerontologist* 28 (1988): 43–50.

52. Sokolovsky, "Bringing Culture Back Home," pp. 201–202, 206; David Maldonado, Jr., "The Chicano Aged," in *Aging, the Individual and Society: Readings in Social Gerontology*, ed. Jill S. Quadagno (New York: St. Martin's Press, 1980), pp. 369–370.

53. Finlay, "Right to Life," esp. pp. 550, 553; Allan R. Meyers, "Ethnicity and Aging: Public Policy and Ethnic Differences in Aging and Old Age," in *Public Policies for an Aging Population*, ed. Elizabeth W. Markson and Gretchen R. Batra (Lexington, MA: Lexington Books/D. C. Heath, 1980), p. 69.

54. David J. Rothman, *Strangers at the Bedside: A History of How Law and Bioethics Transformed Medical Decision Making* (New York: Basic Books, 1991), p. 252; for the DNR quote, see Sam Brody, "We Have Lost Our Humanity," *Newsweek*, September 7, 1992, p. 8; Margaret Pabst Battin, "Euthanasia Is Ethical," in *Euthanasia: Opposing Viewpoints*, ed. Neal Bernards (San Diego: Greenhaven Press, 1989), p. 20; George J. Annas, "Into the Hands of Strangers," *Law, Medicine & Health Care* 13 (1985): 271.

55. Kyriakos S. Markides, "Risk Factors, Gender, & Health," *Generations* 14 (1990): 21.

Chapter 10

1. Pat Moore, with Charles Paul Conn, *Disguised* (Waco, TX: Word Books, 1985).
2. Anthony P. Glascock, "By Any Other Name, It Is Still Killing: A Comparison of the Treatment of the Elderly in America and Other Societies," in *The Cultural Context of Aging: Worldwide Perspectives*, ed. Jay Sokolovsky (New York: Bergin & Garvey Publishers, 1990), pp. 43, 49, 53, 56.
3. James F. Fries and Lawrence M. Crapo, *Vitality and Aging: Implications of the Rectangular Curve* (San Francisco: W. H. Freeman, 1981), p. 93.
4. Joseph Fletcher, "The Courts and Euthanasia," *Law, Medicine & Health Care* 15 (1987): 226.
5. David J. Rothman, *Strangers at the Bedside: A History of How Law and Bioethics Transformed Medical Decision Making* (New York: Basic Books, 1991), p. 252.
6. Quote on *Cruzan* case is from Larry Gostin and Robert F. Weir, "Life and Death Choices after *Cruzan*: Case Law and Standards of Professional Conduct," *The Milbank Quarterly* 69 (1991): 145; Richard Selzer, "A Question of Mercy," *New York Times Magazine*, September 22, 1991; Peter Goodwin, "Illegal Medical Euthanasia Is Not the Way," *Hemlock Quarterly*, No. 45, October, 1991, p. 3.
7. Tish Sommers and Laurie Shields, with the Older Women's League Task Force on Caregivers and Judy MacLean, *Women Take Care: The Consequences of Caregiving in Today's Society* (Gainesville, FL: Triad, 1987), p. 177.
8. R. R. Faden and N. E. Kass, "Bioethics and Public Health in the 1980s: Resource Allocation and AIDS," *Annual Review of Public Health* 12 (1991): 337.
9. Marilyn Waring, *If Women Counted: A New Feminist Economics* (San Francisco: Harper & Row, Publishers, 1988), p. 9.
10. Judith Blake, "Coercive Pronatalism and American Population Policy," in *The Family: Its Structures and Functions* (2d ed.), ed. Rose Laub Coser (New York: St. Martin's Press, 1974), p. 277.
11. Robert M. Veatch, "Comparative Medical Ethics: An Introduction," *Journal of Medicine and Philosophy* 13 (1988): 225–229; quote is from Antony Flew, "The Principle of Euthanasia," in *Death and Society*, ed. James P. Carse and Arlene B. Dallery (New York: Harcourt Brace Jovanovich, 1977), pp. 101–102; also see p. 100; on legalizing physician–assisted suicide and euthanasia, see Robert F. Weir, "The Morality of Physician–Assisted Suicide," *Law, Medicine & Health Care* 20 (1992): 122; James Rachels, *The End of Life: Euthanasia and Morality* (Oxford: Oxford University Press, 1986), esp. Chapter 10; and Margaret Battin, "Voluntary Euthanasia and the Risks of Abuse: Can We Learn Anything from the Netherlands?" *Law, Medicine & Health Care* 20

(1992): 133–143.

12. Goodwin, "Illegal Medical Euthanasia," p. 3; Rothman, *Strangers at the Bedside*, p. 253.

13. Alice Lind, "Hospitals and Hospices: Feminist Decisions about Care for the Dying," in *Healing Technology: Feminist Perspectives*, ed. Kathryn Strother Ratcliff, Myra Marx Ferree, Gail O. Mellow et al. (Ann Arbor, MI: University of Michigan Press, 1989), p. 269.

Index